The Smart Woman's Guide to Midlife and Beyond is a complete, holistic, and state-of-the-art road map for any woman who is motivated to become a more effective steward of her health. The authors' relaxed, personal, and insightful style makes critical health information accessible. This book is a must-have for any woman inspired to improve her health trajectory.

—Mark C. Pettus MD, FACP, medical director of the Kripalu Institute for Integrated Healing and author of *It's All in Your Head*

There is no doubt that women past the age of fifty have different health issues than younger women—a fact often overlooked by many physicians. As a result, these women need to have knowledge about their maturing bodies. Drs. Horn and Miller explore the full spectrum of the mature woman in a candid, conversational manner that integrates the body, mind and spirit. A much needed book.

—Kevin Soden, MD, author and host for the Retirement Living TV network

I have often wished that I had a doctor in my family to ask advice. If you have shared this desire, you'll love this book. It's a practical insider's guide to what maturing women need to be thinking about, and it's written as a concerned friend would discuss it with you. Drs. Horn and Miller have superb training and years of practical experience caring for women patients. It shows on every page of this excellent book.

—Judge Glenda Hatchett, star of the nationally syndicated television program *Judge Hatchett*

More than no-nonsense, the authors' approach is accessible and even entertaining, these are the doctor girlfriends you want to call because they know everything about the area of your concern—not only from practicing their profession but also from their own personal experiences.

—Robin Wolaner, founder and CEO of TeeBeeDee, www.tbd.com, an online network for people over forty, and founder of *Parenting* magazine

This is the girlfriends' guide to taking charge of your health. And these girlfriends are doctors. A winning combination!

—Ari Brown, MD, pediatrician and author of *Baby 411*

The Smart Woman's Guide to Midlife & Beyond

A No-Nonsense Approach to Staying Healthy After 50

Janet Horn, MD
Robin H. Miller, MD

New Harbinger Publications, Inc.

Publisher's Note

Care has been taken to confirm the accuracy of the information presented and to describe generally accepted practices. However, the authors, editors, and publisher are not responsible for errors or omissions or for any consequences from application of the information in this book and make no warranty, express or implied, with respect to the contents of the publication.

The authors, editors, and publisher have exerted every effort to ensure that any drug selection and dosage set forth in this text is in accordance with current recommendations and practice at the time of publication. However, in view of ongoing research, changes in government regulations, and the constant flow of information relating to drug therapy and drug reactions, the reader is urged to check the package insert for each drug for any change in indications and dosage and for added warnings and precautions. This is particularly important when the recommended agent is a new or infrequently employed drug.

Some drugs and medical devices presented in this publication may have Food and Drug Administration (FDA) clearance for limited use in restricted research settings. It is the responsibility of the health care provider to ascertain the FDA status of each drug or device planned for use in their clinical practice.

Distributed in Canada by Raincoast Books

Copyright © 2008 by Janet Horn and Robin H. Miller
New Harbinger Publications, Inc.
5674 Shattuck Avenue
Oakland, CA 94609
www.newharbinger.com

Cover design by Amy Shoup; Text design by Amy Shoup and Michele Waters-Kermes; Acquired by Melissa Kirk; Edited by Kayla Sussell

Printed in the United States of America

Library of Congress Cataloging-in-Publication Data

Horn, Janet, M.D.
 The smart woman's guide to midlife and beyond : a no-nonsense approach to staying healthy after 50 / Janet Horn and Robin H. Miller.
     p. cm.
 Includes bibliographical references.
 ISBN-13: 978-1-57224-556-3 (pbk. : alk. paper)
 ISBN-10: 1-57224-556-5 (pbk. : alk. paper) 1. Middle-aged women--Health and hygiene--Popular works. 2. Older women--Health and hygiene--Popular works. I. Miller, Robin H. II. Title.
 RA778.H78 2008
 613'.04244--dc22

FSC
Mixed Sources
Product group from well-managed forests and other controlled sources
Cert no. SW-COC-002283
www.fsc.org
© 1996 Forest Stewardship Council

                    2008027639

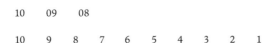

10   09   08

10   9   8   7   6   5   4   3   2   1

First printing

This book is dedicated to our greatest teachers: our patients.

Contents

Acknowledgments

We would first like to thank the two people whose confidence in our book and in us was essential, Sharlene Martin and Melissa Kirk. Ms. Martin, our agent, immediately saw the potential and need for a book geared to our target audience. She reflects what characterizes this group in her intelligence, tenacity, and success. Ms. Kirk, our acquisitions editor, also saw the potential of this book and has guided us with patience, expertise, and insight throughout the project. New Harbinger Publications, with its very creative staff, has been a pleasure with which to work; thanks go to Kayla Sussell for her copyediting expertise, Amy Shoup for the wonderful cover, Earlita Chenault, Leyza Yarkley, Janice Fitch, and Julia Kent for help with promotion, and Jess Beebe for editing assistance early on. We thank Dr. Joanne Perron and Dr. Lori Taft Sours for sharing personal stories with us, as well as those of our patients who allowed us to use their medical stories. We especially thank *all* of our patients—past and present—for being our best teachers and the reason for our work.

Janet's acknowledgments: My husband Alan has always supported my professional efforts, and he enthusiastically did so again with this project. Being the feminist he is, he saw the potential in this book from the very beginning. I thank my parents, who gave me every imaginable opportunity, and only wish they were still here to enjoy this book's publication. My brother Ron encouraged and supported me in my personal and professional endeavors from my childhood on, as did my brother Howard, who was an invaluable consultant for this book. I greatly appreciate the encouragement and advice I received from Joan Cornblath, Jim Magruder, Nan and Craig Duerling, and Anne Fischer. For the chats and laughs in the midst of their work with me, thanks go to Jim Turnbull and Jessica Wescott. My book group, the Literary Ladies of Grafton, provides endless inspiration, great discussions, and laughs. I thank everyone at the Shepherd's Clinic for making it the medical oasis it is; there, against all odds, medicine continues to be practiced the way it should be. Finally, after having been a bridesmaid in Robin's wedding in 1986, I'm thrilled that we could have another collaborative project after twenty-two years, particularly one as significant as this is.

Robin's acknowledgments: I would like to acknowledge the support and patience of my beautiful family, my husband Dr. Peter Adesman (an endless source of laughs and information about the GI tract—his specialty), and my sons, David and Brian. In addition, I would like to thank my wonderful dogs, Tally and Lucy, who were great company throughout the whole writing process, keeping me calm and forcing me to go out and exercise! I am grateful for the advice and encouragement of Jennifer Carr, Dianne Oceana, Doris Roser, Wendy Enneking, Dee Gillen, and Wendy Ortiz. I am grateful to my parents, Burt and Aileen Miller, who have been behind me and supporting me 100 percent (through the process of writing this book as well as through life), along with my brother, Jim, and sister, Janet Cohen. I thank my clinic partners at Asante Health System, who have helped me to create a wonderful work environment, and my many mentors at the National Association of Medical Communicators, including Kate O'Brian, as well as Patsy Smullin, President and owner of KOBI-5 TV, who helped me to find my voice. Finally, thanks to Janet, who has been a great partner, sounding board, and fearless leader in this project.

Introduction

Let us be right up front as you start reading. This book is *not* about becoming young again. Don't get us wrong, we loved our younger years. We had great times back then. But even if we could be young again, that would mean we wouldn't get to enjoy the benefits and wisdom that all our years have given us, or the confidence that comes only with experience. *We want to feel good at the age we are now.* And we want to continue to feel good as we grow older.

Another thing this book is not about is the hot new trend in everything from cosmetics to medicine known as "antiaging." Don't get us wrong about this either. We don't like what aging does to our bodies any more than you do. But like Nora Ephron, in her wonderful book *I Feel Bad About my Neck*, we're tired of everyone chirping about how fabulous it is to get older physically. To the contrary, physical aging can be tough, especially if we're not prepared to deal with it.

Over the years, most of us have had occasion to fight for what we believe in and/or for what we want. And that's good…especially when there's a chance our efforts will yield results. But there are times when being "anti" something can be counterproductive. In other words, sometimes it is better to work with the process rather than against it. Along those lines, we like the Dove commercials and products (not the ice cream, the soap—but we love the ice cream too) that are "pro" healthy aging. So, we feel that we can stay healthy by working along with our bodies as they change with time, not fighting against them. We believe that as our bodies change, we need to change too. After all those years of taking care of everyone else, now is the time to take care of ourselves.

Bottom line: We believe that it's possible to get older and keep feeling good; we just have to be prepared to work at it in the right way with the right tools. And, if in the process of staying fit and maintaining our health, we physically feel much as we did when we were twenty—so much the better!

HOW WE CAME TO WRITE THIS BOOK

We met on the first day of our fellowships at the Johns Hopkins Hospital in 1983, outside the auditorium where the new fellows' orientation was being held. We continued meeting three times a week for sour coffee, greasy food, and long chats at the hospital café for the next several years, talking about everything from the most serious medical issues to the hilarious stories of Dr. R's dates. (Dr. J was already married when we met.)

Now we live on opposite coasts, but our chats have been ongoing for the past twenty-five years, and as we've matured, so have our chats. (Or perhaps more accurately, our chats have become more about growing older—just as we have.) These talks have been about everything—including balancing a full-time career with marriage and rambunctious teens (Dr. R) and balancing the same career with marriage and a rowdy live-in parent (Dr. J).

More recently, our chats have turned to our aging body parts. When comparing notes, we found not only were we feeling surprised by the changes in our bodies brought about by aging, but also that our women patients were feeling exactly the same way. None of us were feeling that we were really any older until our bodies screamed out our age. We now realize that this stage of life is not just a second act, it's a whole new play! So, we thought it might be useful (and possibly fun) to write it all down, and thus, *The Smart Woman's Guide to Midlife and Beyond: A No-Nonsense Approach to Staying Healthy After Fifty* was born.

WHAT THIS BOOK IS ABOUT

This book is written for all women over fifty regardless of your ethnic group or lifestyle. Although the information and recommendations it contains are mostly from the traditional medical world, we also include many recent suggestions from the field of complementary and alternative medicine (CAM). One of our two focuses is on the screening, early detection, and prevention of diseases most common in women of our age group. The other is on recognizing, and taking appropriate action, for the symptoms most commonly occurring at this age.

Since we didn't want our book to be just another long list of orders to exercise, stop smoking, and eat well (although it does suggest those) because, after all, that's your choice, we've also included brief sections on how the individual parts of the body work and what happens to them as they age. We believe that if you understand what's going on with your body as it ages, you'll be much more likely to do the work necessary to stay healthy.

We know that doing that work is not easy. If it were, everyone would be healthy, have a normal body weight, and not smoke nor eat fast foods, and there would be much less heart disease and diabetes. You have to *want* to do the work of becoming and staying healthy so that your long life will also be an active and healthy life.

To that end, we've created a way designed to keep us on the right track of taking care of ourselves, a way to organize and simplify what we need to do to stay healthy, one that works for us as well as for our patients. We call it "the four A's." This stands for awareness, alertness, action, and advocacy. Here's how it works.

- **Be *aware* of how each disease affects your body over time, and what puts you at risk for that disease.**

    Hopefully, using this book will help you figure out which diseases you are at risk for getting, and will guide you to take preventive steps to avoid those and other diseases. It can also teach you how to request the appropriate screening tests to detect disease early, because the earlier you detect it, the greater the likelihood is of curing it. And it will assist you in making your own schedule of recommended screening tests.

- **Be *alert* to your symptoms.**

    We provide you with the tools you need in order to know which of your symptoms are minor, and which indicate an emergency. By maintaining a healthy lifestyle, you can change many of your risk factors for certain diseases, but sometimes, even though you take good care of yourself, you can get sick. It is our hope that when you know how to handle the symptoms and the situation promptly and effectively, you will return to good health in a very short time. We also encourage you to trust your instincts. In our practices, we've learned that women have great "gut" instincts about most things, but especially about their own bodies. Moreover, we've always found that the patients who are most in touch with their bodies stay healthy or recover from illness quickly.

- **Take *action* to get care for yourself when you need it, and to get screened regularly.**
    This is self-explanatory.

- ***Advocate* for yourself.**

    We know that you've long advocated for others—your family, your friends, people who haven't been as fortunate as you have—and now it's time to do the same for yourself. This is an area where trusting your instincts comes into play again, so that, even if a professional in the health care system doesn't find anything "wrong" with you, despite your gut feeling that there is, you will speak up for yourself or seek other opinions.

Just as we didn't want this book to be just a long to-do list of how to stay healthy, neither did we want it to be a dull, dry scientific treatise on diseases and how they're treated. We want you to enjoy what you're reading and feel as though you're sitting in on a chat with a couple of friends. So, you will read about our experiences with the very medical issues we discuss, and how each of us deals with them in her own way. You'll see that we often don't agree on such topics as hormone replacement therapy after menopause; nor are our feelings about vitamins, skin care regimens, or liver and onions similar. You'll learn about Dr. R's schoolgirl love of all things athletic and Dr. J's preference for hiding out in the school gym's locker room—and how those habits matured into Dr. R's killer regimen of daily physical activity and Dr. J's preference for curling up with a book, or napping, over exercise. And you'll find out about all the things we do agree on, particularly those concerning how to be healthy as we grow older.

HOUSEKEEPING ISSUES

There are several things about this book that we want you to know:

+ There are far too many relevant health topics for us to cover in one book. So we've chosen those conditions that are the most common among women our age, and about which there is not a lot of information readily available. For those conditions that we think are important for you to know about but we didn't have room to cover, we've included a Recommended Reading list in the Resources section at the end of the book so that you can find out more about them.

+ We've included real stories of our real patients. Although their names and life details may have been changed at their request, the medical details are absolutely accurate.

+ We've included, in some instances, brand names of specific products and medications that we particularly like, or even that we personally use. Please understand that neither of us has been paid, sponsored, or wooed by any of the companies that make these products.

+ Throughout the book, you will notice we use the word "clinician" when referring to your health care providers. This is in recognition of the fact that there are many capable nurse practitioners and physician assistants providing excellent primary care. When we do use the word "doctor" (or "physician"), we're specifically referring to a specialist (for example, a surgeon, neurologist, or gynecologist) that you may need to see.

+ You will also notice throughout the book that when we refer to your "clinician," we always use the pronoun "she." We did this for simplicity's sake because using the terms "she/he" and "her or him" became too cumbersome and distracting. But please understand that neither of us has anything against male physicians; in fact, male docs are among some of our favorite people (such as Robin's husband and Janet's brother and two nephews)!

HOW TO USE THIS BOOK

There are several ways you can use this book. You can use the table of contents to look up information about specific organ systems and their diseases or about certain symptoms. Or you can read the book from cover to cover. At the end of each chapter we have included a list of what we believe to be the important "take home" points about this particular topic discussed in that chapter; these we call "pearls of wisdom." So you can also flip to the end of a chapter to remind yourself of these pearls.

But no matter how you use this book, please understand we are not just spouting theoretical ideas here or giving you theoretical advice. What we've included in this book is actually what we tell our patients (and ourselves and each other) about how to stay healthy while growing older.

We hope you find it useful and that you will enjoy reading it.

CHAPTER 1

How to Keep Your Memory Vivid
and Stay Stroke-Free

Let's start with a story. You just got home from a busy day of (choose one): work/running errands. You've taken off your purple leather gloves (you got a great deal on them from QVC), and you're busily looking through the mail. Suddenly, your cell phone plays its usual "I Can't Get No Satisfaction," and propping it between your ear and your shoulder while you continue going through the huge stack of letters and catalogs, you answer. It's your (choose one): daughter/best friend excitedly telling you what happened when she asked her boss for a raise today.

As you're listening and looking through the mail, you notice that the table on which you're placing the mail is very dusty. You grab the glove you put there earlier and begin vigorously dusting. The next letter pops up in your stack of mail; you recognize the handwriting on the envelope. The address is printed in block letters written in red ink. It's from your high school crush. At the same time you recognize the handwriting, your daughter/best friend is saying that perhaps she shouldn't have worn the red plaid miniskirt to her meeting with her boss. Suddenly, you realize there's no sound coming from the phone. You go blank. Who were you talking to? How can you not remember who you were just on the phone with? And what was the love of your life's name, anyway, the heartthrob who always printed all his/her letters in red? And, where's your other purple glove? You think, *This can't be happening to me—of all people—I'm a world-class multitasker!*

Sound familiar? We're sure you have your own versions of this story; forgetting why you went into a room once you get there, blanking out the name of your best friend's husband at a party, walking out of a movie and being unable to recall the title, no matter how hard you try. We also know the first thoughts that come into your head after a few of these occurrences: *Am I getting senile? Is this early Alzheimer's disease? Do I have early dementia?* One thing is for sure about your concerns: You're not alone. These days, one of our biggest health concerns is the fear of losing our functioning brains, or literally "losing our minds," due to Alzheimer's disease (AD) or other types of dementia. Or at the very least, we fear losing parts of our mental functioning, such as memory or our ability to reason.

Today, because medical science has advanced so much during our lifetimes, we know more about diseases of the brain than our predecessors knew. And, happily, much of it is good news. For instance, we now know that the deterioration of our brainpower, known for years as "senility," is not a necessary consequence of aging. In fact, the lessening of our brain function as we age is not inevitable. Surprised? Read on.

HOW DO THE BRAIN AND NERVOUS SYSTEM WORK?

The brain is "command central" for the rest of the body. Though each of our organs and body systems plays a unique and important role in keeping us alive and functional, it is the brain that oversees and coordinates them all. It does this by sending signals to, and receiving signals from, the nerves in all parts of the body; these nerves taken together are known as the *nervous system*.

The Brain and Nervous System

One simple way to understand the nervous system is to think of the body as a huge organization. The brain is the very hands-on CEO. The nervous system is composed of three main departments, each having one main function: They are the motor system, the sensory system, and the associational system. Individual nerve cells, the neurons, who are the true "doers" of the organization, group together and are like electrical circuits coursing throughout.

The department that literally takes its marching orders from the CEO to the rest of the body is known as *the motor system*. It is responsible for all of the movement of the body. The second set of circuits (or nerves) carries information from the rest of the body and the outside environment back to the brain to let it know what's going on; this department is known as *the sensory system* and is responsible for our five senses. The CEO of course has her own department, the senior executives if you will, that must operate at their highest level at all times to coordinate and integrate all of the different circuits from the two other departments. This department, including the brain itself, is *the associational system*, and its responsibility is to link the other two; by doing so, it performs the higher functions, such as thinking and feeling, that make us uniquely human.

You can probably guess how the CEO and her department are structured. Different parts of the brain, each in a unique location (some are in a corner office with windows, others not), are responsible for different functions of the body. So, for instance, the temporal lobes, located on each side of the brain, are responsible for recognizing and identifying objects. If one of these lobes is damaged, you will have problems in recognizing and naming familiar objects. This concept is important because certain disease processes, such as strokes, damage only specific areas of the brain, and thus do not result in disability of the entire brain.

What Happens to the Brain as We Age?

The weight of the brain declines by about 2 percent per decade after the age of fifty. This process accelerates the older we get. By age eighty, the average person's brain weight has usually decreased by 10 percent when compared to brains of younger people.

At the microscopic level, approximately 10 percent of our nearly 20 billion neurons die, with the rate of death increasing with advancing age. This death of nerve cells is not uniform throughout the brain; some areas, such as the *hippocampus*, which plays a role in keeping our memory intact, in our navigating through space, and in our sense of smell, are spared in the process of normal aging. Interestingly, however, the hippocampus is not spared in Alzheimer's disease. (This is one of the ways that a normally aging brain differs from the brain of someone with AD.) That the loss of the sense of smell may be one of the first symptoms of AD is also relevant (Drachman 2006).

What Can Happen to Your Brainpower as a Result of Aging?

As our brains age, our reaction time can decrease; this impairment might show up when we drive a car or play a video game. Our short-term, or recent, memory becomes impaired, and the ability to do multiple tasks at once decreases as well (Drachman 2005). Yes, you read that right; you may not be able to multitask as well as you did in your younger years. But at the pace you've been keeping in recent years, that may simply mean that you now can do only three things at once, rather than the six tasks you used to do simultaneously.

Does the Brain Age in the Same Way and at the Same Rate for Everyone?

How the brain function of each individual is affected by the aging process depends on several factors. These include the initial size of the brain before the aging process begins, the person's genetic makeup, and the history of the brain's lifetime experiences, including, for example, whether it has been exposed to trauma, infection, strokes, or poor nutrition. Exciting research has also shown that we, through our own actions, such as exercising regularly or controlling blood sugar, can affect how our brain ages (Drachman 2006). These days, we know that how a person's brain ages is as individual as she and her life experiences are.

For years, conventional wisdom held that the brain completed its development by early adulthood, and that once the nerve cells died, during either the aging process or from trauma or disease, it was impossible for new cells or pathways to grow. We now know that this is not true. Recent studies in mammals have shown that under certain circumstances, nerve cells can be stimulated to grow at any time, even late in life (Fischer et al. 2007). Other research has shown that aerobic exercise actually stimulates the brain to grow new nerve cells, and older brain cells to form new networks that make the brain work more efficiently and faster, no matter how old (Hunsberger et al. 2007; Carmichael 2007).

We can safely say that the deterioration of one's brainpower with age is *not* inevitable. And although the many factors that affect this process are currently being studied, it's a sure bet that how we take care of ourselves now and in the future—getting good nutrition, exercise, and sleep, and managing our chronic diseases—affects how functional our brains remain with age.

MEMORY LOSS

Let's discuss one of the most frustrating signs of aging—memory loss.

What Should You Do When You Begin Forgetting Things?

Many things can cause you to forget what you think you should know; in fact, a memory lapse can happen to anyone at any age. Lack of sleep, an undiagnosed illness, too many things competing for your attention, or a new medication are among the many reasons for memory loss. So, remember that until you see that your memory lapses are occurring regularly, and until other causes have been ruled out, you can't assume that you have dementia. If you are having these episodes frequently, start keeping track of the following: exactly what you're forgetting (a name? a fact? directions to your house?); whether it is a recent memory or one from the distant past (did you forget what you had for breakfast this morning, or where you were born?); what you were doing before and at the time you had the memory lapse (were you multitasking? anxious? tired? recovering from a hangover?); and how you've been feeling physically lately.

If you develop a loss of memory suddenly, and if it is a more comprehensive loss than that of forgetting a name—for example, you don't recognize your daughter—*go to the nearest emergency room (ER)*. For other suspected memory problems, see your primary care clinician. Any information that you can tell her about these occurrences is helpful. She will do a physical exam, including a neurological exam and memory testing; send you to a lab for blood tests; and depending on the results, order a CT (computed tomography) or an MRI (magnetic resonance imaging) brain scan. Based on these results, she may send you to see a neurologist.

Remember this if you are having memory lapses: Don't panic! The anxiety that comes from worrying that you have Alzheimer's disease or another dementia can make your memory problem worse. Before jumping to conclusions and diagnosing yourself with dementia or AD, it is very important that other possible causes for your memory loss be sought. Your memory problems could well be due to an illness, such as thyroid dysfunction. Even if your memory loss is due to age-related changes of your brain, many of these changes are treatable.

Can Memory Lapses Be Treated or Prevented?

As mentioned above, many of the causes of memory lapses can be treated.

TRADITIONAL MEDICAL APPROACHES

The treatment of your memory problems may be as simple as getting more sleep, or changing your cold medication, or getting help for your depression. Once you and your clinician have sorted through all the possibilities and have come to the conclusion that, yes, you really are having some age-related memory changes, then you can think about possible ways to improve your memory or other brain functions. Currently, there are no traditional medications recommended for preventing, or treating, the simple memory loss caused by aging, but there are other ways, mentioned below, that may help.

Just as blood pressure and the health of the heart and lungs are routinely assessed at a medical office, a brief assessment of brain function, including memory, should be done just as routinely. Ask your primary care clinician to perform a "mini mental exam" with your routine physical examination. That way, you can reassure yourself that your brain is still functioning well. It also gives you a baseline against which to compare your brain in the future. If there's even a slight change since your last exam, you can have the problem diagnosed and treated, and, hopefully, prevent its worsening.

COMPLEMENTARY AND ALTERNATIVE APPROACHES TO TREATMENT AND PREVENTION OF AGE-RELATED MEMORY LOSS

There are several approaches to treatment and prevention in the field of complementary and alternative medicine (CAM) that may help with age-related memory loss, including certain herbs, CAM therapies for anxiety, and lifestyle changes. The herb most often studied in the treatment of age-related memory loss, as well as early-stage Alzheimer's disease, is ginkgo biloba (see chapter 13 for a full discussion of this herb).

Because anxiety often follows, or accompanies, the discovery of memory changes, the CAM therapies best for anxiety include massage, biofeedback, breathing exercises, and meditation. It is believed that challenging your brain to learn new things is important for maintaining its optimal level of functioning. Why? The thinking is that by learning something new, the brain may generate new brain cells and form new pathways between cells. The two activities most often mentioned for keeping your brain up to par are learning a new language and doing crossword puzzles. We also recommend that you challenge your brain and increase your vocabulary (and help to decrease global hunger) by going to the website www.Freerice.com.

Our routine recommendations for limiting the effects of aging on your body as a whole apply to your brain as well. Regular physical exercise and proper diet are crucial, as is stopping cigarette smoking, drinking alcohol in moderation, treating your other medical problems, such as high blood pressure, and taking both prescription and nonprescription drugs only as directed.

DEMENTIA

Most people think that dementia is one specific disease. It's not. It is a term that describes a collection of symptoms that can be caused by many disorders in the body that affect the brain. With dementia, a woman not only may suffer loss of memory, but also may have impairment of her intellectual functioning that interferes with her normal daily life. The symptoms of dementia also may include loss of emotional control, loss of language skills, changes in personality, or problems with behavior, to name just a few. The one thing that never occurs with dementia, though, is loss of consciousness. Despite the loss of many other of the brain's functions, the person with dementia is awake and alert.

Just as there are many symptoms of dementia, there are also many types and causes. Alzheimer's disease is the most common type. Others include vascular dementia, caused by diseased blood vessels to and in the brain, such as occurs with strokes; dementia caused by Huntington's disease or associated with Parkinson's disease; and dementia caused by metabolic or thyroid problems, medication reactions, or nutritional deficiencies. Some of these dementias are reversible, such as that caused by a deficiency of vitamin B_{12} or thyroid disease, while others, such as vascular dementia, are not.

However, in some cases, the progression of a vascular dementia can be slowed or halted by controlling the risk factors leading to it, such as high blood pressure.

ALZHEIMER'S DISEASE (AD)

Alzheimer's disease is a specific form of dementia.

What Is It?

Alzheimer's disease (AD) is a specific degenerative disorder of the brain, which progresses slowly and can negatively affect parts, or all, of the brain's cognitive functions; that is, the ability to think, reason, concentrate, and remember. In many cases, these malfunctions can lead to behavioral changes. The definitive diagnosis of AD can be made only by looking at brain tissue under a micro-scope. This is rarely done as it involves taking a biopsy of the brain; therefore, many cases of AD are not definitely diagnosed until autopsy. However, criteria do exist for making the diagnosis of AD based on medical findings. These include a physical examination, a series of blood tests, an MRI of the brain, neuropsychological testing, and the exclusion of all other possible diseases. Taken together these tests can diagnose "probable" AD correctly, approximately 90 percent of the time. There has been ongoing research to find a simpler way to diagnose AD. In fact, recently studies have shown that testing the blood for specific proteins found only in those with AD may be a promising way to diagnose it early (Hye et al. 2006).

This is important because, as with all diseases, the earlier the diagnosis, the earlier treatment can be started to prevent progression of the disease.

What Causes It?

The causes of AD are not fully understood, but since family history is a risk factor, genetics may play a role in some cases. The roles of diet, environment, and education, as well as some of the same risk factors for heart disease and strokes, such as high cholesterol, high blood pressure, and diabetes, are actively being studied.

Who Gets It and What Are the Risk Factors?

AD is the most common cause of dementia of aging in the U. S., affecting more than 5 million Americans. AD usually begins at age sixty-five; it is uncommon for younger people to get it, although it can happen. The most important risk factor is age; the number of people getting the disease doubles every five years beyond the age of sixty-five (Knopman 2008). Therefore, the older one gets, the greater the risk of developing AD.

A long-term study on aging and AD, funded by the National Institute of Aging, that has studied 678 American women, ages 75 up to 106, all of whom are members of the same religious order, began in 1986 and is still ongoing (Snowdon 2003). Known as the Nun Study, it has thus far shown that the main risk factors for AD are age, the presence of specific genetic markers in the blood, and low educational level and/or the inability to skillfully use language in younger years.

The study has also shown that not every participant with risk factors for AD, or with the microscopic findings of AD in her brain at autopsy, developed AD. Whether or not the nun developed the disease clinically depended on other factors, including lifestyle behaviors such as diet, physical and mental activity, cigarette smoking, and, in some cases, attitude, as well as on the presence of other illnesses, especially strokes (Snowdon 2003). (See the Resources section at the back of this book for Dr. Snowdon's book.)

How Do You Know if You Have AD?

AD's onset begins slowly, usually with only a mild forgetfulness, which is why it is so often confused with age-related memory changes. However, most people with mild age-related memory changes don't have AD. As the disease progresses, simple day-to-day functioning may be impaired and behavioral changes may occur.

There are a few interesting differences between the memory loss AD patients experience and the loss that occurs with normal aging. One difference is that the normal mild memory problems associated with aging are related to difficulty in retrieving proper names or recent events, meaning the name you are trying to remember is already stored as a memory and you simply can't find it. In AD, the difficulty is actually in learning something new—before it becomes a memory. In other words, if you were to tell a patient with AD how to do a certain exercise, such as touching her toes, she would not be able to recall this a few minutes later, not because she couldn't retrieve it from her memory, but because she did not learn it in the first place (Knopman 2006).

There is another interesting difference between the memory dysfunction in the AD patient and that in someone whose brain is aging normally. Despite not being able to remember the name you need at the moment, you know that you can't remember it. In other words, you are aware of your memory difficulty. Most people with AD, particularly those past the early stage, do not realize that there's a problem; they simply cannot remember the name or event. This is a loss of self-awareness and insight that shows up as a loss of awareness of one's deficits (Knopman 2006). Because of this, it has been said that AD may be the only disease that causes significant disabilities, but that does not bother the patient or lead her to seek medical help. In fact, most of the time it is the family of the patient that first makes an appointment with a medical provider to have this specific problem evaluated.

What Should You Do if You Think You Have It?

If you are noticing lapses in your memory, there are several things to do, some of which we discussed in the prior section. Observe over time, for at least several weeks, what you are forgetting and how often. If the problems continue or become worse, call for an appointment with your primary care clinician. Remember that anxiety and stress actually can make the memory problem worse; therefore, at the time you can't recall the name you're trying to remember, don't obsess on it.

How Is It Treated?

Currently, AD is thought to be progressive. However, in recent years several medications have been found that slow the progression of the disease in certain AD patients, the most common of which are donepezil (Aricept) and tacrine (Cognex). Obviously, the earlier this type of medication is begun, the better. Also, it is usually recommended that the AD patient take medications to bring relief to some of the other symptoms, such as anxiety, depression, and insomnia. AD treatment continues to be a very active area of research.

How Is It Prevented?

Remember the important lessons from the Nun Study. Make sure your lifestyle is healthy. Stop smoking. Eat a healthy diet. One recent study of AD patients showed that those patients who followed the Mediterranean diet (see chapter 11) had a lower risk of dying from AD (Scarmeas et al. 2007).

Exercise daily. The same studies showing that regular aerobic exercise improves brain function also show that people who do this type of exercise develop AD less often, or at a later age, than do sedentary people (Carmichael 2007). Make sure that any other illnesses you have, such as diabetes or high blood pressure, are well controlled. And regularly exercise your brain. The more you challenge your brain, the healthier it will stay. Also, try to maintain a positive attitude.

OTHER TYPES OF DEMENTIA

There are other causes of age-related dementia, some of which are reversible.

Reversible Causes of Dementia

It is important that a reversible dementia has been excluded before diagnosing one of the more common types of dementia, such as AD. Something as simple as not getting enough vitamin B_{12} in the diet, which may occur with vegetarians, can lead to a dementia with symptoms exactly like AD. The major causes of a reversible dementia include thyroid disease, B_{12} deficiency, late-stage syphilis and other infections, and reactions to medication.

VASCULAR DEMENTIA

Besides AD, the other common type of irreversible dementia is known as *vascular dementia*, formerly called *multi-infarct dementia*. The name refers to the cause: Diseased blood vessels diminish blood flow, and thus diminish the amount of life-giving oxygen that gets to the brain cells. Vascular dementia is caused by strokes, or transient ischemic attacks, which involve exactly the same abnormal processes occurring in the blood vessels that leads to heart attacks. Many people think that strokes only cause paralysis or an inability to talk; they don't realize strokes also can cause a dementia without other symptoms. Which symptoms result from a stroke depends completely on the location in the brain where it occurs. So yes, strokes, especially multiple small strokes, can lead to dementia.

Let's end this section on memory loss and dementia with the same story with which we began. (If you don't remember it, take a minute to go back and read it again.) What should you do while you're propping the now silent cell phone between your ear and shoulder, looking for your purple glove, and

Dr. J's Case of Dementia

My first time diagnosing dementia taught me that it was not a simple thing to do. I was an intern on call in the coronary care unit (CCU) one night, when a patient was admitted for a possible heart attack. This particular patient was in his midforties, intelligent, appropriate in his conversation, and physically healthy. I asked him about the rest of his medical history, his family history, and his social history, including travel. Since he was getting tired, I abbreviated this last question and asked if he had traveled to any exotic places. His answer floored me. I could barely contain my excitement—my first case of dementia! I rushed out of the patient's room to find my supervising resident, told him of my diagnosis, and continued to show my brilliance by spouting which tests the patient needed to have to work up his obvious dementia. The resident quickly pointed out that not only had I left out one very important question in taking the patient's social history—his occupation—but that because of this, my diagnosis was dead wrong. The travel history that convinced me of the patient's dementia? He said he'd been to the moon. His occupation? Astronaut. That night, I definitely learned the importance of not jumping to conclusions when diagnosing dementia!

getting more and more upset because you can't remember who was on the phone or the name of your high school love? First, put down the cell. Then, don't panic!

Remember that a diminished ability to multitask is a normal part of the brain's aging, as is a lapse in recent memory, and that, most likely, you do not have Alzheimer's, or any other type of dementia, for that matter. In fact, this lapse in your memory may not even be caused by the changes in your aging brain; you may have an anxiety disorder or thyroid disease or be overly fatigued. Or it may be simply because you're doing too much.

Be *aware* of your family history and your other risk factors for dementia; be *alert* to the specifics of any changes in your brain's functioning; take *action* to be evaluated and prevent further changes; and *advocate* for yourself. And don't forget to pick up your other glove from under the table!

STROKE

This is a word, and a disease, that is dreaded every bit as much as AD. Stroke ranks second to coronary artery disease as a cause of death worldwide, and as a disability in high-income countries (van der Worp and van Gijn 2007). In the U.S., there are more than 700,000 new strokes each year, with stroke being the third leading cause of death, following heart disease and cancer. Causing more serious long-term disability than any other disease, nearly three-quarters of all strokes occur in people over the age of sixty-five (Kasner and Morganstern 2006). Even more alarming is the recent finding that women ages forty-five to fifty-four are more than twice as likely than men of the same age to have a stroke (Towfighi et al. 2007). Further, obesity has been linked to this increase in strokes among middle-aged women.

What Is It and What Causes It?

A stroke occurs when the blood flow of one of the arteries supplying the brain, either within the brain or in the neck (carotid arteries), is interrupted. Deprived of oxygen, the section of the brain supplied by that blocked artery dies. This is identical to what happens during a heart attack (see chapter 3). In fact, some professionals use the term "brain attack" when referring to a stroke.

There are two types of strokes: ischemic and hemorrhagic. Accounting for almost 80 percent of strokes, *ischemic strokes* are caused by a blockage in an artery supplying the brain. Just as with the coronary arteries that feed the heart, the causes of blockage in one or more of the arteries feeding the brain include blood-clot formation (*thrombosis*), narrowing of the artery (*stenosis*), and movement of a blood clot from another part of the body to the artery feeding the brain (*embolism*).

Hemorrhagic strokes, which are much less common than those of the ischemic type, are caused by the rupture of an artery going to the brain, which then bleeds into the brain. Causes of an artery's rupture include high blood pressure, plaque formation in the vessel wall (as occurs with high cholesterol), and a bleeding aneurysm, which is formed from the ballooning and breakage of a weak spot in a blood vessel.

Are You at Risk for a Stroke?

The conditions that can put you at risk for having a stroke are identical to those that put you at risk for a heart attack. These risk factors include uncontrolled high blood pressure, high cholesterol, smoking cigarettes, diabetes, family history of stroke or heart disease, sedentary lifestyle, and obesity. An additional risk factor for stroke, but not for heart attacks, is the presence of a specific type of irregular heartbeat known as *atrial fibrillation*. In recent years, studies have also found that a history of migraines with an aura may increase the risk of stroke (MacClellan et al. 2007), as may psychological stress (Surtees et al. 2008). Knowing your risk factors and treating those that can be controlled is of utmost importance in lowering your risk of death or disability from stroke. (See chapter 3 for a full discussion of these risk factors.)

How Do You Know if You're Having a Stroke and What Should You Do About It?

Another key step in preventing damage from a stroke is knowing the warning signs.

WARNING SIGNS FOR STROKE

The symptoms of a stroke depend on the location in the brain where it has occurred; because different parts of the brain control many different functions, the symptoms are also many and varied. They are listed in the accompanying text-box.

If you have even one of the warning signs, call 911 immediately and go to a stroke center!

MINISTROKE WARNING SIGNS

Occasionally, one or more of the symptoms of a stroke may occur for only a few moments and then disappear. This brief episode is known as a *transient ischemic attack* (TIA), or a *ministroke*, and indicates a diseased blood vessel in the brain that is not completely blocked. This blood vessel is on its way to causing a stroke at some time in the future, although not necessarily instantly. One review study found that more than 15 percent of patients can be expected to have a stroke within ninety days of having a TIA (Wu et al. 2007). Do not ignore TIAs, even if they last for only an instant. *If the symptoms keep recurring or never quite resolve call 911. Even if the symptoms quickly resolve and do not recur, call 911 and go to a stroke center.* If you remember an episode that happened previously that you think may have been a TIA, call your clinician to let her know of your symptoms as soon as possible. You should be seen within several days after your episode and should wait no longer than a week. Since some hospitals also have TIA clinics, your clinician may refer you there or to a neurologist.

How Is a Stroke Treated?

Once you've arrived at the ER, you will be examined, have blood drawn, and undergo an imaging scan of your brain, such as a CT or an MRI. Any medical abnormalities, such as uncontrolled blood pressure, will be corrected and stabilized at the same time.

USE OF "CLOT-BUSTING" DRUGS

Warning Signs of a Stroke

+ Sudden numbness of the face, arm, or leg—especially on only one side

+ Sudden weakness of the face, arm, or leg—especially on only one side

+ Sudden confusion

+ Sudden difficulty in speaking or in understanding

+ Sudden difficulty in seeing out of one or both eyes

+ Sudden difficulty walking

+ Sudden dizziness, loss of coordination or balance

+ Sudden severe headache, or nausea and vomiting

Once the symptoms of a stroke have occurred, the sooner it is treated, the better the outcome. In recent decades, the use of "clot-buster" drugs, such as tissue plasminogen activator (tPA), can completely reverse, or limit, the brain damage if used *within three hours after the symptoms begin.* The drug does this by cleaning out the blocked artery and allowing blood flow to return to the affected area of the brain. The availability of these lifesaving drugs has made it crucial to do the following three things if you think you're having a stroke.

Do not wait. Call for help as soon as you can after the symptoms begin. Remember, you have a three-hour window of time in which the treatment will work. This means that you must get to the hospital sooner than that; you must get there within one to two hours after your symptoms begin in order to be properly evaluated.

Call an ambulance. If you think you are having a stroke, always call an ambulance. A recent report from the Centers for Disease Control found that more than half of all stroke patients do not arrive at a hospital within the necessary time frame; it also found that those patients who called an ambulance were much more likely to arrive within that time period (CDC 2007b).

Go to a stroke center. Despite the success of clot-busters in treating strokes, fewer hospitals than would be expected actually use them (Schumacher et al. 2007; Kolata 2007). In the Schumacher study, the hospitals most likely to use this treatment were teaching or university hospitals. So you must find out *now*, before you may really need to know, which of the hospitals in your area commonly use tPA, or have a stroke program or "brain attack" program in place. You can do this simply by calling the emergency rooms of nearby hospitals and asking. Because academic centers (university hospitals) almost always use this treatment, you can also call the emergency room of a nearby university hospital.

IF CLOT-BUSTING DRUGS CANNOT BE USED

If you are not eligible to have the clot-busting drugs given to you due to time limitations or your medical history, you will be admitted to the hospital for further treatment and, if needed, physical and occupational rehabilitation. Also, all of your risk factors and their level of control will be assessed in order to prevent another stroke in the future.

How Are Strokes Prevented?

Currently, there are two effective methods for the prevention of strokes.

CONTROL OF RISK FACTORS

As with coronary artery disease, all risk factors must be controlled in order to prevent a stroke from occurring in the first place. For instance, high blood pressure and high cholesterol must be normalized. Because atrial fibrillation, a type of irregular heartbeat, puts you at risk for a stroke by causing blood clots to move from the heart to the brain, your heart rhythm should be controlled as well as is possible; anticoagulation medication (causing the blood not to clot) may also be necessary. (See chapter 3.)

Although the blood vessels within the brain cannot be assessed during a routine physical examination, the carotid arteries in the neck, which supply the brain, can be. Ask your clinician to check your carotid arteries for blockage. She can do this easily and quickly by listening over these arteries for a certain sound (known as a *bruit*) with a stethoscope. Although this exam is not always accurate, if a bruit is found, further studies, such as a carotid Doppler, can be done to make the definite diagnosis of blockage. If you have risk factors for stroke, ask your clinician about getting a carotid study even if no bruit is heard.

FOLIC ACID SUPPLEMENTATION

A recent analysis of eight randomized studies concluded that folic acid supplementation can prevent the occurrence of a first stroke; no advantage, however, was found in preventing strokes for those patients who'd had a prior stroke (Wang et al. 2007). Since the best dose for preventing a first stroke is currently not yet known, we would recommend, particularly if you have risk factors for stroke, that you start with 400 mcg per day; ask your clinician if another dose has been recommended more recently. In addition, many of the studies used other B vitamins in addition to folic acid. You should discuss taking other B vitamins as well as a multivitamin with your clinician as well.(See chapter 13 for more information on folic acid and multivitamins.)

Once again, our mantra of awareness, alertness, action and advocacy applies. Be *aware* of your risk factors for strokes; be *alert* to the warning signs and any new symptoms you might have; take *action* to control your risk factors and seek help if warning signs occur; and *advocate* for yourself by knowing which hospitals are stroke centers, and by asking about evaluation of your carotid arteries and about folic acid supplementation.

Lorraine's Story

Lorraine, a very intelligent sixty-seven-year-old widow, enjoyed her life despite having several medical issues. She had high cholesterol levels that were somewhat controlled on medication, and severe high blood pressure that, despite the use of several medications, was difficult to control. Her biggest issue, though, was her diet; she was a gourmet cook, and she couldn't imagine whipping up her delicious creations without constantly tasting her recipes, despite the fact that this habit made her weight rise right along with her beautiful breads, which made her medical problems worse. Plus, Lorraine hated any exercise other than what she got in her kitchen. She understood that she was at risk for heart disease and strokes, but she felt that since she had never been seriously ill or hospitalized, she would be okay. Then, one day while she was making whipped cream, she suddenly dropped the bowl on the floor and noticed that she couldn't move her right hand and arm. She immediately called 911, and then called Dr. J's office.

By the time she was off the phone, she had to sit because she couldn't move her leg. By the time Dr. J got to the hospital, Lorraine was already able to move her arm and leg after being treated with the clot-buster medication. Today, she's back to normal physically and back to her usual lifestyle, with one exception. She is still known as the best cook in the neighborhood, but now she's using low-fat, low-salt, and low-sugar recipes, and she is delivering her healthy meals—on foot—to people unable to get out of their homes. By the way, her weight is on the way down, and her blood pressure and cholesterol levels are perfect now.

HEADACHES

Since headaches most often begin in our younger years, and since they are so common in women, you probably have had them or know someone who has them. Because of this, we're going to mention two things to know about headaches at this stage of life. First, pay attention and take note of any new headache or, if you have chronic headaches, any change in the pattern of those headaches. Second, if you have migraines, be aware that they may change after menopause; in some people, the migraines become less frequent and less severe, and in others, they increase in frequency and in the severity of the pain.

Why Is It Important to Pay Attention to a New, or Changing, Headache at this Age?

Although, generally, headaches decrease with age, the older we are, the more likely it is that a *new-onset headache* indicates a serious condition. What do we mean by "new-onset headache"? It is a pain inside your head, or on your scalp or face, that you've never experienced before. It may occur only several times or frequently, but it always occurs more than once. If you have had headaches in the past, a new-onset headache is different—in location or intensity—from your previous headaches.

Ninety percent of headaches in younger people are either migraine or tension headaches, neither of which is life-threatening, while only 66 percent of headaches in older people are due to these two less serious causes (Evans 2006). This means that approximately one-third of headaches occurring in older people are due to a serious underlying cause that must be diagnosed quickly.

Some of the conditions that can cause a new-onset headache at this age include uncontrolled and very high blood pressure, an impending stroke, an infection of the brain, a *subdural hematoma* (a blood clot on top of the brain caused by head trauma), or even a tumor. Another worrisome cause of a sudden headache at this age is *temporal arteritis*, which is an inflammation of the temporal arteries, located near the temples on both sides of the face. It occurs almost exclusively in people over fifty years old, and most commonly in women. (See chapter 8.) Because this disease can lead to blindness if not treated, it should always be considered as a possible cause of a new-onset headache.

For a severe headache, particularly if it is of sudden onset, go to the ER. The longer you wait to seek medical help for a new headache, or one that has changed, the longer the delay in diagnosing and treating the potentially life-threatening cause for the headache will be. Are we saying that you should be alarmed by every ache and pain in your head now that you're older? Definitely not, especially if you continue to have headaches in the same old pattern, or have a new headache that is mild, lasts only a short time, and does not recur. But do not ignore a new type of headache or a change in your old pattern of headaches.

THE DOCS CHAT ABOUT
THEIR AGING BRAINS

DR. R: Does taking estrogen replacement after menopause prevent or help memory loss?

DR. J: Good question. For years, it was thought that taking estrogen after menopause helped memory loss. Recently, the thinking is that estrogen may actually worsen it in older women. So, the answer to that question is up in the air. But here we go with our debate! I, personally, will never take estrogen for many reasons, but one reason is the possibility of it worsening my memory.

DR. R: And I'll never stop! Taking bioidentical estrogen, that is. But since we're going to talk about this in chapter 10, on menopause, let's table this disagreement until then. Another question: What do you do when you have memory lapses or can't find the name or word you're looking for?

DR. J: Oh I hate that! I was so used to relying on my memory that I never wrote myself reminder notes and could always remember names of people I just met. Now what happens is that just when I need to remember a specific word or name—it's not there! I know that I know the word, I just can't find it. Sometimes I get so anxious trying to remember that I forget even more names. I finally realized that my anxiety was making it worse. So now, when I can't retrieve a word or name, I make a conscious effort to laugh, stop thinking about it, and quickly move the conversation to another topic, or move on to the next activity. Usually, within a few hours, the lost word comes to me spontaneously.

DR. R: And what do you think of those new studies discussed in this chapter showing that aerobic exercise can improve brain function? Since I love to exercise and you don't, do you think that may be the reason that my memory is better than...

DR. J: Don't you dare go there! I have to admit, though, that the studies about the positive effects of aerobic exercise on the brain will be the one thing to make me exercise more regularly.

DR. R: You mentioned that at the first warning sign of a stroke, we should immediately call 911 for an ambulance. But you also say that we should find out ahead of time which hospitals have stroke centers so that we will know to go there. Don't ambulance drivers make the decision as to which hospital they'll take us? How do we deal with that?

DR. J: Very important question. You're right that the ambulance driver makes that decision. But you can find out before you ever have the first symptom whether the nearest hospital (which is the most likely place you'll be taken by a 911 ambulance) has a stroke center. If it doesn't, then call private ambulance companies (look in the yellow pages) to find out if they will take you to a stroke center even if it's not the nearest ER. Since they usually will take you to the hospital that you request, call a private ambulance rather than 911 if you have symptoms. It is essential to get to an ER that is a stroke center.

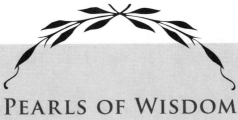

PEARLS OF WISDOM FOR THE BRAIN

○ Loss of brain function is not an inevitable result of aging.

○ Exercise your brain and body regularly.

○ Ask your clinician if you should take folic acid supplements.

○ Find out which hospitals in your area have stroke centers.

○ Know the warning signs for stroke; if you have any of them, call 911 or a private ambulance immediately.

○ Know what a TIA, or ministroke, is. If you think you've had one, see your doctor within one week after the symptoms occurred.

○ Go to the ER for a severe and sudden headache.

CHAPTER 2

How to Keep Your Sight, Hearing, and Balance Intact

We have all seen the caricature portrayed in comics and TV of an older woman with her eyeglasses attached to a plastic chain around her neck, holding a newspaper as far from her eyes as her arms can reach, while she leans to one side and plays with the hearing aids protruding from both of her ears (and buzzing loudly), who constantly complains that everyone around her is mumbling. Of course, this is a bit of an exaggeration, but difficulties with vision, hearing, and balance have always been such common accompaniments to the aging process that we automatically associate getting older with the loss of function in these senses. And although we, who are entering this next phase of our lives in the twenty-first century, may have more stylish chains from which our bifocals dangle, and hearing aids which, when placed in our ears are so tiny as to be invisible to others, will still have to face the insults to our senses that aging inevitably brings. Inevitably? Not necessarily.

Yes, many of our senses do decline with age. But just how much they worsen is not a given. We do have some control over how well we see, hear, and stay upright as we get older. To do this though, we need to be *aware* of what can happen to our organs of sensation; be *alert* to the onset or presence of symptoms that indicate diseases; be *active* in preventing problems with, and in taking care of, our sensory organs; and *advocate* for ourselves if we think we are not getting the care we need and deserve.

THE EYES

Overall, the outlook for our aging eyes is good. There is much new information about how to take care of our eyes to prevent vision loss. Also, as you will read, for several of the major diseases of the aging eye, there are now exciting new treatments to prevent blindness.

The Normal and the Aging Eye

One easy way to consider the eye is to think of it as functioning like a camera. Light from the outside enters the front part of the eye (the lens) and is focused onto the back of the eye (the retina), which then transmits the image, as a signal, through the optic nerve to the brain. The most common changes that occur with normal aging of the eye are discussed below.

Farsightedness. When the shape of the eye does not properly bend the light that enters it, the image sent to the brain is seen as blurry; this is known as a *refractive* vision problem and includes far-sightedness and nearsightedness. The farsightedness that occurs as a natural part of aging is known as *presbyopia*, and it is the most common visual problem to occur with advancing years. You may have already experienced symptoms like blurred vision at a normal reading distance and eye fatigue or headaches when doing close work. And, probably, you've easily corrected it by using reading glasses or changing your regular eyeglasses for bifocals.

Visual difficulty with color, light, and adapting to the dark. Aging may affect the way colors and contrast are seen; for example, it may become hard to tell the difference between the color blue and the color black or green. Remember this when your spouse or partner keeps wearing one green sock and one blue. You may also notice that you need more light to be able to see, and more time to adjust to changing levels of light. The latter is especially important at night and causes you to see less well in the dark after having being inside in bright light. Remember this when you are driving at night, and give yourself enough time for your eyes to adjust to darkness after you go outside from a brightly lit room.

Flashes and floaters. Exactly as their names sound, they are bright flashes of light, specks, or squiggles that suddenly appear in your field of vision. Sometimes they are described as looking like stars, cobwebs, or little bugs. Although floaters and flashes usually disappear quickly, they may persist, but they become less noticeable over time. They always move when you try to look at them, and most of the time they are noticed in bright light. Usually harmless, they are common at any age but become even more so as we grow older.

There is one serious condition, however, that may present with floaters and flashes that can lead to blindness. This is known as a *retinal tear*, or *detachment*. One of the risk factors for a retinal tear is being nearsighted. The warning signs of this include the sudden onset of many new flashes of light and floaters that don't go away quickly or lessen over time, the loss of side vision, and distorted or blurred vision. *If any of these symptoms occur, go to the emergency room.*

Dr. J's Aging Eyes

Although Dr. J has had the same aging eye symptoms as everyone else over fifty, there was one that was particularly bothersome to her. That was the symptom of seeing colors a bit differently than she was accustomed to seeing them. She would occasionally experience "seeing" many large circular yellow spots appearing on solid, light-colored objects. Since she has many dogs who sleep with her and her husband, imagine her distress when those large round yellow spots kept appearing on her white bedsheets!

The Eye Diseases of Age

The three major eye diseases, cataracts, glaucoma, and age-related macular degeneration (AMD) have two things in common: They are all more common as we age, and they can each lead to blindness if left untreated. Since many of their risk factors and warning symptoms are similar, we are going to consider them together.

WHAT CAUSES THESE DISEASES?

These three diseases occur in different parts of the eye and are caused by different mechanisms.

Cataracts. Cataracts are caused by the clumping together of proteins in the lens, almost always related to aging, which results in a clouding, or opacity, in the lens. A cataract may occur only in one eye, or in both eyes at the same time, and develops very slowly over years.

Glaucoma. Glaucoma is the term used for a group of disorders of the optic nerve. It may occur in only one eye, or in both. It is often associated with an increase in the pressure within the eyeball, also known as the *intraocular pressure.*

Age-related macular degeneration. AMD is a degenerative disease of the center of the inner lining of the eye, the *macula*, which is located in the area of the retina, in the back of the eye.

HOW COMMON ARE THESE DISEASES AND WHO GETS THEM?

These diseases all commonly occur with aging.

Cataracts. Cataract disease is the leading cause of blindness in the world and accounts for nearly 48 percent of all blindness (Abraham, Condon, and Gower 2006). Almost 60 percent of all Medicare spending in the 1990s was dedicated to cataract surgery (Ellwein and Urato 2002). In the late 1990s and the year 2000, these costs had decreased, but that was due only to the lower cost of cataract surgery itself (Salm, Belsky, and Sloan 2006). Cataracts occur much more frequently in people over age fifty-five. Nearly everyone who lives long enough will develop the changes of early cataract formation, if not progressive cataracts.

Women get this disease more commonly than men do. African-Americans are at particularly high risk for developing cataracts, though that may be due to the large numbers of this population who have diabetes, a major risk factor for cataract disease. It is also known that African-Americans are more likely to become blind from cataracts (Abraham, Condon, and Gower 2006).

Glaucoma. Approximately 66 million people in the world have glaucoma, with at least 6.8 million of these being blind in both eyes. It is the second leading cause of blindness in the world (Weinreb 2006) and the leading cause of blindness in African-Americans (Sommer et al. 1991). Glaucoma is estimated to affect at least 4 million people in the U.S., where it is one of the leading causes of blindness (Lesser et al. 2001). African-Americans develop this disease more than other ethnic groups; they are also four to eight times more likely to go blind from glaucoma than Caucasians (Sommer et al. 1991).

Age-related macular degeneration. AMD is the leading cause of visual loss in the developed world. Though your chances of getting AMD steadily increase after the age of fifty, the average age of visual loss from this disease is seventy-five. Between 14 and 20 million people currently have AMD in the U.S., where it is the major cause of central vision loss. Also, AMD is much more common in Caucasians than in African-Americans (Clemons et al. 2005).

ARE YOU AT RISK?

Many of the same factors put us at risk for each of these diseases. These factors are as follows.

Advancing age. This is a risk factor for all three diseases.

Smoking cigarettes. This is a risk factor for both cataracts and AMD. In a recent study, people currently smoking had increased risk of developing AMD at an earlier age than the norm and nearly 50 percent more risk when compared to nonsmokers (Klein et al. 2008). In addition, smoking was associated with the progression of AMD over time.

Diabetes and high glucose levels. These are major risk factors for cataracts, and they are being studied for their role in the development of glaucoma.

Overexposure to ultraviolet sunlight. This is a major risk factor both for cataracts and AMD.

Prolonged use of high-dose cortisone. This is a major risk factor for cataracts.

Family history. This is a major risk factor for glaucoma and has been associated with AMD. In 2006, this relationship was further clarified when two genes strongly associated with AMD were found. This particular genetic finding, along with a new and effective medication for the disease, was listed as one of the top ten breakthroughs in science for the year 2006, in the prestigious *Science* magazine's annual list (News Staff 2006).

Elevated intraocular pressure. This causes glaucoma and is a major risk factor.

High blood pressure and high cholesterol. Both of these are risk factors for AMD (Martidis and Tenant 2004).

WHAT ARE THE SYMPTOMS?

Unfortunately, these three diseases may have no symptoms at all in the beginning stages. However, there may be changes in various parts of the eye that your eye doctor can detect, early in the disease process, despite your not having any symptoms. This is why regular and complete eye examinations are so important.

Loss of vision. This is *never* normal! Whether it is a partial or complete loss of vision, located on one side or in the center of the image, occurs in one or both eyes, is of sudden or gradual onset, or is temporary, this is an emergency! *Call 911 immediately or go to the emergency room.* Loss of vision may indicate any one of the three eye diseases discussed above, but it also may be due to a stroke or mini-stroke (see chapter 1) or the eye disease accompanying advanced diabetes (see chapter 11 for further discussion on diabetes). No matter the cause, for you it is an emergency!

Cloudy or double vision. This may occur in the early stages of cataract formation, especially when looking into the distance. One of Dr. J's patients with a newly developing cataract in one eye described it as "like looking through a thin silk or gauze veil all the time."

Sensitivity to bright light. This symptom, common with cataracts and glaucoma, can make driving at night quite difficult due to the glare of the oncoming headlights.

Difficulty seeing in dim light. This may be a symptom of either cataracts or glaucoma.

Yellow tint of visual images. This may occur with cataract development.

Frequent changes in distance vision. With cataracts, you may become progressively more nearsighted, requiring a change in the prescription of your glasses. Since this is the opposite of the farsightedness that normally occurs with aging, be alerted to the possibility of cataracts, especially if you've become more and more nearsighted.

Halos around lights. This may occur with glaucoma.

Painful red eye. This may be a sign of glaucoma.

WHAT SHOULD YOU DO IF YOU DEVELOP ANY OF THE ABOVE SYMPTOMS?

As mentioned, *any loss of vision is an emergency.* In addition, the sudden occurrence of flashes and floaters, or distorted vision that does not resolve or lessen quickly, is an emergency. Call 911 or go to the ER (see discussion below about ERs for eye emergencies). For eye pain and redness without accompanying loss of vision, see your eye doctor as soon as possible. For any of the other symptoms, make an appointment to see your eye doctor.

What to know about emergency rooms for eye problems. Not all emergency rooms have an eye doctor immediately available, and they may not be equipped to deal with all eye emergencies. At one of your regular visits to your eye doctor, ask which ER she would prefer you to go to with an urgent eye problem. Usually, this will be either where she practices or where there is special staff available for eye emergencies. Generally, university hospitals have ophthalmologic staff readily available too. Understand that the ER suggested for your eye emergencies may not be the same one that your cardiologist or family doctor recommends.

The eye exam. Although many of the above mentioned changes in the way you see may not represent a dangerous process, you should still pay attention to new symptoms that develop in either or both of your eyes, and seek advice from your eye doctor. In addition, get regular eye examinations, even if you are having no eye problems at all. We recommend that you see your eye doctor once a year. Obviously, your eye professional may tell you to come in more frequently based on the condition of your eyes.

A complete exam includes a vision check, an intraocular pressure check, and a look into the back of your eye after the pupil has been dilated. Be sure you get all three exams when you have your eyes checked. Most eye doctors do these routinely.

HOW ARE THESE EYE DISEASES TREATED?

Cataracts, glaucoma, and AMD can all lead to blindness if not detected early and treated.

Cataracts. Although some cataracts stop progressing after a certain point, once they have developed, they are never reversible. Surgery to remove the lens of the affected eye is the only treatment that prevents the progression to a complete loss of vision. Fortunately, in the U.S. cataract surgery is a safe outpatient procedure that is usually successful in completely restoring vision within several weeks.

Glaucoma. Although vision that has already been lost due to optic nerve damage cannot be regained, further loss of vision can be stopped with successful treatment. There are three types of therapy with which to treat glaucoma: treatment with medications, laser treatment, and surgery. These may be used alone or in combination depending on several factors relating to your health, and on the opinion of your eye doctor.

AMD. Treatment of AMD has changed dramatically over the past thirty-five years (Fine 2005). In June 2006, a new drug (ranibizumab, or Lucentis) was approved by the FDA. It not only stabilizes vision and prevents further vision loss in all patients with AMD, it also actually improves vision in patients with the more serious form, wet AMD (Stone 2006). This is definitely a treatment you need to know about. Prior to this, photodynamic and laser therapy were the only options for treating AMD.

Another simple approach to halting progression of AMD, and its associated visual loss, was shown in 2001 by a large study that demonstrated the benefit of daily supplementation with antioxidants (500 mg vitamin C, 400 IU vitamin E, 15 mg beta-carotene, 80 mg zinc oxide, and 2 mg cupric oxide). Since then, it is recommended that all patients diagnosed with AMD take these supplements (AREDS 2001).

HOW ARE THESE EYE DISEASES PREVENTED?

Unfortunately, none of these three diseases has been shown to be preventable yet, although stopping smoking may prevent the AMD from occurring at an earlier than usual age. But, as mentioned above, the most serious complication of each—blindness—is preventable through early diagnosis and appropriate treatment. In addition, we provide general recommendations for protecting the health of your eyes below.

Know your risk factors and get regular eye exams. The best way to prevent the long-term complications of any of the diseases is to know that you have it, or are at risk for it. If you have one of the risk factors listed above (and all of us who reach the age of sixty will have at least one of them, sooner or later), you should get a regular eye evaluation yearly without fail.

Change the risk factors that you can. Control your diabetes, blood pressure, and cholesterol, stop smoking, and avoid overexposure to sunlight.

Wear appropriate sunglasses. What about sunglasses? Are those cheap ones from the flea market okay to wear even if your eyes are normal and you don't have risk factors for cataracts or AMD? No! They are not okay. More expensive sunglasses may not even give you adequate protection. You should make sure that the sunglasses you buy are coated with enough ultraviolet (UV) light-absorbing material to prevent cataract formation. Sunglasses that have a label saying "Meets ANSI Z80.3 General Purpose UV Requirements" meet this criterion and are known as "general purpose sunglasses."

If you are at particular risk for cataracts because of having diabetes or having smoked cigarettes, or if your eye doctor has told you that you have early cataracts, wear only "special purpose" sunglasses; these fit snugly on the nose, wrap around the head, and block light from below, above, and both sides of the glasses. They should carry a label that says "the Skin Cancer Foundation's Seal of Recommendation for Sunglasses." Know, too, that polarized glasses cut glare but do not protect against UV radiation. In addition to special purpose sunglasses, a large sunhat will take care of those extra rays.

Supplements. Take daily doses of vitamin C (500 mg), vitamin E (400 IU), beta-carotene (15 mg), and zinc (80 mg) only if a diagnosis of AMD has been made for you. Remember, though, that these supplements haven't been shown to prevent AMD, just to slow its progression.

Although free radicals do play a role in the development of cataracts, antioxidants, such as vitamins C and E, have not been proven to prevent them. Check with your eye doctor before taking any supplements in dosages higher than recommended. (See chapter 13 for further discussion about recommended doses of supplements.)

THE EARS

Did you know that your ears contain sensory organs that govern both your hearing and your balance?

The Normal and the Aging Ear

For descriptive purposes, the ear is commonly divided into three parts: the external ear, those appendages attached to the sides of our head to which we attach our earrings and into which sound enters; the middle ear, housing the tiny bones that aid in sound conduction; and the inner ear, which shelters the organ of hearing, the *cochlea*, which translates sound into electrical signals, and the *semicircular canals*, making up the vestibular system that protects our balance. The information about what we hear, and about the position of our bodies in relation to our external environment, is sent to the brain from the ear via the *auditory nerve*.

All parts of the ear experience some changes with aging. The tiny bones in the middle ear stiffen at their joints, causing sound not to be conducted as well as previously. The sensory cells in the cochlea in the inner ear, and the cells of the auditory nerve, degenerate with age too. As discussed in chapter 1, the aging brain has diminished ability to process some information brought to it, which may adversely affect hearing, causing difficulty in identifying a spoken voice or understanding a spoken sentence, especially when there is background noise (Kashima et al. 2005).

The semicircular canals are also prone to a reduction in sensitivity. The number of sensory hair cells decreases, as does the number of nerve cells going to the brain. These changes may lead to balance problems (Girardi and Konrad 2005). Since the overall maintenance of balance is a function shared with the vestibular system by the brain and the eyes, both of which undergo degenerative age changes as well, you can see why aging itself naturally puts you at an increased risk for falling.

Hearing Loss (Presbycusis)

Another very common condition occurring among older adults is the hearing loss that may accompany aging known as *presbycusis*. It is present in about 25 to 40 percent of people over the age of sixty-five, in approximately half of people over the age of seventy-five, and in 80 percent of those over the age of eighty-five (Bance 2007).

Although presbycusis alone does not usually lead to profound hearing loss, it may occur with other ear diseases, combining to cause severe hearing loss. The exact causes of presbycusis are not known, but the major risk factors are aging and toxic exposures, that is, the sum of all the noise and chemicals to which we've been exposed throughout our life (Kashima et al. 2005). No specific ethnic or gender group is more prone to presbycusis, although once begun, the hearing loss progresses more rapidly in men (Bance 2007).

Presbycusis occurs in both ears simultaneously and progresses slowly over many years. The hearing of high-frequency noises is usually affected first, although some people experience diminished hearing at all frequencies. There are no associated symptoms of imbalance, such as vertigo or dizziness, or ear pain. Therefore, the diagnosis and treatment of this condition is not an emergency. Having said that, if you notice changes in your hearing, tell your primary care provider, who will arrange for the definitive hearing test, an *audiogram*.

The hearing loss of aging may occur at the same time as another, more serious, condition that affects hearing. Consult your primary care provider or your ear specialist immediately if you notice any of the following: hearing loss in only one ear or more severely in one ear than the other; sudden onset of hearing loss; associated dizziness or headaches or ear pain; hearing only low-frequency sounds; or rapidly progressive hearing loss (weeks to months rather than months to years).

Any of these symptoms would indicate that something more is going on than the simple hearing loss of aging. However, whatever this additional problem leading to more hearing loss is, it does not have to be serious; for example, too much wax in the ear pressing against the eardrum can cause loss of hearing.

Although there are currently no treatments to reverse presbycusis, there are two interventions that can improve hearing—hearing aids and cochlear implant surgery. Only 10 to 20 percent of those with presbycusis wear hearing aids, as not everyone needs or benefits from them. There are many different and improved types of hearing aids currently available. Although cochlear implant surgery generally has been done on younger patients, recently, it is has been used more often in older patients, most of whom get good results. Prevention of age-related hearing loss is a very active area of research. Even if you have no hearing difficulties right now, limit your exposure to loud noises (even if that means wearing earplugs!), keep your lifestyle healthy, and ask your primary care clinician to order a baseline hearing test (audiogram) for you so that your hearing can be followed over time.

Dr. R's Story

Recently, since she began having trouble hearing, Robin came to the conclusion that all the hours she spent at rock concerts in her youth, not to mention her stereo blasting in her dorm room, had finally caught up with her. She noticed it specifically when her sixteen-year-old son took his cell phone out of his pocket very abruptly and started talking. This distressed her because she had not heard the phone's musical ring tones, she knew he didn't have the vibrate option on, and she hadn't seen him dial out. She had long thought that he mumbled, but that was his problem, right? Or could she be losing that much of her hearing?

Just as she was trying to adjust to the idea of having hearing loss and wishing she'd had a baseline audiogram when her hearing was still good, she saw an article in the New York Times reporting a new technology that was all the rage of school kids, particularly those in schools that did not allow cell phone use. What was that technology? Someone in Great Britain, knowing that most adults gradually lose their ability to hear high-pitched sounds (high frequencies), had come up with a ring tone for cell phones that was so high-pitched that adults could not hear it at all (Vitello 2006)!

LOSS OF BALANCE WITH AGING

Not only does the organ responsible for hearing, the cochlea, deteriorate with age, but the vestibular system, which maintains our balance, deteriorates as well.

The Problem of Falling

Given how physically active we women born in the twentieth century have always been—vigorously playing tennis, jogging, power walking, snow skiing, white-water rafting, mountain climbing, even bungee jumping—and the many falls we've no doubt suffered throughout our lives, why is falling at this stage of life such a big deal?

Good question. Falls are the most common way that older people get injured. Approximately 30 percent of older people who fall sustain a serious injury, such as a broken bone, which requires them to have help with day-to-day activities for weeks thereafter. A recent study showed that in 2006, approximately 1.8 million Americans over the age of sixty-five sustained an injury due to a fall (Stevens et al. 2008). Even more telling, nearly 40 percent of all admissions to nursing homes—either for long-term care or respite care, are related to falls, mostly for hip fractures (Marchetti and Whitney 2005). On a personal level, we all know at least one elderly person who was doing quite well living independently until a fall caused her entire life situation and health status to go rapidly downhill.

Based on a twenty-five year review of the literature, the American Academy of Neurology recently concluded that the following are definite risk factors for falls: Advanced age, frailty, arthritis, depression, dementia, stroke, and balance disorders (Thurman, Stevens, and Rao 2008). Probable risk factors for falls include: Parkinson's disease, peripheral neuropathy with decreased sensation in the feet, lower extremity weakness, full or partial loss of vision, and a history of falling within the prior year.

Like breathing, maintaining ourselves in an upright position is very easy to take for granted, particularly in our younger years. However, as we grow older, we need to be *alert* to the fact that we may lose our balance more easily due to the aging of our vestibular system, brain, and eyes—all organs keeping us upright; be *aware* of all symptoms that may occur before an unintentional fall; be *active* in seeking medical help for these symptoms, and in doing exercises that help us maintain our balance; and *advocate* for ourselves if someone tells us that "falls are a normal part of aging."

HOW DO YOU KNOW IF YOUR SENSE OF BALANCE IS IMPAIRED? WHAT CAN YOU DO ABOUT IT?

The most well-known symptom indicating a balance problem, or occurring before or causing a fall, is dizziness.

Dizziness. This is a very common symptom. It accounts for more than 8 million visits a year to primary care providers in the U.S. (Sloane, Coeytaux, and Beck 2001). The word "dizziness," however, can mean different things to different people (like a "dizzy" blonde), and is used to indicate different symptoms including light-headedness, the sensation of the room spinning (*vertigo*), and overall body weakness. What these descriptions have in common is that when they are experienced, if not alleviated in some way, a fall will usually occur. Dizziness also can be a warning sign that another, more serious health problem is just around the corner.

The first thing to do when you get dizzy is sit down! If your episode of dizziness is brief, and not associated with either a loss of consciousness or any other symptoms, simply stay seated for a few minutes, drink some water, and wait to see if the dizziness returns. When you get up from sitting, do it very slowly.

Loss of consciousness (fainting). With no previous diagnosis to explain it, loss of consciousness is never normal. How can you know if you lost consciousness if you were alone when you fell? If you cannot remember every part of your fall, if you are confused when you find yourself on the ground, or if you have any question that you may have passed out, proceed as if you actually did lose consciousness. *If you lost consciousness even briefly and have never done that before or been evaluated for it, call your primary care provider immediately; if you cannot get in touch with her quickly, call 911.*

Furthermore, if you have the associated symptoms of chest pain, heart palpitations, shortness of breath, or abnormal sensation in one of your limbs, and/or the episode continues for longer than a few minutes, call 911.

HOW ARE BALANCE PROBLEMS DIAGNOSED?

Once you see your clinician or are in the ER, you will undergo a thorough evaluation including a physical exam, an EKG (electrocardiogram), blood work, and, depending on your symptoms, a CT scan of your head. The goal of this evaluation done so soon after your fall is to exclude the most serious causes of the symptoms, such as a heart attack, a dangerous heart arrhythmia, a seizure, or a brain abnormality, such as a stroke. Once these serious causes have been ruled out, the remainder of the workup can be done at a more leisurely pace with you as an outpatient. If you did not lose consciousness, then your dizzy spells can be evaluated as an outpatient.

WHAT IS THE TREATMENT?

The treatment of dizziness or vertigo depends completely on the cause. Occasionally, no definite cause can be found, and the symptoms are simply observed over time. When it's been established that you're having balance problems as the cause of your symptoms, you may be given medication to stop the dizziness or vertigo itself, as well as some physical exercises.

CAN IT BE PREVENTED?

Tactics to prevent loss of balance are focused on preventing falls and halting the progression of, or reversing, the underlying cause. In recent years it has been found that certain types of physical exercise actually can improve balance. (See chapter 11 for a discussion of this type of exercise.) And, of course (here comes our mantra!) a healthy lifestyle will help.

THE DOCS CHAT ABOUT AGING EYES AND EARS

DR. R: I'm really pleased because the outlook for our aging eyes and ears is much better than I thought it was. Which reminds me, who do you send your patients to for their eye care, an optometrist or an ophthalmologist?

DR. J: An optometrist has studied, and practices, eye care and can examine and diagnose eye disease. But since optometrists don't have MD degrees, they cannot prescribe medication or do surgery. An ophthalmologist has an MD degree and does the same eye exam as the optometrist, but can also do eye surgery and prescribe medication.

DR. R: So, which do you refer your patient to?

DR. J: Both. If my patient needs a thorough eye exam, I will send her to either. If the situation is an emergency or I know she will need medication or surgery, I send her to an ophthalmologist.

DR. R: I know that we didn't have enough pages in our book to cover the nose and mouth. So let me ask you here, are our senses of smell and taste affected by aging?

DR. J: Yes, there is some decrease in the sense of smell itself as we get older, but this is complicated by the fact that many of the medications that we take, and the illnesses that occur with age, such as Alzheimer's disease, and B_{12} deficiency, also may affect our smelling ability. As for the sense of taste, the same thing applies, except that smell declines more than taste. Moreover, those two senses function together so that we often confuse what we taste with what we smell.

DR. R: Is there anything special we should know about our mouth, teeth, and gums as we get older?

DR. J: Absolutely. Many of the mouth structures change with age, making dental and oral care a must, just as it was in our younger years. Also, among the risk factors for gum inflammation are advancing age, smoking cigarettes, smoking marijuana, and poor, or lack of, dental hygiene. In recent years, gum disease has been associated with both heart disease and stroke.

DR. R: Are you saying that gum inflammation causes these diseases?

DR. J: No, just that they are associated somehow; more research needs to be done. In the meantime, regular dental checkups and dental hygiene are crucial for our general health.

Pearls of Wisdom for the Eyes and Ears (and Nose And Mouth)

○ Get regular eye checkups, including a dilated eye exam and a test of the intraocular pressure for glaucoma, once a year.

○ Ask your eye doctor what emergency room to go to for eye emergencies.

○ Any loss of vision, or the sudden onset of any other eye symptom, is an emergency.

○ Protect your eyes from the sun at all times. Make sure your sunglasses give you proper protection.

○ Get a baseline audiogram.

○ Turn down the volume on your TV, radio, and stereo, or use ear plugs if you can't control the volume.

○ Do specific exercises for balance regularly.

○ Get regular dental checkups and maintain your daily dental hygiene.

○ Keep up a healthy lifestyle.

CHAPTER 3

How to Keep Your Heart Healthy and Happy

What is the one disease that women are most afraid of getting? Breast cancer. But just look at these statistics: Approximately 44,000 women will die from breast cancer this year, and 500,000 will die of cardiovascular disease (heart attacks and strokes). Heart attacks alone kill 267,000 women each year and cause six times as many deaths in women as breast cancer. Heart disease is the number one killer of men and women (AHA 2007). Surprised? Most women are.

Until recently, little was known about heart disease in women. Because our unpredictable hormone cycles got in the way, in the past researchers studied only men and then applied their findings to women too. For years, science looked at women as "mini-men" who also had periods. Today, we know that women often experience quite different symptoms of heart disease than men do. We also know now that there are specific factors that contribute to the development of heart disease in men that may affect women differently, such as smoking cigarettes, diabetes, and lipid levels. It is important to understand all we can about these differences and how to prevent heart disease in the first place.

THE NORMAL AND AGING HEART

Let's talk about the basics. First of all, what is the heart…really?

The Normal Heart

The heart is an organ made completely of muscle, roughly the size of your fist. In a lifetime, it can pump enough blood to fill three Olympic-sized swimming pools. If you have ever wondered whether a higher power existed, seeing a heart beating inside the chest would make you believe. This miraculous organ is linked to an intricate system of blood vessels, the arteries and veins, which together are known as the *circulatory*, or *vascular*, system.

The *heart*, the driving force of this system, is actually a two-sided pump. The right side of the heart pumps the "used" blood (without life-sustaining oxygen but with carbon dioxide, the body's waste product) it receives from the body to the lungs. The left side of the heart receives the "fresh" blood (with oxygen but without carbon dioxide) from the lungs and pumps it to the body and the blood vessels, including to the blood vessels that feed the heart, known as the *coronary arteries*. All this pumping of the heart, also known as "contracting" or "beating," is done in an orderly and synchronized way, creating your pulse.

What keeps the heart beating? An electrical system, influenced by the brain and nerves, regulates the rate and rhythm of the contractions. When the electrical system becomes damaged or doesn't work properly, the contractions of the heart may become irregular, too fast, or too slow, or a contraction may be skipped; all of which will be experienced as an abnormal pulse. It's important to know that an irregular pulse does not always mean there is a problem with your heart; some pulse rhythms or rates that are abnormal for others may be normal for you. That's why it is imperative to learn what is normal for your body.

Because the heart is made up of muscle tissue, it needs to be treated just like any other muscle in your body: kept in shape in order to stay healthy so that it maintains a good, strong blood flow. When this blood flow is compromised, disease occurs. Compromise of the blood flow to the heart itself results in a heart attack.

The Aging Heart

How an individual's heart ages is as unique as she is and depends on many factors, including genetic risks for heart disease and the sum total of her lifetime experiences and choices. Physical activity, body weight, diet, smoking history, presence of other diseases and how well they are managed, and stress levels are among the many factors that influence the aging of the heart. Therefore, from one person to another, there is much variability in how the heart ages.

Having said that, the heart and blood vessels, with no disease, do very well with aging. Some changes in this system related to aging include stiffening of the blood vessels, which causes the systolic blood pressure (top number) to increase and the heart to pump harder. A decrease in the number of muscle cells causes the heart itself to stiffen; and, as in the aging brain, the death of some of its nerve cells results in changed electrical transmissions and a slowed, or irregular, heartbeat.

Despite these changes brought about by aging, the heart continues to function well in "normal" times. It is only when the heart is stressed, for instance, during a sudden emotional upset or when running or rushing up the stairs, that you may notice more difficulty than when you were younger; you may become short of breath or tire more quickly, or you may need to stop and catch your breath. However (and you can guess what's coming next), if you've kept your heart muscle in shape with regular physical activity, both aerobic and strength training exercise, your heart will not show signs of aging even when stressed—yet another reason to exercise.

The Healthy Heart

For a healthy heart, you need healthy blood vessels, a healthy electrical system, and healthy heart muscle. Since diseases of the blood vessels and the electrical system are common in our age group—women over fifty—we'll discuss how to keep these two components of the cardiovascular system healthy in this chapter.

CORONARY ARTERY DISEASE (CAD)

The most common cause of problems with the heart is coronary artery disease.

What Is It? What Causes It?

Disease of the arteries that feed the heart itself, the *coronary arteries*, evolves over a long period of time. It occurs as a result of *atherosclerosis*, which means the hardening, or narrowing, of the arteries. Over time, many things can injure your arteries, such as high blood pressure, high cholesterol, high blood sugar, or chemicals from cigarette smoke, to name a few. After the arteries are injured, inflammation occurs, which results in the body's response of depositing a *plaque* (think of a plug), made of protein, fat, and calcium, in the wall of the damaged arteries. These plaques can be of various sizes; they start out small and enlarge as time goes by. They may grow so large that they block off the coronary artery in which they originated, or they can break off from a distant artery and be carried by the bloodstream to a coronary artery. Both of these processes result in acute coronary syndrome.

What Happens Next?

Acute coronary syndrome is the name for what can happen immediately after a coronary artery gets blocked off. One of three events occurs: angina, a heart attack without EKG (electrocardiogram) changes, or a heart attack with EKG changes. An *EKG* is a recording of the electrical activity of the heart.

ANGINA

Angina, or chest pain, occurs when there is an incomplete blockage of the coronary artery; this means that some blood can still flow through that artery. What results from the inadequate blood flow is pain in, but no damage to, the heart muscle. Think of this pain as like a cramp in your heart muscle. There are two types of angina.

Stable angina. Pain that occurs only with certain activities and remains at the same intensity each time it occurs is known as *stable angina*. It is your body's warning signal for you to rest and to seek help.

Unstable angina. When the pain increases in intensity and frequency, or occurs when you are at rest, it is called *unstable angina* and can soon lead to heart muscle damage. This is an emergency.

HEART ATTACK WITHOUT EKG CHANGES

The second possible occurrence, caused by a total coronary artery blockage, is heart muscle damage, known as a *myocardial infarction*, or heart attack. Despite the muscle damage to the heart, there are no changes in the EKG. It's important for you to know that you can be having a heart attack but show no EKG changes.

HEART ATTACK WITH EKG CHANGES

The third event that may occur, also due to total coronary artery blockage, is a heart attack with EKG changes. This is the most common form of heart attack.

Who Is at Risk for CAD?

There are many factors that increase the chances that a woman will develop coronary artery disease. We call these *risk factors*; the more you have, the greater your chance of getting CAD. Some of these risk factors cannot be changed; others can be. We discuss the risk factors, and what you can do to modify them, at the end of this section on CAD.

How Do You Know if You Are Having a Heart Attack?

The symptoms of a heart attack are not always the same for men and women. The typical symptoms in men are crushing chest pain that radiates down the left arm or up into the neck, accompanied by shortness of breath and/or sweating lasting for more than a few seconds. For women, the symptoms *may* be the same, but often they are more subtle. Women more often experience shortness of breath, a feeling of weakness or overwhelming fatigue, cold sweats, and/or dizziness. Women may also experience chest heaviness, indigestion, nausea, and discomfort in the arm or jaw.

A study on heart attack in women done by the National Institutes of Health found that 95 percent of the women studied had experienced symptoms that they knew were *unusual for them* about one month before they had their heart attack. The most common symptoms reported were unusual fatigue, sleep problems, shortness of breath, indigestion, and anxiety (McSweeney et al. 2003).

Because many of these symptoms are vague, we may ignore them. But they are important warning signs. Even with an increased awareness of the differences of heart attack symptoms between men and women, there is still a problem getting women to seek help early. And when we do seek help, the medical evaluation is either not done or is delayed because the clinician thinks that the symptoms are not typical for heart disease. In this situation, you must be your own advocate; you know more than the clinician that the symptoms you're having are not normal for you. Moreover, now you know that these abnormal symptoms may be caused by heart disease.

As we've mentioned in several other chapters, we've noticed that women are very intuitive about their bodies. If you have a sense that something is wrong with your heart (or your body), you are most likely right. If you visit your clinician and are not taken seriously, go to another doctor, or go to the emergency room. Insist on an evaluation. Remember our mantra: Be *aware* that you are at risk for heart disease; be *alert* to all of your symptoms; take *action* by getting a thorough medical evaluation; and *advocate* for yourself!

Ellen's Story

Ellen, a charming sixty-year-old Caucasian professional chef who previously had been healthy except for having high blood pressure and a "weight problem," woke up one morning with severe jaw pain. So sure was she that the cause of the pain was a bad tooth, she went to her dentist twice in one day when the pain continued to get worse. He could find nothing wrong with her teeth or mouth at either visit. Out of frustration and still with severe jaw pain but no other symptoms, Ellen called Dr. R, who saw her immediately and did an EKG.

Ellen was having a massive heart attack. Her jaw pain was her only symptom. Despite having several risk factors for CAD, including her age, high blood pressure, and being overweight and sedentary, it didn't occur to her that she could be having heart problems. But she knew something was wrong, followed her gut instincts, and pursued the cause of her pain until she got the correct diagnosis.

What Do You Do if You Think You Are Having a Heart Attack?

If you think you are having a heart attack and you are not allergic to aspirin, call 911 and chew an aspirin; time is of the essence here. Do not wait, just call and take the aspirin! Either adult or baby aspirin will do. (It is always good to have a small bottle of aspirin around for just this purpose.) The aspirin will help to break up the clot that is plugging the artery and prevent further clotting from sticking to the plaque. Chewing the aspirin makes it dissolve faster than swallowing it whole, so it gets into the bloodstream more quickly.

How Is a Heart Attack Diagnosed and Treated?

Once you are in the ambulance or at the hospital, you will be given oxygen through a mask or nasal prongs and be connected to a heart monitor immediately; you will also have an intravenous line (IV) started. You may be given medication immediately as well, depending on your symptoms and examination. You will have an EKG done in order to look for changes indicating a heart attack, and blood will be drawn to look for certain heart enzymes that are released when the heart is damaged.

IF YOU ARE HAVING A HEART ATTACK

If you are in the midst of a heart attack, the cardiologist will be called to see you. In many cases, it will be necessary to see which artery is blocked so it can be opened to prevent permanent heart damage. If the blocked artery can be opened within three hours, there is a good chance that the heart muscle affected by the blocked artery can be saved. In certain cases, thrombolytics, or clot-buster medications, will be used.

Coronary angiogram. In order to see and possibly open the blocked artery, you will be taken to the cardiac catheterization laboratory, where the cardiologist will inject dye into your coronary arteries through a catheter that is placed into your groin artery and moved up to your heart. This procedure is known as an *angiogram*. With it, all of the arteries of your heart can be seen. If there is a blockage, the dye won't go through. This sounds scary, but it has become almost a routine procedure and is relatively safe. However, it is always best to have a cardiologist who has a lot of experience with this procedure do your catheterization.

Coronary angioplasty and stent placement. Once the blockage is detected, it can be opened with a little balloon that presses the side of the blockage to open the artery. Next, a *stent*, which looks like a little metal cage, is placed in the area to hold the artery open permanently. After this procedure is completed, or if it is decided that you don't need the angiogram, you will be taken to the coronary care unit (CCU) of the hospital, where you will receive further treatment.

IF YOU ARE NOT HAVING A HEART ATTACK

For patients with chest pain who are found not to be having a heart attack, several causes and treatment recommendations are possible.

For unstable angina. If your chest pain is getting worse and is unstable, it usually means that you are on your way to having a heart attack, even if it has not yet occurred. The cardiologist will most likely recommend an angiogram to look at your coronary arteries. Depending on how they look, you may need angioplasty and stent placement, or even bypass surgery.

For stable angina. If the pattern of your chest pain is stable, one of the less invasive tests will be recommended. All of these tests involve observing your heart function during and after exercise; the difference between the tests lies in the method used to determine how your heart is functioning. If you are found to have a stable blockage, there are many options for long-term treatment as an outpatient.

One of the tests that may be recommended is known as a *thallium stress test.* You will be placed on a treadmill or a stationary bicycle and asked to walk or cycle. At the peak of the exercise, a small amount of a radioactive dye called thallium is injected through the IV into your vein. After this, you will lie down on a special table to have an x-ray machine take pictures of your heart muscle, which will show a lack of blood flow to the heart if you have a blockage of a coronary artery when you exercise. The pictures are taken again after two to three hours of resting; these will show whether that lack of blood flow persists.

Another similar test is the *stress echocardiogram.* Again, you will be placed on a treadmill and asked to exercise; in this test, an ultrasound of your heart (the same type of machine used to look at babies in the womb) is done. Just as with the thallium stress test, the cardiologist can tell whether your heart is getting enough blood to function normally by watching your heart muscle movement on the echocardiogram.

You may be asked to undergo an even simpler type of test, a plain *stress test*, in which you are hooked up to an EKG machine during exercise. Abnormalities in the EKG are then evaluated, which can be related to changes in the blood flow to your heart. It is important for you to know that in women, this test is not as accurate for detecting CAD as it is in men. The chances that the test isn't really positive (known as the *false positive rate*) are high. There is a false positive rate with the imaging studies described above as well, but it is not as high as with the plain stress test.

Be aware that the coronary angiogram is the gold standard test for finding out if there is blockage in one or more coronary arteries.

How Is CAD Treated?

We have just discussed the treatment of an acute, or ongoing, heart attack. What about treatment for stable angina or the treatment recommended *after* a heart attack? In other words, how is coronary artery disease treated in the longer term?

MEDICATIONS

There are many medications that are used alone, or in combination, to treat CAD. The three standard medications given after a heart attack include either a beta-blocker or an ACE inhibitor (both have been found to protect the heart muscle), a statin drug (to lower the LDL cholesterol and reduce inflammation in the blood vessel walls), and medications such as aspirin or Plavix (clopidogrel) which act to reduce platelet clumping and attachment to plaques. Other medications may be added to this regimen that can help with smoking cessation, lowering blood pressure, or treating diabetes if present.

Even though the medications mentioned below are standard recommendations for CAD and thus should be given to everyone with CAD, *studies have shown that they are often underprescribed (or not prescribed at all) to women, and especially to women of color.* That is why it is so important for you to know what these medications are, as well as when and why they should be taken (Bell and Nappi 2000). Again, this is another situation in which you need to advocate for yourself!

Aspirin. If a woman has had a heart attack or is at risk for a heart attack, aspirin at a dose of 81 to 325 mg daily is recommended. Aspirin in a dose between 81 and 100 mg prevents strokes in women under sixty-five (whose blood pressure is controlled) and heart attacks in women sixty-five or older by making platelets less sticky, and thus preventing their clumping and attachment to plaques. For this reason, aspirin causes the blood to clot less easily, in essence "thinning" the blood. However, because of this effect, the main risk of taking aspirin is bleeding, especially in the gastrointestinal tract.

If you have an aspirin allergy or a bleeding problem, do not take aspirin and discuss what you should do instead with your doctor. If you are at high risk for a first or second heart attack and cannot take aspirin because of an allergy, often clopidogrel (Plavix) is recommended. Like aspirin, it "thins" the blood and can cause bleeding as well.

Beta-blockers. This class of medication includes such drugs as atenolol (Tenormin) or propranolol (Inderal). They blunt the effects of adrenaline on your system, such as a rise in heart rate or increased anxiety, and thus protect your heart. In women who have had a heart attack, beta-blockers have been found to reduce the chances of having a second heart attack, and to reduce the chances of dying after a heart attack. Since some formulations of these drugs can cause wheezing, specific types of beta-blockers that are safer for women with asthma may be prescribed. Other medications that may be recommended for treatment of CAD include ACE inhibitors, such as quinapril (Accupril); angiotensin receptor blockers (ARBs), such as losartan (Cozaar); aldosterone blockers, such as spironolactone (Aldactone); and nitrates, such as nitroglycerin which comes in pill, patch, and spray form.

NUTRITIONAL SUPPLEMENTS

In addition to prescribed medications, certain supplements are recommended.

Fish oil. The American Heart Association (AHA) has recommended that those with CAD, or at risk for developing it, either add fish into their diet two to three times a week or use fish oil, both of which contain omega-3 fatty acids. For her patients, Dr. R often recommends between 1 and 3 grams a day. Fish oil has been found to decrease the risk of heart disease and has also been shown to decrease triglyceride levels in the blood. It may, however, increase the chance of bleeding in some patients. It's important to look for distilled fish oil that is free of heavy metals like mercury.

Vitamins. Though previously recommended, vitamins such as vitamin E are no longer recommended for prevention of heart disease. (See chapter 13.)

How Are Heart Attacks Prevented?

Lifestyle changes to decrease your risk of having a first or second heart attack, or a stroke, are just as important as taking the recommended medications. These changes really do work, as shown by the precipitous decline in heart-related deaths between 1980 and 2000. Rapid treatment at the time of a heart attack and improvements in risk factors accounted for the major part of this drop (Ford et al. 2007).

RISK FACTORS FOR CAD THAT CANNOT BE CHANGED

Some of us have factors that put us at risk for CAD that we cannot change. However, knowing what those factors are can help us make healthy choices and also help us change those factors that we do have control over. Risk factors that cannot be changed include the following.

Increasing age. Growing older is a major risk factor.

Gender. Men have a greater risk of having a heart attack than women prior to menopause. Once menopause hits, we catch up.

Heredity. If your parents or a sibling had a heart attack, your chance of having one increases.

Race. Premature death from heart disease is highest in Native American, Alaskan native, and African-American women. Their increase in the risk of CAD is due to the fact that these ethnic groups have more risk factors such as diabetes, obesity, and high blood pressure. This also accounts for the increased risk in Asian Indians.

A history of previous heart attack or stroke. Having had either of these in the past increases a woman's risk for having another. This is why it's so important to modify all the risk factors that you can, even if you have already had a heart attack or if you have known heart disease.

RISK FACTORS FOR CAD THAT CAN BE CHANGED

Many factors that can be changed may increase our risk for heart disease. These include the following.

Cigarette smoking. Smokers have two to four times the chance of developing heart disease as non-smokers. Smoking isn't an equal opportunity risk factor either. It appears to have a more deleterious effect on women than men. A woman who quits by the age of thirty-nine will add three years to her life; a man who quits will add five years to his life (Njolstad, Ameson, and Lund-Larsen 1996).The good news, however, is that once you quit smoking your risk goes down right away.

Cigarette smoke damages the lining of blood vessels and can cause the plaque to erode, become unstable, and break off. Smoking also leads to CAD by raising blood pressure and lowering "good" cholesterol (HDL) levels. When combined with birth control pills, smoking is particularly deadly, increasing the risk of both heart attacks and strokes by increasing the risk of blood clots. (See chapter 15 for more on smoking.)

High blood pressure. This is a powerful risk factor for all vascular disease: CAD, stroke, and *peripheral vascular disease* (atherosclerosis of the arteries supplying the legs). *Normal blood pressure* is defined as less than 120/80 mm Hg (millimeters of mercury, the measurements on a blood pressure machine). The top number is known as the systolic pressure. The bottom number is known as the diastolic pressure. A blood pressure that is between 120/80 mm Hg and 140/90 mm Hg is considered *prehypertension*. A blood pressure of 140/90 mm Hg or greater is considered *hypertension*.

The researchers in the Women's Health Initiative study found that 40 percent of postmenopausal women have prehypertension (Hsia et al. 2007). This puts them at an almost 70 percent higher risk of cardiovascular death than women with normal blood pressure. Even within the prehypertensive group, the higher the blood pressure, the greater the risk (Conen et al. 2007). So, small elevations in blood pressure above what is considered to be normal can be risky.

There are definite ethnic differences in both prehypertension and hypertension rates. As of 2004 in the U.S., 46.6 percent of African-American women, 31.9 percent of Caucasian women and 31.4 percent of Mexican-American women had high blood pressure. What is frightening about this is that over two-thirds of those people who had had a first heart attack and 77 percent of those who had had a first stroke had high blood pressure (AHA 2007).

The good news is that, like stopping smoking, when you control your high blood pressure, the risk for heart attacks and strokes goes down substantially. So, the key is being *aware* that you have it. Many women have no idea what their blood pressure is at all, much less if it is high. Because most often high blood pressure has no symptoms, it is important to have it checked at least once a year, and if you have a family history or other risk factors for high blood pressure, such as being overweight, have it checked more often.

High total cholesterol. *Cholesterol* is a type of fat, also known as a *lipid* or *lipoprotein*, that is needed by every cell in the body. However, when there is too much of it, there are problems. When your doctor checks your cholesterol level, she is also checking your entire lipid profile. One type of cholesterol is good to have and the other… not so good. The following lipids are those found on a standard blood test:

LDL (low-density lipoprotein) is called the "bad" cholesterol. It can build up along the walls of the arteries and cause narrowing or hardening of those arteries. High levels of LDL are considered a major risk factor for CAD.

HDL (high-density lipoprotein) is called the "good" cholesterol. It acts like a scavenger and picks up extra cholesterol in the body and carries it back to the liver, where it is packaged and released when the body needs it. Low levels of "good" cholesterol, or HDL, are a more powerful predictor of heart disease in women than in men. That is, if a woman has low amount of the good cholesterol, her risk of having heart disease is greater. The flip side is that the higher a woman's HDL level is, the less likely she is to have coronary artery disease. Even in the face of high LDL, or "bad" cholesterol, HDL is important for protection. The higher the HDL, the better (Barter et al. 2007). Before menopause, women's HDL levels tend to be high; afterward, they tend to drop (along with a few other things!)

Triglycerides (TG) are circulating fats that are used for energy and in making hormones. They appear to play a bigger role as a risk factor for heart disease in women than men. High TG levels are part of what make up metabolic syndrome, discussed in chapter 11.

Lp(a), or *Lipoprotein a*, is another type of fat in the body, for which there is currently no treatment recommendation. High levels of Lp(a) are considered a risk factor for heart disease; there is a strong genetic link to this risk factor. It is not included on the routine lipid profile blood test but is ordered separately if you have a family history of heart disease.

How do you know if your lipid levels are healthy? There are guidelines based on risk of heart disease (NHLBI 2004). Acceptable levels of each lipid are those that put you at a low risk of developing heart disease. It is recommended that your total cholesterol be no greater than 200 mg/dl (milligrams/deciliter).

+ Your HDL should be greater than 50 mg/dl.

+ Your LDL should be less than 100 mg/dl.

+ Your triglycerides should be less than 150 mg/dl.

Since it is almost impossible to know if your cholesterol levels are high without testing your blood, it is important that every woman over fifty have these blood tests at least once a year.

Diabetes. Diabetic women are three times more likely to develop CAD when compared to those that don't have diabetes, and it is more of a risk factor for CAD in women than it is in men. Diabetes can cause blood pressure to rise and the good cholesterol (HDL) to fall—not a healthy combination. Diabetes is another of those conditions like high blood pressure and high cholesterol that often have no symptoms. As with the other two risk factors for CAD, you should be checked for diabetes yearly, in this case by having a fasting blood sugar test. (Diabetes is discussed in chapter 11.)

Obesity. Being overweight or obese is a risk factor for CAD for two reasons: It is a risk factor for heart disease in and of itself, and it can lead to the development of several other risk factors for CAD such as diabetes, high blood pressure, and high cholesterol. In addition to being overweight, an "apple" body shape (the midsection of your body is larger than the lower portion), or a waist circumference greater than 35 inches, puts you at increased risk for CAD. The definitions and risks of being overweight or obese, including those unrelated to heart disease, and what to do about excess pounds, are discussed in chapter 11.

Sedentary lifestyle. Being inactive on a regular basis increases the likelihood of developing obesity, diabetes, high blood pressure, and hardening of the arteries, thus making it more likely that you will get CAD. Regular exercise helps keep your blood vessels open and flexible, and your blood pressure and HDL cholesterol in the normal range. Therefore, exercising regularly is as important for the inside of your body as it is for your external appearance. Because physical activity is so important in protecting against CAD and heart attacks, doing it routinely should be viewed as necessary and every bit as important as taking prescribed medications. (See chapter 11 for more on exercise.)

Stress and depression. Although stress and depression have not been studied as extensively as other CAD risk factors, your mind and your spirit definitely have an impact on your heart. Depression has been found to affect how fast and regularly the heart beats. It can also increase the buildup of plaque in the arteries. People who are depressed often have poor eating and exercise habits that contribute to the risk of heart disease as well. Depression also increases the risk that a person who has had one heart attack will have a second (Zellweger et al. 2003).

One powerful example of how the emotions can affect the heart is called the "broken heart syndrome." Researchers at the Johns Hopkins Hospital found that the body often releases a big surge of adrenaline for days at a time when a person is confronted with an overwhelming and stressful event (Wittstein et al. 2005). When this happens, the heart acts like it was hit with a stun gun, causing the patient to develop an abnormality in the movement of the heart muscle. This occurrence can look and act exactly like a massive heart attack. Middle-aged women are particularly prone to this syndrome. The good news is that patients with this syndrome do not develop permanent damage to their heart muscle; they can recover quickly in a few days, and return to normal in a few weeks.

Hostility also plays a role as a risk factor. Other psychosocial factors that affect the heart include job and/or marital stress, social isolation, and the effects of poverty.

Hormone replacement therapy (HRT). Since the release of the results from the Women's Health Initiative (WHI) study (Writing Group for the Women's Health Initiative Investigators 2002), there has been much confusion regarding the safety of HRT when it comes to the heart. This study and what it means for our health are discussed in chapter 10, but we briefly mention the results related to heart disease here.

Remember that one of the major reasons HRT had been recommended to menopausal women for years was that it was thought to prevent heart disease. The WHI study seemed to show the opposite. In fact, the study had to be stopped early when an increase in heart attacks, strokes, and breast cancer was found in the group of women taking hormones, as compared to the group who were not taking them.

When the data was analyzed looking only at the younger women in the study, there was no increased risk of heart attack in those who began using HRT within ten years of going through menopause; in fact, it now appears that their risk was diminished (see chapter 10). The increased risk of heart attack appeared to be present only in the older women taking HRT. Therefore, HRT may pose a risk for heart attacks only in older women and in those who already have heart disease. Obviously, more studies on the issue of HRT are needed.

Decreasing Your Risk for CAD

Once you are aware that you have risk factors for CAD and know what they are, there are two ways to decrease your chance of it developing, or progressing (if you already have it): screening for the presence of CAD and modifying your risk factors.

SCREENING

Remember that CAD can develop over a long period of time without causing any symptoms until the blocked coronary artery prevents blood flow to the heart. That's when you either get angina or have a heart attack. Therefore, if you have a risk factor for heart disease, such as a strong family history or diabetes, or several risk factors, your clinician may recommend that you have a screening test to look for the disease, even if you are feeling well. If disease is found, then treatment can be started to hopefully prevent a heart attack.

Because plain EKG stress tests can be inaccurate in women, screening for CAD often will involve your having a thallium stress test or a stress echocardiogram in addition to, or instead of, the plain stress test. There is a newer test, not involving exercise, that may be recommended. Known as the *coronary calcium screening test*, or *rapid heart CT* and it involves a special CT scan that shows if there are calcium deposits in the coronary arteries. Although this test is simpler than the others, there is concern that it may increase the risk of cancer, particularly in women, due to the increased radiation exposure. This is currently being studied (Einstein, Henzlova, and Rajagopalan 2007).

So, when should you be screened for CAD? This depends on your individual risk factors and should be discussed with your clinician. It is important that you advocate for yourself and ask your clinician about being screened for CAD if you have risk factors.

MODIFYING YOUR RISK FACTORS

Now that you know what your risk factors are, it should be fairly straightforward to move ahead and modify those factors that can be changed. But that doesn't seem to be what most of us are doing. A recent article in the *New York Times*, one of a well-researched series on the major health problems in America today, pointed out that most Americans know the risk factors for CAD and know how to modify them, but most of us are not using this knowledge (Kolata 2007). In other words, we are not changing our habits to help our hearts stay healthy. We're not giving up cigarettes, eating healthy foods, exercising regularly, checking our blood pressure, having blood studies done, or taking prescribed medications. And we're not taking these preventive measures in spite of knowing that these habits lead to CAD. Don't let this be you! Use your knowledge to change your habits. Read on to learn how to specifically do this.

Quit smoking. The addiction to cigarettes/nicotine is as powerful as the addiction to heroin. Even when people are able to quit, they often relapse. However, the more you try, the more likely you are to succeed. See chapter 15 for a discussion of ways to stop smoking.

Avoid high blood pressure. Women from our generation take for granted that there are many treatments available for high blood pressure. At the time of our thirty-second president, Franklin Delano Roosevelt, very little was known about it, including the fact that it is dangerous. FDR suffered from severe hypertension and heart disease. His blood pressure was 226/118 mm Hg at the time of the invasion of Normandy in 1944. Doctors advised rest and time away from work. Since his death, which eventually occurred as a result of this problem, doctors and researchers found better ways to combat hypertension and CAD.

The change in lifestyle recommended to FDR still applies. Exercise (such as thirty minutes of brisk walking a day), and eating a heart-healthy, low-salt diet with olive oil, fish oil, fruits and vegetables (such as the Mediterranean diet) can reduce blood pressure (as well as improve LDL or the "bad" cholesterol; Fito et al. 2007). Beware of hidden salt in processed foods; the salt you add may not be the problem. Foods such as prepackaged soups can have 1,000 mg of salt per cup! Most doctors recommend 2,400 mg of salt a day for patients with normal blood pressure, and 1,500 mg of salt a day for those with high blood pressure. Small amounts of dark chocolate can lower blood pressure slightly. The operative word here is "small," or about 30 calories worth. A half cup of soy nuts eaten throughout the day can also lower blood pressure (Welty et al. 2007a). (See chapter 11 for further discussion of healthy eating habits.)

Another potential way to lower your blood pressure is through the practice of meditation, a mind-body technique that fosters a relaxed state and a different level of awareness. Research has shown that meditation can lower blood pressure in men and women. Since high blood pressure affects more African-Americans than Caucasians, research using meditation is ongoing specifically in this group. In fact, one study found that in older African-Americans, meditation reduced systolic blood pressure by 10 points and diastolic blood pressure by more than 6 points (Schneider et al. 1995). (See chapter 14 for more on meditation.)

If diet, exercise, and meditation do not work, you may require medication to lower your blood pressure. (See the section above on medications used to treat CAD; many of these are also used for high blood pressure.) For a mild elevation in blood pressure, a water pill, or diuretic, is enough to lower it. If you do not respond to a diuretic alone, you may need an additional medication, such as a beta-blocker, ACE inhibitor, or ARB. Two other classes of antihypertensive medications are the calcium channel blockers, such as verapamil (Isoptin) and nifedipine (Adalat), and the class that includes clonidine (Catapres).

Lower Your Cholesterol if It Is High. It is extremely important to lower your total cholesterol level, LDL level, and/or triglyceride levels if they are higher than recommended, and to raise your HDL level if lower than recommended. As with high blood pressure, diet and exercise can have a huge impact on decreasing these levels. Exercise can also increase the HDL level. If you are unable to effect a big enough change in your cholesterol levels with these measures, the next step is medication.

The most commonly used are niacin (Niaspan) and the statin drugs, such as atorvastatin (Lipitor). The statins are very effective in lowering total cholesterol, LDL cholesterol, and triglycerides, and in slightly raising HDL cholesterol. Statins help to prevent stroke and heart attack as well. The most serious, though unusual, side effect of the statins is muscle damage; less serious, though more common, is a rise in the blood tests that reflect liver function. It is important to have your clinician follow you closely when you take statins, or any medication. We recommend taking the supplement CoQ10 along with a statin drug to potentially prevent muscle injury.

Herbs and supplements have become popular for treating high cholesterol. Red yeast rice is a natural statin drug, and must be monitored the same way. It is effective for lowering moderately high cholesterol. If you are going to take it, have your doctor monitor your liver; if you get muscle pain, stop taking it. The supplement, policosanol, which comes from sugarcane, has shown impressive results at lowering cholesterol, although no one is quite sure why it works. More studies are needed. Coenzyme Q10 does not lower cholesterol; however, studies suggest that when it is taken with statins, there is less muscle pain and injury. As discussed earlier in this chapter, fish oil, rich in omega-3 fatty acids, has been found to lower triglyceride levels. Before you start any of these supplements on your own, discuss with your clinician whether they are right for you, especially if you are taking prescription medications. (See chapter 13 for more information on supplements and their risks and benefits.)

CONTROL DIABETES

Because diabetes is such a big risk factor for CAD, especially in women, controlling high blood sugar is of major importance. This is discussed in chapter 11.

PAY ATTENTION TO YOUR MENTAL AND SPIRITUAL HEALTH

It is important to pay attention to your mental and spiritual health. We often forget that they can have an impact on our physical well-being. Putting yourself last on the list is a risk factor that you won't find in any conventional medical literature; but it is at the top of our personal lists. Women almost always care for others before taking care of themselves, which puts us at risk for getting a serious illness. Why? Because we're so busy or distracted that we often neglect our own health and ignore worrisome symptoms. Please think about this: If you don't take good care of yourself, how can you successfully care for others? Ways to decrease stress and relax are discussed in chapter 14.

STROKES

The risk factors for stroke and heart disease are the same. Thus, when you modify your risk factors for heart health, you also improve the health of your brain. Strokes are discussed in detail in chapter 1.

ARRHYTHMIAS: A "SHORT" IN THE ELECTRICAL SYSTEM

When there is a problem with the electrical system of the heart, a conduction abnormality can occur, resulting in an arrhythmia, or abnormal heart rhythm. Arrhythmias are classified in several ways, but mainly by where in the heart they originate. Because there are so many of them, we cannot discuss them here, but we will give you general recommendations for how to deal with an abnormal pulse.

General Recommendations for an Abnormal Pulse

Many people have abnormal heart rhythms and never notice it. Others may be very symptomatic, with heart palpitations, dizziness, a "fluttering" sensation in the chest, shortness of breath, and/

or fatigue. If you experience any of these symptoms for longer than a few minutes, feel your pulse. If it is irregular or very rapid (greater than 100 beats per minute), or seems to skip a beat, you probably have an arrhythmia. It is important to have this evaluated. Some arrhythmias are harmless and may be your norm. This is why it is important to take your pulse when it's normal, so that you'll be able to tell if or when it becomes abnormal. Get into the habit of checking your pulse regularly.

For a rapid, slower than usual (for you), or irregular pulse rate with no associated symptoms (dizziness, fainting), call your primary care doctor for an appointment as soon as possible. *If you have fainted or are constantly dizzy along with a pulse rate that is abnormal for you, go to the emergency room or call 911.*

Usually, arrhythmias can be diagnosed with an EKG. If the irregular rate or rhythm is intermittent, and thus not seen on a routine EKG, you will need to have your heartbeat monitored for several days. This can be done as an outpatient. Some arrhythmias need no treatment. Others are treated with medications, or, in some cases, with surgery that may do away with the need for medication.

THE DOCS CHAT ABOUT
THE HEART

DR. J: I've read that one way to raise a person's HDL, or good cholesterol, is to drink red wine. Does that work? Should we all be drinking it? And how much?

DR. R: It does work. Red wine, and grapes of course, are loaded with compounds called flavonoids, and another called resveratrol. These are antioxidants that may be responsible for raising HDL. If you have a low HDL and either don't like to drink or cannot drink for medical reasons, I wouldn't recommend starting just for the sake of a higher HDL. However, if you do drink wine, I'd suggest you limit it to one glass a night. That will give you some benefit and limit the risk of other problems related to increased alcohol, such as breast cancer.

DR. J: You said to watch out for mercury in fish oil. What brands do you recommend?

DR. R: There are a couple of brands I like: Nordic Naturals or Eskimo Oil.

DR. J: I love chocolate and I've read that it's good for the heart. What do you think?

DR. R: A lot of studies are finding that dark chocolate may lower blood pressure and protect blood vessels from inflammation. Remember though, we are talking about small amounts and the type of dark chocolate that tastes bitter. That is, chocolate without sugar and milk added, because that would defeat the purpose.

DR. J: Guess that does away with my regular deliveries from Hershey's!

PEARLS OF WISDOM
FOR THE HEART

○ Anyone can have CAD—even you.

○ Women may have different symptoms of CAD than men; these symptoms can be vague.

○ If you have chest pain or other symptoms that make you think you are having a heart attack at that moment, call 911 immediately and chew an aspirin tablet. (Do not take aspirin if you are allergic to it.)

○ If you have a gut instinct that something is wrong with your heart, even if a medical professional tells you there isn't, insist on having your heart evaluated.

○ If you have CAD or have had a heart attack, be sure to ask your clinician about the standard medications you should be taking.

○ The only cure for heart disease is not getting it in the first place. Know your risk factors and modify those that you can.

○ If you have risk factors for CAD, ask your clinician about screening tests.

○ If you pass out or feel palpitations or chest pain, especially with an irregular or rapid pulse, call 911 or go to the emergency room.

○ Learn how your pulse feels normally so that you will recognize when it is abnormal.

CHAPTER 4

YOUR LUNGS: HOW TO BREATHE EASIER

Of all the life-preserving processes that go on in the body, what is the one we take most for granted? Breathing. Though we don't tend to think much about this process, or the organ system responsible for it—unless there's a problem—the lungs are critical to our health and well-being. And because lung disease in women is on the rise in this country, it is particularly important to understand the risk factors, symptoms, and treatment for it.

LUNG FUNCTION

Since the lungs are so delicate, knowing how they work will help keep them disease free.

Normal Lung Function

We breathe in air through our mouth and nose, after which it goes into the main breathing tube, the *trachea*. From there, the air flows down the branches of the trachea, first into two main tubes, one to each lung, the *bronchi*, and then on to more tubes that branch twenty-two times into 100,000 smaller and smaller tubes, the *bronchioles*. The air then flows from the bronchioles into the 300 million air sacs of the lung and then into the blood vessels bathing the lungs. In the opposite direction, carbon dioxide, coming back from the body into the lungs as waste, flows out from the blood vessels into the sacs and is expelled into the air from the lungs. So, the process works like this—oxygen comes in and carbon dioxide goes out.

Mucus coats all the bronchial tubes of the lungs, helping to trap dust and bacteria. The bronchi are also covered with tiny hairs, known as *cilia*, that move the mucus up the trachea and toward the mouth so it can be coughed up or swallowed. As disgusting as mucus is at times, it's actually a very useful substance.

Lung Function as We Age

As we age, our lungs become less elastic, and the cilia beat more slowly. Moreover, our immune system starts to weaken. These changes set us up for bacterial infections that might not have bothered us in our younger days. Because we become more susceptible to infections with age, we need to get a pneumonia vaccine around the age of fifty-five (see chapter 15) and a yearly flu shot.

Common Symptoms as We Age

Shortness of breath and coughing are two symptoms that occur more frequently as we age. Although these symptoms often indicate a lung problem, they can also be due to the malfunction of other organ systems.

SHORTNESS OF BREATH

Remember when you were little and you were tackled on the playground and had the wind knocked out of you? Shortness of breath can be terrifying.

What are the main causes of shortness of breath? Most of us have experienced shortness of breath at some point in our lives. This symptom can indicate the presence of many conditions, including asthma, emphysema, heart disease, arrhythmia, pulmonary embolism, neurologic diseases such as Guillain-Barré syndrome, and even a panic attack.

Is your shortness of breath dangerous? What should you do? Sometimes shortness of breath has a simple explanation, such as exercising too much when you are out of shape. Other times it is a sign of something serious. It is important to have it checked out if it persists. *If your shortness of breath begins suddenly, and/or is severe, and/or does not resolve within a short period of time (minutes to an hour), it is an emergency: call 911.* If you have shortness of breath that you experience on a regular basis that is not severe and has not been evaluated, it is important to see your clinician. She will do a physical examination, order appropriate blood work, and if necessary order a chest x-ray. Treatment will be based on the cause of the symptom.

CHRONIC COUGH

As we get older, it becomes common for a cough to linger.

What causes a cough that lasts and lasts? There are many common causes of a persistent cough, categorized by how long it lasts. The cough that develops over a few days and lasts less than three weeks is known as an *acute cough* and is most often due to a respiratory infection, either bacterial or viral. If your cough lasts more than three weeks, it is called *chronic* and could be due to many things, including asthma or other lung diseases, acid reflux, smoking, postnasal drip, allergies, or even a medication you're taking, such as the ACE inhibitors or beta-blockers used for high blood pressure or heart disease. It's also possible that your chronic cough indicates a more serious condition, such as a lung abscess or lung cancer. The good news is that, most often, the causes of a chronic cough are treatable.

Is your chronic cough dangerous? What can you do about it? If a cough leads to severe shortness of breath, it is an emergency; it is also an urgent situation if you are coughing up blood in quantities larger than small specks in your mucus. For either of these situations, call 911, or go to the ER. A chronic cough without associated symptoms needs to be evaluated, but not immediately. Treatment of the cough is based on the cause.

The Chronic Cough Experiences of Dr. R and Dr. J

Dr. R's husband, always healthy previously, developed a constant cough that went on for weeks and weeks. As it was driving Dr. R crazy—both with worry and in general—she had him undergo an extensive evaluation including visits to lung, allergy, and ENT (ear, nose, and throat) specialists, as well as blood tests and a CT scan. Ultimately, the diagnosis made was gastroesophageal reflux disease (and Dr. R's husband is a gastroenterologist!); the cough went completely away after he started an acid-blocking medication. When Dr. R recently mentioned this to Dr. J, Dr. R was surprised to hear that Dr. J's husband had just been through the same thing and was now on acid-blocking drugs as well. Moral of the story: A cough caused by reflux is more common than you might think and is usually easy to fix. Be sure to get a chronic cough checked out before it drives you crazy! (The other moral of the story: Sometimes doctors can overdo a medical evaluation on members of their own family just a bit!)

ASTHMA

Asthma used to be thought of as a disease of childhood, but in recent years it is frequently being newly diagnosed even after the age of fifty. This is especially true for those of us who love to run outside, and seems to be due to the increased air pollution in many places (Reynolds 2007). Another cause of new-onset asthma at our age is occupational exposure to substances that damage the lungs. Asthma often coexists with chronic obstructive pulmonary disease (COPD or emphysema), discussed below.

Between 1982 and 1994 the number of asthma cases nearly doubled in the U.S. Some speculate this rise is caused by a combination of better diagnostic procedures, environmental pollution, and possibly the rise of consumption of trans fats (American Lung Association 2006). As of 2004, the National Center for Health Statistics estimated that 20.5 million Americans had asthma. Another scary fact is that about 64,000 women die of emphysema each year, and 65 percent of those who die from asthma are women (CDC 2001). Asthma is not just a diagnosis for kids anymore!

What Causes Asthma? Are You at Risk?

Asthma is a chronic lung problem caused by inflammation of the airway tubes, the bronchi and bronchioles. The inflammation makes them sensitive and "twitchy," eventually leading to a spasm of the bronchial tubes; this is what makes it difficult to move air in and out of the lungs, that is, to breathe. Dust, cold air, cigarette smoke, emotional upset, chemicals, reflux stomach acid, and even exercise are just a few of the factors that can initiate asthma.

Women with a family history of asthma, and those who have had early lung infections or exposure to secondhand smoke, are at the greatest risk for developing asthma. Air pollution contributes to the risk. More African-American women have asthma than any other group. They are also more than twice as likely to die from the disease as Caucasian women.

Do You Have Asthma? What Can You Do About It?

When the airways become irritated during an asthma attack, wheezing, coughing, and difficulty breathing can occur. It is like trying to breathe through a narrow straw. When it is severe, patients describe the feeling of an actual "air hunger." Because many of the above symptoms are often attributed to aging, the proper diagnosis may be missed. On the other hand, the diagnosis may also be missed because many clinicians think that only children can develop asthma.

Some people with asthma have only a chronic dry cough. Others have the symptoms of asthma only when they have a respiratory infection or a flare-up of their seasonal allergies; after the infection or allergy resolves itself, the asthma symptoms also go away. Still others develop the symptoms only with exercise; this is known as exercise-induced asthma, and can be easily managed so that you don't have to give up being physically active.

If the shortness of breath is severe and doesn't go away, especially after you've tried your usual inhaler or other treatment, go to the ER. When asthma doesn't respond to treatment, it is considered a medical emergency. Otherwise, if you have only recently developed any of the above symptoms, see your clinician as soon as possible. Asthma is usually diagnosed with pulmonary function tests (PFTs), or breathing tests.

Can Asthma Be Treated?

There is no cure for asthma, but there are medications that help to reduce the inflammation in the lungs and open the bronchiole tubes so that the symptoms are lessened or completely gone. This treatment may also prevent the long-term complications of asthma, particularly that of developing emphysema.

MEDICATIONS

There are several types of medications used to treat asthma. These include steroid inhalers, such as Flovent (fluticasone) or Azmacort (triamcinolone), which help reduce inflammation in the airways and are usually used as a frontline treatment; long-acting *bronchodilator inhalers*, such as Serevent (salmeterol), which open up the bronchial tubes; short-acting bronchodilator inhalers, such as Proventil (salbutamol), which are known as "rescue inhalers" because they are the best for treating acute asthma symptoms; leukotriene inhibitor inhalers, such as Singulair (montelukast), which help to prevent asthma attacks; Intal (cromolyn), which helps to prevent exercise-induced asthma; theophylline tablets, which used to be the mainstay of treatment before inhalers were available and can help to prevent asthma; and Xolair (omalizumab), a new injectable treatment that is used to treat allergic asthma.

HERBS AND SUPPLEMENTS

Herbs and supplements for treating asthma have been popular through the ages. Because the traditional medications for asthma are so effective, you should not try herbs unless you have discussed it with your clinician. Quercitin is a phytochemical found in red wine and green tea that may help some people with allergic asthma, but it shouldn't be taken by pregnant or nursing women. Butterbur is a European herb in the ragweed family similar to the leukotriene inhibitors mentioned above. The plant contains pyrrolizidine alkaloids (PAs), which are toxic to the liver, so it is important to find butterbur that is PA free. Obviously if you have an allergy to ragweed, you shouldn't take this.

Can Asthma Be Prevented?

Despite the fact that good treatments are available, 86 percent of women in one recent study reported that they still had symptoms fifteen years after being diagnosed (Vonk et al. 2003). Why? Only a third of them were taking their regular medication. Clearly, although it seems obvious, the medications are effective only if you take them!

If you have asthma and know what makes it worse, the key is to avoid those things; the exception to this is exercise, for which you should take preventive medication. If acid reflux sets off your asthma, take medications that decrease the acid, such as Prilosec (omeprazole) or Prevacid (lansoprazole). If dust and pollens cause an asthma flare-up, consider buying HEPA filters for your house and office to remove the irritants from the air. If you know that seasonal allergies set off your asthma, be ready with inhalers and antihistamine drugs.

Left untreated, asthma can have serious consequences, including the development of emphysema, and even death. The key is to be *aware* of what your triggers are, *alert* to when those triggers may occur and to your symptoms, and to take the appropriate *action* by always having your medications readily available. And, of course, *advocate* for yourself if anyone tells you that only kids have asthma.

CHRONIC OBSTRUCTIVE PULMONARY DISEASE (COPD)

Even Marlboro Men Can't Fight the Ravages of Smoking

Do you remember the Marlboro Man? Handsome, virile, and take-charge, he was every woman's fantasy male. One of the original Marlboro men was Wayne McClaren; he died of lung cancer at the age of fifty-one. The other original Marlboro Man, David McClean, developed severe emphysema and died of lung cancer at seventy-three. There is a great documentary about the Marlboro Men. Dr. R used it when she taught medical students about smoking. It is called "Death in the West."

One major reason that lung problems in women are increasing is that the number of women (particularly teenagers) who smoke cigarettes is also rising. Remember those seductive cigarette commercials of the 1960s? "You've come a long way baby…" At that time, cigarette smoking was equated with women's liberation and being cool. Looking further back, remember how sophisticated Lauren Bacall and the other actresses of her day looked with a cigarette in one hand and a martini in the other?

Unfortunately, those ads and the portrayal of smoking as a glamorous habit did women a huge disservice. We now realize that cigarette smoking is *not* cool and is, in fact, very dangerous to the smoker's health and to those around her. Earlier, we talked about why smoking cessation was important for the heart. Now we'll discuss why it is important for the lungs. How to stop smoking is discussed in chapter 15.

What Is COPD?

COPD is a term that describes what happens in several lung conditions, such as chronic bronchitis and emphysema. It results from a blockage of the bronchiole tubes and damage to the delicate air sacs in the lungs. Since we rely on the elasticity of these air sacs to help the air move out of the lungs, when they are damaged and the tubes are blocked in COPD, air can't get out; it is trapped. For asthmatics, it is also hard to get air into the lungs. Once this damage is done, it is irreversible. Further damage can be prevented by stopping smoking, treating asthma, and removing or avoiding pollutants.

What Causes COPD? Are You at Risk?

According to a report of the Surgeon General in 2004, smoking is the number one cause of COPD, and is responsible for 80 to 90 percent of all deaths caused by this disease (USDHHS 2004). Exposure to chemicals, urban pollutants, and dust may also cause COPD. A genetic condition, alpha-1 antitrypsin deficiency, for which a blood test is available, is responsible for approximately 3 percent of COPD cases. Allergies, asthma, and chronic bronchitis also increase the chances of developing COPD.

How Do You Know if You Have COPD? What Can You Do About It?

Initially, there are no symptoms. Eventually, however, there will be a persistent cough, increased mucus, shortness of breath, wheezing, and/or an increased susceptibility to lung infections, all of which progress to dependence on oxygen supplementation and eventual lung failure. If any of the above symptoms lasts longer than three weeks, see your clinician.

Can COPD Be Treated?

There is no cure; however, treatment is given to help prevent the condition from worsening and to improve the symptoms.

Smoking cessation. Smoking cessation is crucial to keep COPD from worsening.

Asthma medications. Many of the asthma medications, such as the long-acting steroid inhalers and bronchodilators, are also used for COPD.

Antibiotics. When bacterial respiratory infections occur in people with COPD, antibiotics should be started quickly.

Oxygen supplementation. Many COPD patients benefit from using oxygen taken through a mask or nasal prongs from a tank.

Pulmonary rehabilitation. Exercise can be very helpful in COPD. It is best done through a pulmonary rehabilitation program, in which a supervised exercise plan focused on improving lung health is specifically tailored to the individual. For instance, playing the harmonica can be therapeutic for some patients with COPD!

Can COPD Be Prevented?

To prevent COPD, never smoke. If you do, then quit! (See chapter 15.) If you are exposed to pollutants as part of your job, wear a respirator or mask and ask your doctor to give you routine pulmonary function tests to monitor your lung function. If you have asthma, seek proper treatment and take your medications.

PULMONARY EMBOLISM (PE)

In 2003, David Bloom, a healthy, young NBC correspondent covering the war in Iraq, died of a *pulmonary embolism*, or blood clot to the lung. This focused national attention on what it is and, potentially, how to prevent it. According to the National Heart, Lung, and Blood Institute, each year 600,000 people develop a pulmonary embolism. One-third of those will die as a result if it is not treated quickly (NHLBI 2006).

Are You at Risk for a PE?

A PE occurs when a blood clot forms in a leg, an arm, or in the pelvis (known as a *deep venous thrombosis* or DVT) and then breaks off suddenly and travels to the lung. Therefore, you are placed at risk for a PE by anything that allows blood clots to form in your legs or, less frequently, your arms or your pelvis. The main factor that promotes clots in the legs is prolonged immobilization, such as being bedridden for a long while, or taking a long car trip or airplane flight. The most common causes of clots in the pelvis are infection or surgery of the pelvic organs. The most common cause of a clot in your arm is having had an intravenous (IV) line there recently. After a hospitalization for either an illness or surgery, you are at increased risk of having a PE for up to three months (Spencer et al. 2007).

In addition, recent trauma to the lower extremity, pelvis, thorax, and spinal cord can lead to a PE within forty-eight hours or longer (Menaker, Stein, and Scalea 2007). Other risk factors include birth control pills (especially in combination with smoking); the oral form of hormone replacement therapy (as opposed to the patch or gels, which do not increase the risk of clotting); certain surgeries such as those involving the hips or legs; a blood disorder that increases blood clotting; cancer (which causes the blood to clot more easily); obesity; being over sixty; and certain medical conditions such as varicose veins, cellulitis of the legs, or chronic leg edema.

If You Think You Have a PE, What Can You Do About It?

Symptoms of a PE include the sudden onset of shortness of breath, chest pain, a bloody cough, light-headedness, sweating, and/or a rapid heartbeat. Some people who have had a PE remember having had a sudden strange feeling of "doom and gloom." All of these symptoms may not always be present; the main feature is that symptoms start suddenly.

If you experience the sudden occurrence of any of these symptoms, especially if you have a swollen leg or have been sitting or lying down for a prolonged period of time, call 911. This is crucial; a PE can be fatal.

How Is a PE Diagnosed and Treated?

Once you are at the hospital, you will immediately have your oxygen level checked with the arterial blood gas test, and then will be placed on supplemental oxygen; blood is obtained for this test from a wrist or groin artery. Depending on your physical exam, you may have a Doppler study (sonogram) of your leg or arm veins. You will get a chest x-ray and an imaging test known as a ventilation/perfusion scan or a special CT scan; depending on what these show, you may still need more tests.

Treatment depends on the severity of the symptoms. If the PE is life threatening, doctors may treat the blood clot with a clot-buster drug or with a procedure to remove or dissolve the clot through a venous catheter. In less urgent circumstances, a PE is treated with an intravenous or injected anticoagulant, heparin, which thins the blood immediately. An oral blood thinner, Coumadin (warfarin), will be started at the same time so that it can build up in your system. After about two to three days, heparin can be stopped.

If the cause of the PE was a DVT, Coumadin will be continued for at least three to six months. For other causes of a PE, such as an inherited blood disorder that increases clotting, cancer, or a previous history of blood clots, the treatment will be longer.

Can a PE Be Prevented?

To prevent a PE, you must first prevent the development of clots in your legs, the most common site for clots to form without prior trauma or infection.

Prepare for long car or airplane rides. If you are on a flight for longer than four hours, your risk of getting a blood clot increases greatly; it is recommended that you move your legs vigorously *at least every hour.* If on a plane, get up and walk around. If in a car, stop and do some walking. If you are at high risk for a blood clot, you may need to take a blood thinner before taking any long flights or car rides. Be sure to discuss this with your clinician.

Practice prevention if you need prolonged bed rest. Remember about prevention. If you've been given *prophylaxis* (preventive medicine or device) to prevent blood clots in your legs, such as special inflatable leg wrappings or blood thinner injections, be sure to use them. If you have not been given any, *ask for them!*

Wear support stockings. If you have chronic swelling or edema in one or both of your legs, wear support stockings all the time.

Drink plenty of fluid to prevent dehydration. Getting dehydrated causes the blood to thicken, and thus be more likely to form a clot.

Exercise regularly. This may help prevent blood clots.

Take seriously *any* calf or thigh pain that lasts longer than a few days, and any swelling that occurs only in one leg. Take seriously any arm pain or swelling if you have recently had an IV line or trauma there. Although the pain may be due to a pulled muscle, it is possible that you have a blood clot in your leg or arm vein; getting that diagnosed and treated before it breaks off and forms a PE could save your life.

The best way to treat this problem is never to have it in the first place. Be *aware* of the risk factors for a PE and leg and arm blood clots; be *alert* to the symptoms of DVT and PE; take *action* to prevent blood clots; and *advocate* for yourself by asking for the appropriate prophylaxis if you are bedridden. For a discussion on lung cancer see chapter 12.

THE DOCS CHAT ABOUT THE LUNGS

DR. J: Is there any special diet that may help asthma patients?

DR. R: There is, and it may help both allergies and asthma. It is called the anti-inflammatory diet, and is similar to the Mediterranean diet discussed in chapter 11. It helps by reducing inflammation in the body. I'm a believer!

DR. J: I've heard that the type of inhaler used for asthma medications has changed. Talk about that.

DR. R: This change was actually mandated by the U.S. federal government in 2005. It requires that by January 1, 2009, the manufacturers of all types of inhalers stop using chlorofluorocarbons (CFCs) as the propellant in order to protect the earth's ozone layer, because CFCs are harmful to the environment. The new types of propellant used in inhalers now are called hydrofluoroalkanes (HFAs).

DR. J: Will the change to the HFA inhalers make any difference to the inhaler users?

DR. R: Yes. There are differences between the old and new inhalers in the force, feel, taste, and the cleaning and priming that users should definitely know about. Unfortunately, the public and many clinicians have not been made aware of these differences yet. For instance, the propellant force with which the medication comes out is not as strong as it was in the old inhalers, and the feel of the spray is softer.

Not being aware of this, many patients have thought that their new inhaler wasn't working right, and didn't use it again. You can see how this could be dangerous for someone with asthma in an emergency.

DR. J: Any other differences?

DR. R: Yes. Before the new inhaler is used for the first time, it must be primed (pumped) at least four times, depending on what the package insert says. The old inhaler did not need to be primed as much. Also, the spray of the new inhalers is stickier than the old ones and, therefore, the inhaler itself must be cleaned more often or the sticky residue will prevent the medication from coming out smoothly. Another concern is the fact that the new inhalers are more expensive than the old ones.

DR. J: I'm sure we'll be hearing more about these issues. One more question about inhalers. Do over-the-counter inhalers work?

DR. R: Do you remember hearing about a seventeen-year-old model named Krissy Taylor, who died of asthma in 1995? She had been treating herself with an over-the-counter epinephrine inhaler for her wheezing. These inhalers may work only for very sporadic episodes. They help the symptoms, but do nothing to stop the inflammation that makes the asthma worsen. For that reason they're dangerous because they mask what's really going on in the lungs. Anyone with asthma who needs to use an inhaler regularly—even if it's just once a week or once a month—needs to be monitored medically and to be on long-acting treatment.

DR. J: One last question. Do you have any more special advice about avoiding a pulmonary embolism (PE)?

DR. R: Yes. Before you get a massage or even a pedicure (because many times the pedicurist will massage your calf muscles during the process), let your masseuse or pedicurist know if your leg is sore, especially if it's been sore for more than a few days. It's possible you could be developing a clot there, and the last thing you want is for it to be massaged. That's because a blood vessel might break off and be pushed up into your lungs.

DR. J: So, this is another example of how important it is to be aware of our risk of a blood clot, be alert to any pain in our legs or arms, take action to get it evaluated, and advocate for ourselves, right?

DR. R: Absolutely!

PEARLS OF WISDOM FOR CARE OF THE LUNGS

○ Sudden onset of severe shortness of breath is an emergency. Call 911.

○ Asthma can and *must* be treated to prevent complications.

○ You can develop asthma for the first time, even at your current age.

○ Never take up smoking cigarettes!

○ If you do smoke, it is time to quit. (See chapter 15.)

○ COPD can be prevented by treating your asthma and stopping smoking.

○ If you have pain or swelling in only one leg or arm that lasts longer than a few days, get it checked out.

○ Prevent DVT in your legs, and a PE, by moving your legs and taking walking breaks during long airplane or car trips, staying well hydrated, and making sure you are given either special stockings or a blood thinner during prolonged bed rest.

CHAPTER 5

How to Keep Your
GI Tract on Track

The gastrointestinal (GI) system fascinates children, and continues to intrigue, and at times frustrate, many of us throughout our lives. Children are bewitched by what goes in and, especially, what comes out, be it gas or solid. For aging adults, the workings of the GI tract become more a cause for concern. In fact, 60 to 70 million American adults suffer from chronic GI disorders.

THE GI TRACT AND THE NORMAL DIGESTIVE PROCESS

When food enters your mouth, you chew it. At the same time, your salivary glands make and send substances known as *enzymes* into your mouth to help break down food so it is easier to digest. When you swallow, the partially broken-down food products enter your *esophagus*, the muscular tube that propels the food toward your stomach through a valve called the *lower esophageal sphincter* (LES).

This sphincter, or valve, allows food to go into your stomach and then closes, so that the food cannot splash back up into the esophagus (that is, if it is working properly).

Once in the stomach, the food is churned and further digested by more enzymes and by strong hydrochloric acid. Due to mucus that coats and protects the stomach, the acid is not able to damage the lining. The food in the stomach then empties into the *small intestine*, also known as the small bowel, which is not really small at all. It is about twenty to twenty-three feet long and provides the surface through which the fluids and nutrients are absorbed, then utilized, by the body.

The small bowel then empties into the *colon*, or large intestine, which is about five feet long. The colon acts like the "trash compactor" of the body. What's left of the food, or the waste, enters here, where bacteria work on it to break it down further. These bacteria have their own digestive systems, which give off gas. This gas accumulates and results in (you guessed it!) *flatus* or, as your kids might say, "farts." Everyone has his or her own unique components of gas. Some people produce methane gas (which is flammable if lit by a match) others produce nitrogen or carbon dioxide gas. As the waste becomes more and more compact, the muscles of the colon push it toward the anus at the end of the digestive tract. This results in a bowel movement.

If you look at the cells of the intestines under a microscope, they look like brain cells. Dr. Michael Gershon, who made this observation and is studying the connection between the brain and the gut, has called the gut the "second brain." We now realize that the gut is in constant communication with the brain. This makes sense when you think about what a gut reaction feels like, or butterflies in your stomach when you are nervous, or why some people get diarrhea and even throw up when they are upset (Gershon 1999).

Although the liver, gallbladder, and pancreas are not part of the food passageway, they are essential to the proper functioning of the GI tract and digestion. The *liver* produces bile that is important for absorbing fat. It also is important for processing nutrients, getting rid of certain wastes, and metabolizing many of the substances you take into your body. The *pancreas* provides essential enzymes for digestion. The *gallbladder* holds the bile, and then squirts it into the small intestine when you eat. When all the parts of the GI tract work well, everything is fine. But, as you can see, digestion has many steps where problems can arise.

THE AGING GI TRACT

As we age, everything starts to slow down—from the mouth to the end of the GI tract. The amount of saliva diminishes, making it tougher to swallow pills. The lower esophageal sphincter may weaken and not close, allowing acid to reflux back up the esophagus. The overall amount of stomach acid may diminish, which can increase our susceptibility to the infection that can lead to ulcers. Furthermore, with more aches and pains, we may be taking more anti-inflammatory medications, which increase the likelihood of developing inflammation in the stomach and esophagus and can also cause ulcers.

The muscular contractions in the lower intestine that push food through the system can slow down, causing constipation to occur more often. Knowing what can happen to your gut with aging is half the battle; finding out how to protect and defend it is the rest. Read on.

GASTROESOPHAGEAL REFLUX DISEASE

Twenty percent of the U.S. population suffers from gastroesophageal reflux disease, otherwise known as GERD (Adams, Hendershot, and Marano 1999). According to the American College of Gastroenterology, 60 million Americans experience this at least once a month, and 15 million experience it daily (2006). That's a lot of TUMS and other antacids being consumed.

What Causes GERD?

GERD occurs when the lower esophageal sphincter between the esophagus and the stomach doesn't stay closed, allowing acid and food to come back up into the esophagus, and sometimes even into the mouth. This can result in "heartburn," or a burning feeling, along with the taste of acid coming into the throat and mouth.

A *hiatal hernia* is a common cause of GERD. This occurs when the stomach pops up through the hole in the *diaphragm* (the muscle that separates the chest from the stomach), which normally helps the lower esophageal sphincter do its job. Hiatal hernias allow acid to go up, rather than down, and are very common in people over fifty.

Certain behaviors increase the chances of having reflux, including cigarette smoking, drinking alcohol, and overeating. Gaining weight or being pregnant also can lead to reflux because of the increased fat or the enlarged uterus pushing up against the stomach, causing an increased pressure that displaces and pushes the acid up into the esophagus. Wearing constricting clothes, pantyhose with a tight "control top," or a girdle can do the same thing. Some foods trigger reflux as well, including spicy foods, tomato-based foods, caffeine drinks, chocolate, fatty foods, fried foods, garlic, onions, mint, and citrus foods.

How Do You Know if You Have It?
What Can You Do About It?

There are many ways that GERD can make itself known. Some people with this problem may wake up in the mornings with a sore throat, hoarseness, and a cough. Others may have a chronic cough. Still others may have trouble swallowing or a burning sensation all the way down their esophagus; sometimes this burning feeling occurs only with spicy foods or alcoholic drinks.

The most worrisome symptom that reflux can cause is chest pain, which is easily confused with a heart attack or anginal pain. This type of pain is due to the esophagus having a spasm in reaction to the acid coming back up, it is actually called "esophageal spasm." It is even relieved by nitroglycerin, which is used to treat angina, causing more confusion as to where the pain is coming from—the heart or the esophagus.

Remember, too, that women are known to have different symptoms with heart disease than men; women may not have the classic "chest pressure" and may instead experience heart problems as a burning in the chest. That's why it is so important to be checked out for any chest pain. If you have heartburn that either doesn't go away or keeps recurring, it is important to see your doctor for two reasons: First, it may be your heart causing the pain, and not heartburn; sometimes it is hard to tell them apart. Second, if your pain is due to GERD, the continuous acid bathing of the esophagus that occurs with reflux disease can cause long-term damage, leading to scarring and narrowing of the esophagus. In rare cases it can even lead to cancer. Though men are more prone to this type of cancer than women, it can happen to us. To prevent this, you must have a diagnosis made and get started on treatment.

If you have chest pain, regardless of what you think may be causing it, check it out as soon as possible. (See chapter 3 for specifics about chest pain.)

Can It Be Prevented and Treated? (Do You Really Have to Give Up Chocolate?)

There are many things you can do if you have reflux, and no, you don't have to give up chocolate. You might have to eat only 30 calories worth instead of 30 pieces though!

Lifestyle changes. Here are some simple tips that can prevent and treat GERD: Quit smoking cigarettes; avoid the foods that you know trigger your heartburn; avoid alcohol; give away those control top pantyhose (and maybe those Spanx, too); lose weight if you are overweight; stop eating two hours before you go to bed; and put the head of your bed up on blocks so that it is about six to eight inches off the floor, which will cause the acid to flow downward simply because of gravity.

Medication. If these measures fail or are not enough to stop your symptoms, there are medications available. Antacids, such as Tums and Maalox, neutralize the acid and can work quickly. If your reflux is mild, taking these meds as directed by your doctor for a few days to a week can relieve your symptoms. If you are popping them all day long, however, not only can they give you diarrhea or constipation, depending on which one you take, but that is a sign you may need a longer-acting, or stronger, medication.

A stronger class of medications for GERD, called H_2 blockers, includes drugs like Tagamet (cimetidine) and Zantac (ranitidine). These reduce the amount of acid made in the stomach. They can be effective but may not be strong enough to get rid of the symptoms for some people. More potent than the H$_2$ blockers are the proton pump inhibitors (PPI), such as Prilosec (omeprazole) and Nexium (esomeprazole), which also decrease the production of acid in the stomach, but by a different mechanism than the H$_2$ blockers. If GERD is a chronic problem that is not resolved with lifestyle changes, you may need to take either H$_2$ blockers or proton pump inhibitors for life.

Acupuncture. Although the PPI medications are effective treatments for GERD, sometimes the usual dosage may not be enough. When patients continue to have symptoms, the medication is often doubled. Based on a recent study, acupuncture, when given two times a week for four weeks, improved GERD symptoms and eliminated the need for increased doses of medication (Dickman et al. 2007). This may be an alternative for some patients. Dr R has a patient who has been able to control her GERD with the usual dosage of medications and acupuncture treatments once a month.

Herbs and supplements. Deglycyrrhizinated licorice comes from licorice root and can help with reflux symptoms. (See chapter 13 for further discussion, including recommended dosage.)

ULCERS

Ulcers are open sores that can occur in the lining of the esophagus, the stomach, or the first part of the small intestine, the *duodenum*.

What Causes Ulcers? Who Is at Risk?

Two-thirds of ulcers are caused by a bacterial infection with *Helicobacter pylori* (Blaser 1990). The other common cause of ulcers is medications such as aspirin and nonsteroidal anti-inflammatory drugs like ibuprofen. Cancer is rarely a cause of ulcers. A family history of ulcers, age greater than fifty, cigarette smoking, and heavy use of alcohol can all increase your risk for developing ulcers. Spicy food and stress do not cause ulcers, but they can make them worse.

What Are the Symptoms? What Can You Do About Them?

People with ulcers usually experience pain that is described as a dull ache or a burning or gnawing sensation. This pain can occur anywhere in the abdomen but usually is localized to the area right below your sternum (the center of your rib cage), a few inches above your belly button. It also may be located anywhere in the middle of your abdomen. This discomfort usually comes and goes, and often starts two to three hours after a meal. It also can happen at night when the stomach is empty. Food usually makes it feel better, although some people actually experience the pain while eating. Other common symptoms include nausea, vomiting, and even weight loss.

If you experience this type of pain, call your health care provider for an appointment to be scheduled as soon as possible. *If the pain is sudden, severe, and doesn't go away within a few minutes, or if you vomit blood or have black, tarry stools, call 911 or go to the ER.*

How Are Ulcers and GERD Diagnosed?

The doctor can see if you have an ulcer or GERD by looking down your esophagus into your stomach with a special lighted tube known as an *endoscope*. Sometimes imaging studies or a type of x-ray known as a barium swallow or an upper GI series is used to diagnose ulcers, but endoscopy is better for the following reasons: It can diagnose GERD, which the x-ray studies cannot; it allows the doctor to take a biopsy of the ulcer, which is necessary for detecting the presence of cancer or of *H. pylori*; and the x-ray studies may occasionally miss ulcers. Since *H. pylori* is such a common cause of ulcers, your doctor may want to confirm the presence of this bacterium also through a blood, breath, or stool test.

How Are Ulcers Treated?

Ulcers are treated with one of the medications used to treat GERD, such as an H_2 blocker or a proton pump inhibitor. The other part of the treatment is based on the cause. For instance, the treatment for ulcers caused by aspirin or ibuprofen is to stop those and all similar medications immediately, and also to take a proton pump inhibitor. If the cause of the ulcer is *H. pylori*, antibiotics are also used.

Since the H_2 blockers and proton pump inhibitors are so good at treating ulcers, and at relieving the symptoms, why should you bother to take antibiotics, even if *H. pylori* is found to be responsible? Many patients ask this question because the recommended antibiotics may initially cause an upset stomach. It is important to treat *H. pylori* infections not only to completely cure the ulcer, but to kill the bacteria. It has been found that this infection increases the risk of getting some types of stomach cancers (Uemura et al. 2001), as well as other cancers of the GI tract. In addition, it is important that the bacterium is killed to prevent other people from becoming infected with it. No one is quite sure how *H. pylori* is spread, but being in close contact with an infected person and being exposed to infected vomit seem to increase the likelihood of getting it. In the future a vaccine may be designed to prevent this infection.

Dr. R's Painful Morning in the Hospital

When I was a resident in Internal Medicine a long, long time ago, I once got up in the middle of the night and remembered I needed to take the antibiotic for my skin called doxycycline (Vibramycin). I took it and was half asleep, so I didn't use much water. I went right back to sleep. The next morning, I had a horrible pain in my chest. I thought I was having a heart attack. It turned out I had a pill ulcer. Tagamet (the first H$_2$ blocker) had just come out on the market. It helped take the edge off, but I was hurting for at least a week. I learned that if you don't take an antibiotic, or any medication for that matter, with a lot of water, it can get stuck on the wall of the esophagus and cause an ulcer. Aspirin, ibuprofen, and other anti-inflammatory medications can do the same thing. So, always remember to take all pills with a full glass of water!

GAS (FLATUS)

Here is Dr. R's childhood gas memory: "I lived a good part of my childhood thinking that my parents never passed gas. They never talked about it and I never detected any in their vicinity. My mother to this day denies that she passes gas! We know that this isn't true, however, because the average person passes one to four pints of gas a day, with an average of fourteen 'gas passages' (or, farts, as my children say) a day."

What Causes Gas?

As mentioned above, flatus is composed of an array of gases that results from the bacteria in the colon eating various undigested foods. Gas also comes from swallowed air, such as when you chew gum, eat or drink too quickly, or smoke cigarettes. If that swallowed air doesn't come back up as a burp, it can flow down through your GI tract and add to your gas load. In addition, certain foods cause gas to form.

Sugar is one of the biggest culprits in causing gas. Raffinose, a type of sugar found in beans and broccoli; fructose, another sugar found in fruits and in certain types of corn syrup; and sorbitol, also found in fruits and used as an artificial sweetener—all cause gas through their breakdown by the bacteria in the colon. If you eat a lot of the above-mentioned foods, or diet foods, you may expect to have some gas.

Due to the sugar and lactose which they contain, milk and milk products are a big source of gas for many people. In our digestive system, most people have an enzyme called *lactase* that helps break down lactose. As we age, this enzyme level decreases, making it harder to digest milk products. That is why so many of us have problems with gas now when we eat ice cream that we didn't when we were younger. In fact, for years Dr. J thought of ice cream as a laxative, as that was how her mother always used it.

Other foods like starches (potatoes, corn, and oatmeal) cause gas. Foods with soluble fiber, such as that found in vegetables, are broken down in the colon and cause gas. Insoluble fiber, in wheat bran for example, is not digested and goes right on through.

How Do You Know You Have It?

This is one symptom that we don't have to describe. We all have it. It's a normal part of digestion. When it becomes excessive (meaning if it bothers you—this is all relative), there are ways that the amount of gas can be decreased. However, it is important to know that it's not dangerous by itself, unless accompanied by massive diarrhea or bloody stools. Actually, passing gas means that your entire GI system is open and working.

How Is It Prevented and Treated?

You cannot prevent gas because it is part of the process of digestion. However, you can control the quantity to some degree; that is, if you want to. Some people don't mind it. (You probably already know this since you were sitting next to one of them at the movies last week.)

ELIMINATE GAS-PRODUCING FOODS FROM YOUR DIET

If you cut out some of the foods that contain the sugars named above, you will cut down on the amount of gas your body makes. Unfortunately, that also means cutting out vegetables and some fruits, both good for you. So we suggest, rather than cutting out all vegetables or fruits at once, try removing just one type of food at a time, for instance, broccoli; see if that makes a difference. If it doesn't, remove another specific food from your diet, then a combination of foods. That way, hopefully, you can cut down the amount of gas your GI system produces, and still eat nutritious foods.

SIMETHICONE, DIGESTIVE ENZYMES, AND BEANO

Antacids such as Mylanta Gas and Maalox antigas contain simethicone, which can help with gas in the stomach but doesn't help with gas in the intestine. In addition, simethicone is available by itself in an over-the-counter preparation known as Gas-X. Other over-the-counter medications such as digestive enzymes can help, including lactase, which is available for those who are lactose intolerant.

One of these is Lactaid; to work, it must be taken just before a meal. Beano, another product, helps to digest the sugars in vegetables and also should be taken before eating.

Bottom line: It is possible to cut down on the amount of gas you have, but you will still make enough to pass. Remember, everybody farts, even Dr. R's mother! (Sorry Mom! Love, R)

IRRITABLE BOWEL SYNDROME (IBS)

Approximately 20 percent of the adult population has symptoms of irritable bowel syndrome, known as IBS. It is more common in women (Adams, Hendershot, and Marano 1999).

What Causes IBS?

No one really knows what causes IBS. It is generally thought of as a motility disorder of the muscles in the entire GI tract, resulting in erratic contractions, or spasms, that alternate with absence of contractions. This then results in abdominal pain and cramping, constipation and/or diarrhea, and bloating. We may not know what causes IBS, but we do know what factors worsen it. These include caffeine, large meals, chocolate, milk products, wheat, rye, barley, stress, and emotional upset.

How Do You Know if You Have It?
What Can You Do About It?

Patients with IBS usually have a change in frequency of their bowel habits, a change in the look of their bowel movements, mucus in the stool, new-onset abdominal pain, bloating, a sense of urgency with bowel movements, or some combination of these symptoms. To make the diagnosis, these symptoms need to be present for at least three months (not necessarily consecutively) out of the year. Fever or blood in the stool are *not* usually seen in IBS and indicate a more serious problem, such as inflammatory bowel disease (Crohn's disease or ulcerative colitis), and must be evaluated as soon as possible. Although persistent severe abdominal pain *may* occur with IBS, it can also indicate that a more serious problem is present.

Since IBS involves the motility of the entire GI tract, the esophagus may react as well. If this occurs, you can have esophageal spasms, experienced as chest pain, which can mimic heart disease.

If you have any of these symptoms and they either persist for longer than three months or recur and are present three months of the year, see your clinician. There is no emergency unless the abdominal pain is severe and unremitting (see chapter 6 for what to do about abdominal pain), the diarrhea is so frequent or of such a large amount that you are having trouble staying hydrated, or you are having esophageal spasms showing up as chest pain.

How Is IBS Diagnosed?

Since there is no specific test to diagnose IBS, it is what we call a "diagnosis of exclusion." This means that it is necessary to exclude other, more serious diseases, as a cause for your symptoms. If no other disease or cause for your symptoms is found, such as inflammatory bowel disease or cancer, then it can be said that your symptoms are due to IBS. Therefore, your doctor will want you to have a thorough evaluation of your GI tract, including a colonoscopy.

How Is IBS Treated?

Many people with IBS try to ignore their symptoms and never seek help, thinking that there is nothing that can be done. This is a mistake. Once properly diagnosed, there are many options for treatment.

Medications. There are a variety of medications that may help. If you have constipation, laxatives may help. If you have diarrhea, Lomotil (diphenoxylate and atropine) or Imodium (loperamide) may help. For painful bowel spasms, there are relaxants; our favorite is Levsin (hyoscyamine) sublingual. If you have a combination of symptoms, you can learn how and when to take a variety of medications to keep your symptoms in control.

Diet. It is important to find the right diet. Some IBS patients do well with a lot of fiber, others have problems with it. Finding that happy medium is important, as is drinking enough water. Talk to your clinician about a diet good for your specific symptoms, or ask to be referred to a nutritionist.

Exercise. Regular exercise is a must. Sitting or lying around with little activity can cause the bowels to become sluggish.

Herbs and supplements. There are several types of herbs and supplements that can help with the various symptoms of IBS. Probiotics, available over the counter contain the "good" bacteria that are normally present in our GI tract, and that can occasionally be decreased due to the use of antibiotics, dietary changes, infection, illnesses such as diabetes, and even stress. Taking probiotics can restore the proper balance of "good" bacteria in our guts. The better types of probiotics contain at least 1 billion live bacteria. The most effective are *Lactobacillus* GG (used in the popular product known as Culterelle) and *Bifidobacterium*. Probiotics can be obtained in food in lesser amounts. Yogurt with live bacterial cultures, acidophilus milk, kefir, sauerkraut, and natural pickles all contain probiotics. Some gastroenterologists believe that the majority of their patients should be taking them on a daily basis.

Peppermint oil can help with irritable bowel symptoms if taken fifteen to thirty minutes before each meal. Dr. R took peppermint oil right after she had a Caesarean section in order to get her bowel moving and get out of the hospital. It worked like a charm! Peppermint can make acid reflux worse, so you might want to avoid or limit it if you have GERD. Slippery elm can soothe irritated innards. It is available in both pill and powder form. Carob powder can slow down diarrhea and be very soothing to the gut. It is typically mixed with applesauce. Tea can act as a potent laxative in people who predominantly have constipation with their IBS. Dr. J thinks that Stash green tea is great for this use.

Stress reduction. Stress can either result from IBS or it can set IBS off. Either way, it is important for IBS patients to learn to deal with stress. Exercise, yoga, and psychotherapy are among the many ways that help. See chapter 14 on the complementary and alternative (CAM) methods that help.

A FINAL THOUGHT ON IBS

Remember that, although it can be uncomfortable and stressful, IBS is not life-threatening and does not lead to more serious illnesses. It is just a pain in the butt! But there's no need to suffer with it either. Be *aware* of what the symptoms are, be *alert* to your own symptoms, and take *action* to get it diagnosed and other causes excluded, and to get treatment. (Also see Dr. J's story about IBS below and in chapter 6 under "Pain: Pelvic or Abdominal.") Abdominal pain, a very common symptom, is discussed in chapter 6.

Dr. J's Painful Night in the ER

A few years ago, during a very stressful time, I was having nightly episodes of squeezing chest pain which were getting worse. I went to the ER, where the docs on call were convinced I was having a heart attack, especially since nitroglycerine tablets relieved the pain. The tests showed that I hadn't had a heart attack, nor did I have CAD. I was ultimately diagnosed with esophageal spasm due to irritable bowel syndrome, and placed on Levsin. The chest pain had fooled all of us. And I was shocked at the eventual diagnosis because I had never had a problem with my GI tract before. But I knew that it's better to be safe than sorry when it comes to chest pain. Remember to always get your chest pain checked out.

THE DOCS CHAT ABOUT THE GI TRACT

DR. J: You mentioned the liver as being important to our health. Talk more about that.

DR. R: When I think about the liver, I remember, growing up, how my mother used to cook it (smothered in onions) once a week. I was totally grossed out by its slimy appearance and awful taste. I still remember how it made me gag.

DR J: I actually loved it (but smothered in ketchup)! I bet a lot of our readers have similar memories. Maybe that's why the liver is one of the most underrated organs. We never hear as much about it as we do about the heart or the brain. Don't you think?

DR. R: Absolutely. The liver performs over 500 important jobs for us. Like removing toxins from the blood, helping to make agents that boost our immunity, making proteins that help our blood to clot, producing bile that allows us to absorb fat, making cholesterol, and helping to metabolize much of what we take into our bodies. Without it, we couldn't survive.

DR. J: Anything special we need to know about liver diseases, or taking care of our liver, as we grow older?

DR R: The main thing to know is that many things can inflame the liver, and once it is inflamed, the healthy tissue can become replaced by scar tissue, a disease process called cirrhosis, which is the twelfth leading cause of death in this country (Kochanek et al. 2004). When too much of the liver becomes scarred, it stops functioning. However, many times the inflammation is reversible if caught early enough.

DR. J: What are some of the common causes of liver inflammation?

DR. R: Of course, a common cause of liver inflammation is alcohol; how much it takes to cause disease is different for different people. But we do know that women need to take in less alcohol than men to cause the same amount of liver disease. Another cause of liver disease that a lot of people don't know about is metabolic syndrome (discussed in chapter 11). This occurs along with obesity, both of which can lead to fatty liver disease, which can progress to cirrhosis. Viruses can cause liver inflammation; these are discussed in chapter 6. Also, certain inherited diseases, such as Wilson's disease and hemochromatosis, can lead to it, which is why it's important to let your clinician know if there's a family history of liver disease. Certain medications, like Tylenol (acetaminophen) and even aspirin, can cause inflammation. There are two other conditions, more common in women than men, that also can lead to liver disease, they are known as autoimmune hepatitis and primary biliary cirrhosis.

DR. J: What can we do to prevent liver disease and keep our liver healthy?

DR. R: Being aware of the above-named causes is a first step. Obviously, it's important to drink alcohol in moderation, or not at all. And it's just as important to keep your weight down. Knowing if one of the medications you take can cause liver damage is important, so that your clinician can follow your liver tests. And, of course, maintain your healthy lifestyle and, especially, follow a health-maintenance schedule so that your doctor checks your liver tests and your liver on a routine basis. Many times, liver problems can be caught early with routine blood tests.

DR. J: What do you tell your patients about constipation?

DR. R: Constipation is a symptom and not a disease. It occurs when either the colon gets sluggish and doesn't move things along quickly or the stool gets dried out and hard to move. Since there can be many medical causes of constipation, a woman should never ignore this symptom; she needs to be evaluated by her clinician for medical causes, such as hypothyroidism. Her clinician can then advise her on what is available for treatment. This may include exercise, fluids, fiber, and the elimination of certain medications or milk products. Also, she shouldn't just grab a laxative to treat herself if the constipation is a new symptom for her; laxatives can, in fact, be dangerous if the cause of the constipation is not yet diagnosed.

PEARLS OF WISDOM FOR GASTROINTESTINAL HEALTH

○ If you have heartburn that doesn't go away with antacids, or if you are using loads of antacids, don't ignore it—get it checked out.

○ Don't forget that what you think is heart*burn* may really be heart *disease*.

○ Always, always, always take your pills with a full glass of water.

○ Everyone passes gas; it is a bigger problem if you can't pass it.

○ Constipation is only a symptom, not a disease; if it is new for you and not easily treated, see your clinician.

○ IBS may be annoying, but it does not result in serious illness. On the other hand, you don't have to suffer with it.

○ If you have a change in bowel habits, see your doctor.

○ You have only one liver; take good care of it. Drink alcohol in moderation, know if your meds can affect your liver, get your liver function tested regularly, eat a healthy diet, avoid trans and saturated fats, exercise, and ask your clinician about the viral hepatitis vaccines.

○ Know your family history, especially if a family member has a history of liver disease or ulcers.

CHAPTER 6

How to Take Care of Your Uterus Now That You Don't Need It

By now, you've seen (and probably knew before) that each organ system of the body has at least one unique function that it performs beautifully, until diseased or damaged, of course, and that no other organ system can perform. So why even talk about the reproductive system since we know that at our age we really don't need it? In fact, what's there to discuss besides menopausal symptoms? As it turns out, quite a lot.

Even though the reproductive tract is no longer functional in the creation of another human being, medical science is not entirely convinced that parts of that system, like the ovaries, do *not* have other functions. Further, those organs are still present in our bodies and can become damaged or diseased. Just by their location in our lower abdominal cavity, also known as the *pelvis*, and the fact that they are close to our bowel and bladder, the uterus and ovaries can make their presence known. For instance, ovaries can twist and cause pain. Those common benign growths in the uterus, called *fibroids*, can grow, causing pain and bleeding.

In addition, that entire area of our body is not as nonfunctional as you might think. Did you know that many postmenopausal women continue having sex well into their eighth decade?! (Of course you know this. We have our tongues embedded in our cheeks here.) This was confirmed by a recent study of sexuality among older adults in the U.S. (Lindau et al. 2007). Also, did you know that older adults with health problems are less sexually active? (We could've told the researchers that!) And, were you aware that the declining sexual activity in some older women does not always have to do with cooling passions, but instead is due to an acute shortage of older men? (We could've told the researchers that too!) This "new" information is another reason that you need to read this chapter.

The aging reproductive tract was never even an issue for women before and during the nineteenth century because their life spans usually did not exceed their reproductive years. Our grandmothers and great-grandmothers never had to think about this area of the body—and didn't, or at least they never *talked* about it—after their childbearing years. So continuing to take care of our reproductive organs is a new issue thanks to the privilege of living longer. In this chapter, we cover all of these issues as well as the topics of the hysterectomy and sexually transmitted infections. The symptoms and treatment of menopause and the issue of sexuality after menopause are discussed in chapter 10. Care of the breasts is discussed in chapter 15, and cancers of the reproductive organs and breast are discussed in chapter 12.

MAKE AN APPOINTMENT FOR A PELVIC EXAM AND PAP SMEAR

We need to continue taking care of our reproductive organs even after our childbearing years. An important way to do so is to routinely have a pelvic exam.

The Different Parts of the Exam and Why You Need Them

Since you have been getting (or should have been getting) a pelvic exam and Pap smear for years, you should know that they are two different exams. The *Pap smear* is a sample taken from the tissue of your cervix (the mouth, or opening, of the uterus) with a wooden spatula and a tiny soft brush, which is used to detect precancerous or cancerous cells. At the same time that a cell sample is taken for the Pap smear, your clinician may also take samples from the cervix, with separate swabs, to look for infections, such as chlamydia, gonorrhea, herpes, and, more recently, human papillomavirus. Usually, these additional samples are obtained very quickly, with little or no discomfort. In fact, you may not even know extra samples have been taken. (But always ask.)

The *bimanual exam* is the way in which your gynecologist examines your reproductive organs manually and thus may be able to detect any abnormalities of your uterus or ovaries. A rectal exam is usually included. So, you can get a bimanual exam without having a Pap smear, and vice versa, although usually both are done at the same visit.

What about those of you who have had a hysterectomy? You too still need to get yearly pelvic and rectal exams to look for recurrent or new cancers in the pelvic area—even if your uterus and/or ovaries have been removed. You don't need to have a Pap smear after a hysterectomy *unless* your cervix was left when your uterus was removed or *unless* you had cervical cancer in the past or have had abnormal Pap smears of the vaginal cuff, which is that tissue left in the vagina after the hysterectomy.

Other Reasons You Need a Yearly Pelvic Exam

Having a yearly pelvic exam, rectal exam, and (maybe) a Pap smear is important not only because they screen for cancer, but because you will also have the opportunity to discuss with your clinician any symptoms or other concerns you may have, including your current sexual activity and your sexual history. She then can assess whether you currently are at risk for having a sexually transmitted infection or acquiring one. At these exams, you also will have your blood pressure, pulse, and weight checked, as well as a breast and thyroid exam, and you can discuss your need for a mammogram and any other screening tests. You should also know that many clinicians other than gynecologists do these exams. If you're more comfortable with your primary care clinician, ask her if she will routinely perform your pelvic exam.

Many of you are probably thinking that our recommendation to have a regular pelvic exam is obvious. We thought that too until we had taken care of lots of women currently our age and older (that is, over fifty), many of whom told us that they hadn't had a Pap smear or seen a gynecologist since their last baby was born, ten to fifty years ago! So, now that you know that some older women don't know the importance of having a regular pelvic exam, you should make sure your friends and relatives get their exams. Don't let anyone, expert or not, tell you that postmenopausal women no longer need this exam.

POSTMENOPAUSAL BLEEDING

One of the most common symptom occurring in our reproductive tract after menopause is postmenopausal bleeding. What exactly is the definition of postmenopausal bleeding? You probably know that the medical definition of *menopause* is when you've had no period for one year. Therefore, postmenopausal bleeding is any bleeding, even spotting, that occurs after one full year of no menstrual periods, or after one year of hormone replacement therapy.

With regard to bleeding after menopause, any bleeding from the uterus through the vagina is considered abnormal and must be taken seriously. One of the reasons is that up to 10 percent of all cases of postmenopausal bleeding are due to cancer, and as is always the case with cancers, the earlier found, the better the outcome (Shwayder 2000). But before you convince yourself that you have cancer if you have postmenopausal bleeding, remember that the majority of cases are not due to a malignancy. In most situations you may even be able to prevent the development of cancer by seeking help early.

What Causes Postmenopausal Bleeding?

There are many causes of bleeding after menopause due to abnormalities of the reproductive tract, including *fibroids* (benign growths of the uterine lining); *polyps* (small growths) on the cervix or in the uterus; a hormonal imbalance, particularly if you are taking estrogen replacement therapy; infection of the cervix; atrophy of the vaginal wall (the thinning and drying of the vaginal lining due to lack of estrogen); or, more seriously, cancer of the cervix, uterus, or ovaries. Illnesses of other parts of the body may also lead to bleeding after menopause. They include disorders of blood clotting, thyroid disease, and liver disease. Certain medications also may cause this, including blood thinners, prednisone, and tamoxifen, which is used to prevent a recurrence of breast cancer.

How Do You Know if You Have It?
What Can You Do About It?

After menopause, *any* bleeding that seems to come from your vagina must be taken seriously, even if it is just a spot or two of blood on the toilet paper or your underwear. Because the bleeding may be coming from your bladder or rectum, rather than your uterus, it may be difficult for you to know the origin of newly appearing bloodstains. One way to find out exactly where the bleeding is coming from is to place a tampon in your vagina for a few hours, or even a day. If you still notice blood on your underwear, even with the tampon in place, then you can assume the bleeding comes from either your bladder or rectum. Most often, blood from the rectum or bladder doesn't have a serious cause and may be due to hemorrhoids or a urinary tract infection. But it still needs to be checked out.

Therefore, always see your primary care clinician or gynecologist when you first notice the bleeding. It is not an emergency, however, unless the bleeding is very heavy. When you see your clinician, she will want to know the history of your bleeding, such as when you completed menopause; the pattern of the bleeding—if it has been a heavy constant flow or just a few spots on one occasion; and the duration of the bleeding. She will ask if you've had other symptoms, such as abdominal swelling or pain, or weight loss or gain. Then she will want to do a pelvic exam and will probably order a pelvic sonogram or CT (computer tomography) scan. If the cause of bleeding is still not found, she will want to do further tests.

Can It Be Treated or Prevented?

The treatment depends on the cause of the bleeding. There may be no treatment other than to have you come back for more frequent exams, or you may need the medication that is causing the problem to be adjusted, or you may need a hysterectomy. There is no way to prevent postmenopausal bleeding itself, but you can prevent the complications, such as the progression of a cancer, by being aware that the bleeding is abnormal and not falling into the trap that many women our age do who consider bleeding a mere nuisance, and then ignore it.

Don't let anyone tell you that a little vaginal bleeding after menopause is normal. It's not.

ABDOMINAL BLOATING

Although not as common as bleeding or pain, abdominal bloating is another symptom that may indicate a serious problem with your reproductive organs. In this situation, we use the term "bloating" of the abdomen to mean the same thing as "swelling."

What Causes Abdominal Bloating?

Short-lived abdominal bloating is a common symptom of a buildup of gas in the bowel. Bloating due to gas is relieved by antigas medications, having a bowel movement, or passing gas; it never lasts longer than several days at most. (See chapter 5 for more on gas.) One cause of persistent abdominal bloating, other than bowel gas, is the buildup of fluid confined within the abdominal cavity, in which, normally, there is very little fluid. This abnormal fluid is known as *ascites*. Although the late stages of chronic liver disease can cause ascites, the more common cause in women of our age is ovarian cancer. As with all other cancers, the earlier it is discovered, the more successfully it will be treated.

How Do You Know if You Have It?
What Can You Do About It?

If your jeans or belt that fit you perfectly yesterday cannot be buttoned or buckled today, you most likely have abdominal bloating. Note that it's very important to observe over what period of time this change has occurred. It's the most worrisome when it has occurred over a short time period (days to weeks) and is not due to gas. It is unlikely that your belt isn't fitting today, when it did yesterday, because of weight gain, because it is impossible to gain weight, other than from fluid, in that area of the body that quickly.

Another symptom you may experience is from the effect of the bloating, that is, the increased pressure it causes on internal organs, particularly on the stomach. When this happens, you may experience a sudden loss of appetite, nausea, vomiting, and heartburn, or feel full immediately after eating just a small amount. You also may feel that you need to urinate urgently or frequently because of the increased pressure on your bladder from the swelling.

You may have recently read the announcement that there are several symptoms related to ovarian cancer that should cause a woman to see her gynecologist quickly (Gynecologic Cancer Foundation 2007). Two of the four symptoms mentioned are abdominal bloating and difficulty eating or feeling full quickly. The other two are abdominal pain and urinary frequency or urgency. Ovarian cancer is discussed further in chapter 12.

The most common mistake women make about abdominal bloating is to think that it is due to a localized weight gain in the abdominal area and thus write it off. Not a good idea. Although most women do tend to gain weight first, and most noticeably, in the abdominal area as they age, a newly and rapidly protruding abdomen is cause for concern. So, if you've recently had to buy pants with an elastic waist for the first time ever (even though you swore you never would because they remind you too much of your _____ [fill in the blank here: mother-in-law, choir director, math teacher]), don't attribute these signs to middle age. Weight gain, if it is truly that, is usually somewhat more evenly distributed on your body or, at the very least, should have occurred over weeks to months, rather than over days to weeks.

WHEN SHOULD YOU SEEK HELP IF YOU HAVE BLOATING?

If the bloating has occurred daily for more than a few weeks, or if it is not relieved by one or several bowel movements, an antigas medication, or actually passing flatus, seek help. Make an appointment for an exam with either your gynecologist or your primary care clinician, as soon as possible. Bloating is not an emergency unless accompanied by severe pain or so much vomiting that you cannot hold any fluids down. If this occurs, call your doctor immediately or go to the nearest ER.

How Is It Diagnosed? Can It Be Treated or Prevented?

When you see your clinician, she will want to do a full exam, including a pelvic exam, blood work, and an imaging study such as a sonogram or CT scan. Most often, this combination of studies will give the diagnosis. The treatment, as with bleeding, depends upon the cause of the abdominal swelling.

PAIN: PELVIC OR ABDOMINAL

Another common symptom occurring in the area of our reproductive tract is pelvic or abdominal pain. What's the difference between pelvic and abdominal pain? *Pelvic pain* refers to symptoms originating from the area of the pelvis, which is in *the lowest part of the abdomen*, below the belly button and just above the pubic bone. *Abdominal pain* usually refers to symptoms coming from anywhere in the area of the belly, from the bottom of the rib cage all the way down to the pubic bone. So yes, lower abdominal pain and pelvic pain can both refer to pain coming from the same location. This is important to know as different health care providers may use these terms interchangeably. If you can't remember these terms, it's okay—just point your finger to where it hurts! But when you point, be as specific as possible.

What Causes Pelvic and Abdominal Pain?

It can be confusing to figure out what is causing the pain because so many organs are in the abdominal cavity: the lower portion of the stomach, the small bowel, large bowel, liver, gallbladder, spleen, urinary bladder, uterus, and ovaries are all enclosed within this area. (The kidneys are positioned closer to your back, although in some cases they may be causing the abdominal pain.)

If the pain is in the upper abdomen, you could have a stomach or *duodenal* (small bowel) ulcer, a gallstone or infection of the gall bladder, or an obstruction of your small or large bowel. Pain in the lower abdomen on the right side could be due to appendicitis, a ruptured ovarian cyst or twisted ovary, a large fibroid on that side of the uterus, or even a bowel spasm (see "Dr. J's Pain" below). Pain in the lower left side could be due to an inflammation or infection of a small sac in the large bowel, known as *diverticulitis*, or a problem with the left ovary or the left side of the uterus. A urinary tract infection also can cause symptoms in the lower abdomen.

Don't forget that heart disease in women can have unusual symptoms, such as upper abdominal pain, with or without nausea, vomiting, and sweating. Once again, it is very important that you take notice and be able to describe your abdominal pain as specifically as possible.

What Should You Notice About Your Abdominal Pain? What Can You Do About It?

Just as with chest pain and, in fact, all types of pain, try to describe the character of the pain (sharp or dull?), its main location, as well as whether it travels to another location, and how long each episode lasts if it is intermittent, or how long it has been present if it is constant (duration). Tell your clinician how severe you think it is. Often, care providers will ask you to rate the intensity of the pain on a scale of 1 to 10, where a rating of 10 is the worst pain you've ever had. Notice if there are other symptoms accompanying the pain, such as nausea, vomiting, diarrhea or constipation, urinary burning, or fever and chills.

Most important is the severity of the pain and whether it's a new pain. *Any pain that is new for you and that doesn't go away within a few hours must be evaluated.* If it's severe (say, an 8 to 10 on a scale of intensity), or of lesser intensity (a 5 to 7), but is accompanied by nonstop vomiting such that you cannot hold fluids down, go directly to the ER. If it's of lesser intensity, without accompanying symptoms, but has not gone away within a few hours, call your clinician and have an evaluation that day.

If you have had the same pain before, or have gotten it on a regular basis for months to years, this is known as *chronic pain*, and most times, it can be safely evaluated within a few days to weeks, unless it is getting worse or changing in any way. In any case, let your clinician know exactly what's going on to get her judgment of how quickly you need to be seen. Once you see your clinician and she has asked you to describe the pain, she will want to do a physical examination and possible an imaging study, most often an ultrasound or CT scan. If the cause still is not clear, further tests will be needed.

How Is It Treated?

Just as with abdominal bloating and postmenopausal bleeding, the treatment of abdominal pain depends on the cause. Since there are so many possible causes of abdominal/pelvic pain, it would be difficult to advise on preventive methods effective for all of them. However, the same things you do for diseases of the other organ systems, already discussed, will work here. That is, be *aware* of the many diseases that can cause abdominal pain; be *alert* to your own body, its symptoms, and any change in those symptoms; take *action*, both to seek help when you have the symptoms, and to take care of this part of your body routinely with regular pelvic exams and Pap smears; and if you're told that "nothing is wrong," *advocate* for yourself.

Dr. J's Pain

For years, I had pain in my right lower abdomen when I ovulated each month; this is not uncommon, and is known as mittelschmerz. *How did I know that was what my pain was due to? Simple. Exactly two weeks later I would always get my period. At the time I began going through menopause but had not completed it (I was still having occasional periods), this chronic pain changed. It became more sporadic, completely unrelated to any menstrual bleeding, more severe in intensity, and lasted longer. Initially, I ignored it, thinking it was the result of my changing cycles and menopause. Because of the severity, I soon worried that it could possibly be something else, like cancer of the right ovary. I saw my physician, who did a pelvic exam and sonogram, which were normal. She sent me to a GI doctor who, after performing a colonoscopy on me, diagnosed my pain as due to spasm of the bowel that lies in the right lower abdomen and told me that I had irritable bowel syndrome (IBS; see chapter 5). I was floored. In my entire life I'd never had any GI problems, or had I? Had I misinterpreted some of the pain I got as being from ovulation? I definitely learned something from that experience: How important it is to pay attention to all aspects of your symptoms, even if you've had the same symptoms before, and to be able to describe them. And of course, not to self-diagnose!*

REMOVAL OF THE REPRODUCTIVE ORGANS: THE HYSTERECTOMY

There are approximately 600,000 hysterectomies performed each year in the U.S., making it the second most frequently performed surgical operation. (The most frequently performed is the caesarian section.) In a survey between 1994 and 1999, it was found that there were approximately 20 million American women who'd had hysterectomies (Keshavarz et al. 2002). Dr. R has had this procedure and tells her story later in this chapter.

The issue of how many hysterectomies are performed in the U.S. is controversial. The reason is many experts believe that too many hysterectomies are performed in this country; in other words, that many of the hysterectomies performed are not medically necessary. Since so many of us already have had the procedure and many more may need to have it, it's important that you know the specifics about this surgery and its aftereffects.

What Is a Hysterectomy?

As you know, surgical removal of the uterus is known as a *hysterectomy*. When the cervix is left in place, it is called a *subtotal* or *partial hysterectomy*. In recent years, when a hysterectomy is done by using a laparoscope, part of the cervix is sometimes left. When the cervix is removed along with the body of the uterus, the surgery is called a *total hysterectomy*. If one or both ovaries and fallopian tubes are removed with the uterus, the procedure then becomes known as a *hysterectomy* with either *unilateral* or *bilateral salpingo-oophorectomy*.

If the procedure is done through an incision made in the abdomen, it is called an *abdominal hysterectomy*; if done through an incision in the vagina, it is known as a *vaginal hysterectomy*. In the past, this was called a blind hysterectomy, as the surgeon cannot see the organs at certain points during the surgery. Dr. J once had a patient ask very seriously how the gynecologist could do the procedure blindfolded because he told her he was doing a "blind procedure"! These days, the more common type of vaginal hysterectomy is done with a laparoscope and is called *laparoscopy assisted vaginal hysterectomy (LAVH)*.

Why You Need to Know the Medical Terms

If your doctor recommends a hysterectomy, it's important that you know if only your uterus is to be removed, or if one or both ovaries are also being removed. Occasionally, the surgeon will take out your appendix as well, even if it is healthy, since it is prone to infection. You need to know that too. These issues may seem obvious to you. But we've had patients who did not realize there was a difference between the surgical procedures, and, for example, they could not tell us if their ovaries were still present after their hysterectomy, or whether they'd had their appendix out as well. Knowledge of exactly what surgery you've had performed can become very important if, for example, you end up in the ER with pain in your right lower abdominal area—the area where the appendix normally is located. If you know that your appendix was removed when you had your hysterectomy, you could possibly save yourself from exploratory surgery. If you're worried that you won't remember what was involved in your pelvic surgery, even after your surgeon tells you, request a copy of the operative report. That way, you will always have close at hand a record of exactly what was removed. Remember: Ask questions. And keep records of your health care.

How Do You Know if You Need a Hysterectomy?

What are the common conditions for which a hysterectomy (with or without removal of the ovaries) is recommended in our age group? These include uterine fibroids (benign growths), endometriosis (uterine lining tissue outside of the uterus causing pain and bleeding), chronic pelvic pain, abnormal and heavy bleeding, uterine prolapse, and cancer of the uterus or ovaries. Remember this: A hysterectomy is done as a last resort in all of the above conditions except cancer. The usual nonsurgical treatments (such as a pessary for prolapse or hormone therapy for abnormal bleeding), and less invasive procedures (such as endometrial ablation for fibroids) are always tried first. For your specific condition, ask your doctor what the alternatives to a hysterectomy are.

What Should You Expect After the Surgery?

In our experience, many women are as worried about the aftereffects of a hysterectomy as they are about the surgery itself.

IMMEDIATE EFFECTS

Although it may sound obvious because this is such a common procedure, a hysterectomy is major surgery with expected aftereffects, including soreness in the area of the incision and fatigue for up to several months afterward. Usual physical activities are resumed gradually over the month or two after the surgery. Sexual activity should be avoided for at least four to eight weeks postoperatively. Women who have had a laparoscopic hysterectomy may have a quicker recovery time.

LONG-TERM EFFECTS

The larger issues that concern many women include the long-term effects. One surprising finding in recent years is that women who have had their ovaries removed, even after menopause, have a higher incidence of heart disease. The reason for this is not known, but is possibly due to the ovaries' lifelong production of tiny amounts of estrogen, or of a substance other than estrogen, as yet undiscovered, both of which may protect against heart disease (Kritz-Silverstein, Barrett-Connor, and Wingard 1997). More recent studies have noted an association between removal of both ovaries before menopause and Parkinson's disease and dementia (Rocca et al. 2008; Rocca et al. 2007). These latter two associations need further study. The possibility that our ovaries continue to keep us healthy even after menopause is the reason why it's important to discuss with your surgeon if there is a medical need to remove your ovaries during your hysterectomy.

Sexual functioning. The most common concerns of women undergoing this surgery are the physical impact on sexual response and enjoyment, and the psychological effects of having their reproductive organs removed. It is now commonly accepted that the surgery itself does not affect sexual functioning (National Institute on Aging 2005). In fact, many women report improvement in their sexual functioning after the surgery, probably because the condition for which the surgery was performed, such as chronic pain, has been removed as well. It is not uncommon, however, for women to experience painful intercourse due to vaginal dryness, or a decrease in sex drive, after having had their ovaries removed, just as occurs after menopause. Some do well using topical estrogen for the vaginal dryness and testosterone cream for low sex drive (see chapter 10). Those who develop depression related to the removal of their reproductive organs usually do well with counseling and/or short-term use of antidepressants.

Why Shouldn't All Postmenopausal Women Have a Hysterectomy?

Why do you need your uterus or ovaries anymore anyway? Aren't they useless and just sitting there waiting to cause trouble or develop a cancer? Interesting question, and not surprisingly for our generation of inquisitive women, one that does come up, especially given how blasé we Americans have become about having surgery. Although removal of the uterus and ovaries may be recommended for some women with a healthy reproductive tract (for those with a specific genetic predisposition to cancers, see chapter 12), it is not performed routinely on healthy postmenopausal women. And for one good reason: *It is major surgery.*

Yes it is relatively safe surgery. But all major surgery has risks: The risks related to the surgery itself, such as damaging nearby organs or a blood vessel in the area; the risks related to the anesthesia, such as fatal allergic reactions; and the risks related to the immobilization of the body during and after the procedure, such as blood clots in the legs or to the lung. If you have a condition for which the surgery is needed, then it should be true in most circumstances that the risk of leaving your uterus and/or ovaries intact is greater than the risks of the surgery.

If a hysterectomy is recommended to you, even by your longtime doctor whom you trust, and you're not sure you really need it, get a second opinion. Remember to always be your own advocate.

Dr. R's Story

Everyone has her own "normal" when it comes to her body. For me, it was normal to have extremely heavy periods. Maybe that's why, when I started going through menopause, it didn't strike me as odd that I was having a period every two weeks, and that I was getting really tired and really pale. Or maybe I was in total denial that something was wrong. It finally got so bad that I called my doctor, who ordered an immediate ultrasound and, with a very worried face, told me that something was growing in my uterus and the whole thing had to come out. Was it an alien? A fibroid? Of course, I panicked and was sure I had cancer. Fortunately, the biopsy of my uterus proved me wrong. It was a benign fibroid gone wild. But, my uterus still had to come out, because it had grown into the shape of a soccer ball fourteen inches in diameter! Because of the large size of the uterus, I had to have an abdominal hysterectomy rather than the laparoscopic type. In addition to my uterus, the doctor wanted to take my ovaries and my appendix. I saw no reason to do either because from my reading I knew that the ovaries still provide a function after menopause, and my appendix was just fine (thank you very much).

I prepared for surgery using guided imagery and acupuncture (my doctor looked at me cross-eyed when I told her). But they worked! Both helped to reduce my pain and speed my healing. After the surgery I had very little pain and was able to get by with Tylenol or Advil for any discomfort that I had. Within two weeks I was doing my regular walking route. (This was against the rules, but I couldn't help myself. It felt so good to be out and about.) The strange thing is that I didn't realize how badly I was feeling prior to my hysterectomy as a result of the growth of the fibroid and all that bleeding. Although I feel nostalgic about my uterus that hatched my sons and served me well for fifty-three years, I am glad that it is gone and I am feeling so much better!

SEXUALLY TRANSMITTED INFECTIONS (STIs)

"Finally," you say. You've navigated the reproductive years successfully—after putting up with nausea and vomiting and weight gain on the Pill, or having had the equivalent of a Brillo pad put in your uterus. (Remember that Dalkon shield IUD?) Now that many of you have gone through menopause, you've already found that sex can be wonderful without the ever-present worry of pregnancy or worrying about the need for protection, or so you thought. But you need to be aware that there are other risks of unprotected sex, namely the risk of sexually transmitted infections (also known as sexually transmitted diseases, STDs, or venereal diseases, VDs). They are still around, and you can still get them at this age, even after menopause.

In fact, you may be even more prone to getting infected with some of the sexually transmitted bacteria or viruses due to the effects of menopause. Even those of you who have had a hysterectomy and both ovaries removed can become infected. If you're newly single and sexually active, or if you or your partner is not sexually monogamous, you need to be informed about these infections. And even though you may have known a lot about VD when you were younger, there are a lot of new facts *and* newly discovered infections. This information is not just for your teenagers anymore.

What Causes STIs?

Sexually transmitted infections are just that: infections transmitted by sexual contact. The infectious agents can be bacteria, viruses, or parasites, and they have something in common besides the way they are transmitted: They all require a specific type of environment in order to flourish. As you might expect, that environment must be moist, warm, and enclosed, as is found in the vagina, the cervix, and the male and female urethra, anus, mouth, and throat.

Although they are all transmitted through sexual exposure, these organisms may infect your body in different ways. Some can be transmitted *additionally* in ways other than sexually, and others can infect parts of the body in addition to the sexual organs. Some of these infectious agents, like herpes, syphilis, and human papillomavirus (HPV), are transmitted by direct contact, or skin touching skin, and then cause infection in the exact area with which they come into contact. Others of these organisms, such as the hepatitis viruses, human immunodeficiency virus (HIV), and syphilis, can actually enter into the bloodstream through tiny tears in the lining of the vagina, cervix, or rectum, and then infect other organs in the body, remaining inactive, or becoming active, inside the body for the individual's entire life.

How Common Are STIs?

Chlamydia is the most commonly reported STI in the U.S. Gonorrhea is the second most commonly reported STI (Weinstock, Berman, and Cates 2004). Both of these STIs continue to increase anually in the U.S. (CDC 2007c). Hardest hit populations include young women, gay and bisexual men, and African-Americans. It is estimated that at least 45 million Americans over the age of twelve have been infected with the virus that causes genital herpes (Patel and Rompalo 2005); that is one out of every five adolescents and adults in the U.S.! Infection with genital human papillomavirus (HPV) is also quite common. Approximately 20 million Americans are currently infected with HPV. In the 2003-2004 National Health and Nutrition Examination Survey, approximately 27 percent of the nearly 2,000 women surveyed, who were between the ages of fourteen and fifty-nine, tested positive for HPV (Dunne et al. 2007).

You may not have heard much about syphilis in recent years because the number of new infections in the U.S. had dropped so dramatically by 1998 that this STI was considered to be rare, especially in women. However, the U.S. syphilis rate increased for the seventh consecutive year in 2007, primarily increasing in gay and bisexual men (CDC 2008b). As troubling is the fact that the number of cases in women and African-Americans had increased.

The hepatitis viruses that are sexually transmissible are hepatitis B (HBV) and hepatitis C (HCV). There are an estimated 1.2 million Americans infected with HBV (Buccolo 2005). Currently the highest rate of infection occurs in those aged twenty to forty-nine. A study conducted between 1988 and 1990 showed that the number of Korean-Americans (first and second generation) with HBV was about thirty times higher than that in the general U.S. population (Hann, Hann and Maddrey 2007). Hepatitis C virus is more often transmitted by sharing infected needles than by sexual contact, which is thought to account for only 10 to 15 percent of all cases (Bialek and Terrault 2006). In fact, the risk of sexual transmission of HCV between monogamous heterosexual partners is quite low, unlike that of HBV. HCV is more common in people of color than in Caucasians, and more common in men than women. All ages get HCV.

HIV is discussed in a separate section below.

Are You at Risk for STIs?

The well-known factors that put you at a higher risk for becoming infected with an STI include young age (teens and twenties), a history of being sexually active with multiple partners, and a history of having had even one STI in the past. Before you breathe a sigh of relief here or feel happy for the first time in years that you're no longer young, look again at the risk factors, other than the first one, and know that they can apply to you, and to your partner, no matter what age either of you are. You are still at risk for STIs even if you are in monogamous relationship now but had multiple partners in the past. Remember that these same risk factors apply to your partner, either male or female.

Can you get an STI even though you are not sexually active right now? The fact is, you may already have an STI of which you are not aware. Certain STIs (especially genital herpes, syphilis, HPV, the hepatitis viruses, and HIV) may cause no initial symptoms to alert you that you've been infected, and can live silently in your body forever. And though they may hibernate in your body, causing you no trouble, they still can be easily transmitted to your sexual partner—even years after you were initially infected, and even without you knowing it. Further, these same organisms can cause you to have symptoms, such as a genital ulcer or a wart—out of the blue and even years later. Talk about sneaky biological weapons.

Can you get an STI even at this age? Traditionally, statistics have shown that the age group that gets STIs the least frequently is the "older generation," that is, the age we are now. This finding was based on studies of previous generations, who, when they reached this age, either didn't have sex as often as when they were younger (doubt that) or didn't talk about it, particularly to their doctors (more likely). And since it was during our younger years that VDs, as we called them then, became rampant owing to our practicing "free love" and to the introduction and widespread use of the birth control pill, we were more exposed to these infections than previous generations. Which means that the herpes infection you got back then, you still have now, and can still pass along. So the statistics about older folks not getting STDs very often are about to change, now that *we* are the older folks. With respect to HIV, the statistics are already changing. (See the section on HIV below.)

Can you get an STI if you have sex with women only? You are much less likely to get certain STIs (syphilis, gonorrhea, and chlamydia) if you have sex with women only. There are several possible reasons for this difference, including the fact that these infectious agents are probably far less prevalent in the lesbian community than in the rest of society, and that the infectious agents are simply not as easily spread by the forms of sexual contact most common among lesbians, such as mouth to genital contact.

You are not completely safe though. There are some STIs—such as herpes and HPV—that do occur in lesbians (Bailey 2004). In addition, a recent study has shown that bacterial vaginosis (BV), a vaginal infection caused by a mixed population of bacteria previously thought not to be sexually transmitted, is more common in sexually active lesbian women than in sexually active heterosexual women (Evans et al. 2007). This is important since BV is considered a risk factor for HIV transmission and pelvic inflammatory disease. Because there are few studies comparing diseases in lesbians to those in heterosexual women, this is a field needing more study. Even so, you should be aware of the possibility of acquiring these infections and discuss it with your partner. Female condoms and dental dams will decrease the risk in the appropriate situation. Obviously, these facts do not apply to women who are bisexual: You have the same risks as women who are solely heterosexual.

What Do You Need to Know About STIs in General?

Here are some general principles that apply to *all* STIs.

Male-to-female transmission of STIs occurs more often than female-to-male. Why this is so should be obvious by thinking about the mechanics of intercourse. Male-to-female sexual contact is designed to be efficient for reproductive purposes, and this efficiency of transmission applies also to STIs. As for those infections transmitted through direct skin-to-skin contact, the fact that the male has a larger external surface area of his genitals makes male-to-female transmission of these organisms efficient as well. (We know there's a joke lurking in that last sentence...) We women are at greater risk of getting an STI than we are of giving it. Sadly, in this case, our anatomy is truly our destiny.

Many of the STIs cause no symptoms initially, or ever. The fact that we females are highly likely to acquire an STI through intercourse with an infected male partner is even more frightening when one considers that we may not even be aware that we've been infected.

Several sexually transmitted agents may, and do, infect one person at the same time. This is the reason that knowledgeable clinicians never test a patient for only one STI, but recommend screening for several STIs. Be sure to ask your clinician to check you for all STIs, even if you think you've been infected with only one.

Some of the STIs can remain inactive in your body forever but can still be passed to your partner. These include HIV, the hepatitis viruses, HPV, genital herpes virus, syphilis, and, often, chlamydia.

The STIs that can remain inactive in your body may also flare up and cause you to have symptoms at any time—even fifty years later. Because of this, if you break out with a genital herpes ulcer for the first time, it is possible you didn't get the infection from your current partner, but from a past partner.

Both partners need to be treated for the STI when one is diagnosed with it, even if there are no symptoms. Yes, this means what you think. You're going to have to talk to your partner about your infection because he/she needs to be treated, even if there are no symptoms. If you're the only one treated, then your partner will continue to reinfect you, and he/she will also be at risk for the long-term complications of the infection. (You may be mad enough to wish the latter on him/her, but be nice.)

Barrier contraceptives are no longer considered 100 percent effective in preventing STIs. Regular use of condoms can greatly decrease the risk of transmission of the organisms. But it is known that even with correct condom use, people have become infected with the STIs. It is also important to know that only latex or polyurethane condoms should be used; other types have been found ineffective in preventing transmission.

How Do You Know if You Have an STI?

As already mentioned, you may have no initial symptoms after being infected with an STI, or the symptoms can be quite subtle. In addition, the symptoms may mimic other problems you've had in the pelvic area that are not caused by STIs. The symptoms occurring in the genital area due to an STI include vaginal discharge; burning on urination; frequency of or difficulty urinating; swelling or pain of the vulva or labia; an open sore (ulceration) that may or may not be painful; a new small growth that looks like a wart or is larger; and/or pelvic pain. If you practice oral or anal sex, some of the same symptoms may occur in the mouth or anus, as well as a sore throat or ulcerations in either the mouth or anal area.

The symptoms caused by the two sexually transmitted hepatitis viruses (B and C) include nausea, profound fatigue, loss of appetite, darkened urine, and jaundiced (yellow) skin. However, remember that there may be no symptoms at all after infection. The symptoms caused by HIV are discussed below.

Are There Long-Term Consequences of STIs?

Infection with chlamydia or gonorrhea may lead to pelvic inflammatory disease, scarring (which can cause infertility), and chronic pelvic pain if not treated. Genital herpes infection can cause recurrent painful ulcerations, but otherwise does not cause long-term complications other than discomfort. If untreated in its initial stages, syphilis can lead to symptoms in the entire body, and eventually can lead to heart and brain problems. In recent years, certain types of HPV have been shown to cause cervical cancer.

In a small percentage of people infected, the hepatitis viruses can cause chronic liver disease, which can lead to cirrhosis and death. Hepatitis B can also lead to cancer of the liver. Both of these complications are unusual; more likely you'll recover with no further problems.

How Are STIs Treated?

The STIs that cause symptoms mainly in the genital or pelvic area are treated with medication. Antibiotics are used to cure chlamydia, gonorrhea, and syphilis. The antivirals used for herpes infection do not cure the infection, they simply shorten the course of the symptoms. If taken on a regular basis, these medications can prevent recurrences of herpetic ulcer outbreaks. There is no treatment to cure HPV infection, but the warty growths it causes can be treated locally with liquid nitrogen,

Mathilda's Story

Dr. J's longtime patient, a lovely seventy-six-year-old named Mathilda, was very healthy and active. And though she still dearly missed her husband (she had been a widow for the past seven years), she was ready to realize her dream of living in California, where she'd be able to enjoy her favorite outside activities—hiking and running her dogs—year-round. Her final checkup with Dr. J before her move proved that her good health continued, and she was off. Three months after she had left, Mathilda called Dr. J, saying that she would be in town shortly and urgently needed an office visit. At that visit, Mathilda told the following story.

She had found a wonderful retirement community in California and had immediately made new friends, including a very special man; she had instantly felt she had known him always. And though she'd been a bit nervous—she hadn't had sex since her husband died—she now had a wonderful physical relationship with him as well. So, what was the problem?

About one month after she began having sex with him, she noticed painful blisters in her vaginal area. Since her husband had been her only sexual partner previously and had never had any genital problems, and since she had never had any gynecological complaints before, she was totally puzzled. Initially, she thought that the sores were just due to irritation because they went away within a week, but now that they had returned, she was worried.

Her exam proved the sores to be caused by the herpes virus. This shocked Mathilda. But not being afraid to confront sensitive issues, she spoke with her new partner immediately on returning to her new home. He admitted that he was infected with genital herpes, and had been for many years, but hadn't told her because he had not had an outbreak of the infection when they had had sex. He had wrongly assumed that the only way this STI could be transmitted was if he had an active outbreak at the time of intercourse. Though still dealing with her surprise—that she could even get an STI at her age and that he had herpes and hadn't told her—Mathilda handled the situation well. He agreed to be tested for other STIs, including HIV and all of his tests came back negative.

Mathilda takes medication for her outbreaks of herpes now and knows that she has to get more information from future sex partners before having sex. And she now insists on her partner wearing condoms. She recently had a private laugh one day when she was visiting her grandson and noticed in his bathroom a bottle of the same herpes medication that she takes and thought how surprised he'd be if he knew!

laser therapy, or topical medications; they are treated, however, only if they are causing discomfort or bleeding as, in many cases, the growths recur after the treatment.

There is no treatment for the acute phase of viral hepatitis, but there are medications available for the chronic stages. There is a vaccine for hepatitis B virus that is effective in preventing it, and that is routinely recommended for all babies at birth, for children through age eighteen not vaccinated at birth, and for those people older than eighteen whose behavior or job puts them at risk for getting hepatitis B, including sexual partners of people who have the infection, health care workers, and intravenous drug users who are not already infected. The vaccine is also recommended immediately after exposure to hepatitis B in order to, hopefully, prevent long-term infection.

If you think you've been exposed to viral hepatitis B through sexual or injected-drug use contact with someone who is infected, *see your clinician immediately to receive treatment that may prevent you from becoming infected.* Although there is no vaccine for hepatitis C, see your clinician if you think you may have been exposed to it as well.

Methods to prevent all STIs are discussed at the end of the chapter.

HUMAN IMMUNODEFICIENCY VIRUS (HIV)

HIV is the most serious of the STIs for the following reasons: It involves the internal organs of the body, and not just the genital area, thus causing serious illnesses; it remains in the body forever, causing the infected person to stay infected forever, despite treatment; and it causes the body fluids and blood of the infected person to be infectious. These facts are also true for the hepatitis viruses, although the effects of these viruses are not as widespread throughout the body as are those of HIV.

Since there is too much information concerning HIV to discuss here, and because the virus and the disease it causes are so deserving of our respect, we will not try to cover all the facts about HIV. However, we don't want to leave you with the idea that this virus is irrelevant to you either—quite the contrary. You are still very much at risk to acquire this infection if you are sexually active now, or plan to be.

Who Is at Risk for HIV in Recent Years

The latest estimates show that by the end of the year 2003, there were an estimated 1.1 million people in the U.S. living with HIV infection with approximately 25 percent undiagnosed, and unaware of their infection. Of those, men who have sex with men made up the largest proportion of the total (CDC 2008a). Before you breathe a sigh of relief, thinking that you're not at risk for HIV, read on.

Although few women were diagnosed with HIV early in the epidemic in the 1980s, the HIV/AIDS epidemic today is a very real threat to the health of American women, particularly young women, African-American women, and Hispanic women. Between 1981 and 1995, women made up 15 percent of the total population with HIV/AIDS in the U.S.; between 2001 and 2004, the percentage had increased to 27 percent (Schneider et al. 2006).

This next set of facts is very relevant to our age group: In 2003, 30 percent of all the reported AIDS cases in the U.S. were in people over the age of forty-five! These studies also showed that in women over the age of forty-five, the most common way of acquiring HIV is through hetero-sexual contact, and that among women over fifty who are HIV-infected or have AIDS, 70 percent are women of color. Currently, approximately 19 percent of all people with HIV/AIDS in the U.S. are age fifty and older (National Institute on Aging 2008). So this infection is definitely of concern to all of us.

How Is HIV Transmitted?

Although the major mode of spreading HIV is through sexual contact, as with the hepatitis viruses there are other behaviors that can transmit HIV, including sharing needles with an infected person when using drugs intravenously; a needlestick exposure from a needle used previously on or by an infected person (both of these are due to the possible exposure to the blood of the infected person in the needle, and not from the needle itself); and an infected mother passing the infection to her baby during birth and/or breastfeeding. HIV and the hepatitis viruses used to be spread via infected blood transfusions in this country, although this is no longer the case. Donated blood here is now screened, and if these viruses are found, that blood is not used. In developing countries, however, it is still possible to acquire these viruses through a blood transfusion.

Can you give HIV to, or get it from, your female partner? There are no confirmed cases of female-to-female transmission of HIV, although it is thought that female sexual contact should be considered a possible means of transmitting the virus, since female-to-male transmission is known to occur. If you are sexually active with a female partner, keep the following facts in mind: Menstrual blood and vaginal secretions are potentially infectious; and having the linings of your mouth or vagina exposed to these infected fluids, particularly if these linings are not intact (as with mouth sores or vaginal ulcers), can potentially lead to HIV infection (CDC Divisions of HIV/AIDS Prevention 2006).

Why does being postmenopausal put you at risk? You already know, or will know in the near future, that one of the major discomforts of menopause is the lack of moisture in the vagina caused by the absence of estrogen. The lining of the vagina in this condition is easily torn, and that tear becomes a perfect entry portal into the body for HIV or the hepatitis viruses (Kojic and Cu-Uvin 2007).

What other sexual practices put you at risk? What about transmitting HIV through sexual contact other than vaginal or anal intercourse? The risk of acquiring HIV through oral sex is much lower than that of vaginal or anal sex. Oral sex becomes more of a risk for acquiring the virus if the membranes of the mouth are disrupted, such as with bleeding gums. How about kissing? Closed mouth kissing poses no risk for HIV infection, although there is a potential for infection with French kissing, particularly if there are open sores inside the mouth of either partner.

How Do You Know if You Have HIV? What Can You Do About It?

Once infected with HIV, there may be absolutely no symptoms at all for up to ten years, although some people get a nonspecific illness within the first two months.

Initial symptoms. If there are symptoms upon initial infection, they may include fever, night sweats, enlarged lymph glands, and a sore throat. You can see why this is called a "mono-like illness," since it is similar to the infectious mononucleosis you, or one of your high school or college classmates, may have had. These symptoms last only a short time, and then disappear. Infection with HIV does not become acquired immunodeficiency syndrome (AIDS) until the advanced stages of the infection, at which time the immune system is damaged and thus unable to fight certain infections.

Later symptoms. Women in the later stages of infection get some of the same symptoms as men, such as profound fatigue, weight loss, night sweats, short-term memory loss, and persistent skin rashes. In addition, they also get symptoms specific to female anatomy. Among these are recurrent vaginal yeast infections, menstrual irregularities, increased frequency or severity of long-standing genital herpes infection, abnormal growth of genital warts, and increasing symptoms of PID (pelvic inflammatory disease).

How the later symptoms of HIV can be confused with menopause. As you read the symptoms above, were you able to see why a woman might not suspect that she had been infected with HIV years before? Or why she might completely overlook—particularly at this age—irregular menses and night sweats? Many of the symptoms of HIV infection are exactly the same as those for menopause, which could lead a woman to attribute all new symptoms to the wrong diagnosis.

For that reason, you should ask to be tested for HIV, even if you have no symptoms, as soon as you discover from a sexual partner that he/she has HIV, or if you suspect it. The diagnosis is made with a simple blood test. If you find out early enough after you have been exposed (had sex with that person), there are medications you can take immediately that may prevent the infection from taking hold in your body, even if you have been exposed to it. (This is discussed below.) Also ask to be tested for HIV if your partner tells you he/she has another STI, or if you develop symptoms of another STI after having sex. Many of the other STIs, such as chlamydia and genital herpes virus, increase the likelihood that you will become infected with HIV if you are exposed. The safest thing to do, obviously, is to ask any new partner to be tested, although we realize that this can be a difficult thing to do. (See the discussion about open communication below.)

In these situations, if you are unable to get an immediate appointment with your clinician, go to an urgent care center. In many cities, the public health department operates clinics that can test you for all the STIs without you needing to make an appointment.

Can HIV Be Treated?

No doubt you've read about the large group of new drugs that have decreased the number of deaths from AIDS over the last decade. This is true. But, as with the drugs used for hepatitis viruses, they do not rid the body of HIV. When the patient stops taking them, the virus and the disease flare up again. So the fact that there are good medications available, and people are living well with this infection, should not make you blasé about becoming infected.

Can HIV Infection Be Prevented?

Obviously, the best way to prevent becoming infected with HIV is to prevent being exposed in the first place. However, if you are exposed, there are several medication protocols that, when taken *within seventy-two hours* of either sexual exposure or injected-drug-use exposure to HIV for a *full twenty-eight days*, can, in many cases, prevent you from becoming infected with HIV (Smith et al. 2005). This regimen includes several anti-HIV medications and is the same treatment recommended for hospital workers exposed to HIV by a needlestick, and for women who have been raped. Therefore, *contact your primary care provider or your gynecologist within seventy-two hours after you think you've been exposed.* You can also call your local public health department or emergency room.

HOW CAN YOU PREVENT OR REDUCE THE RISK OF GETTING ALL OF THE STIs?

There are several ways to lower the risk of getting STIs. They are discussed below.

Abstinence. If this works for you, it is a surefire solution.

Condoms. If abstinence isn't for you, then use condoms. Latex and polyurethane condoms used consistently and properly during vaginal, anal, and oral intercourse have been shown to greatly reduce the risk of acquiring or transmitting the STIs. It is important to emphasize that only latex and polyurethane condoms are effective; natural membrane condoms and those made of other materials are not effective. (Trojan makes condoms of both materials; Durex Avanti is a popular polyurethane condom.) Spermicides have been shown in some instances to cause genital ulcerations, which then increase the likelihood of acquisition of HIV infection, and thus are no longer routinely recommended for use with condoms. Female condoms should be considered in those instances in which a male condom cannot be used, as well as for women having sex with other women.

Dental dams. A dental, or oral, dam is a six-inch square piece of thin latex that is placed over the entire vulva or anus to prevent the transmission of the sexually transmitted viruses from mouth to vagina or anus, and vice versa, during oral sex. Also called vaginal dams, they are available at most pharmacy chains or medical supply stores.

Anti-HIV medications and/or the HBV vaccine. Don't forget that these two options are available to, hopefully, prevent HIV or HBV from taking hold in your body, even after you've been exposed to these viruses. Time is of the essence here; the anti-HIV medications must be started within seventy-two hours of exposure (when you had sex), and the HBV vaccine must be given as soon as possible after the exposure too.

Open communication between partners. Another way to protect yourself from STIs is to have a long-term, monogamous, mutually exclusive sexual relationship with a partner who has been tested and is negative, and with whom you can talk freely. At the very least, before you have sex with someone, be aware of his/her risk of having STIs and ask him/her to get tested. And, of course, if you are heterosexual, ask him to use condoms all the time, since they at least decrease the risk of your getting infected. We know how excruciatingly difficult this conversation can be, but this is one of those times when advocating for yourself could save your life. With STIs, as with all of the other diseases we've discussed in this book, ignorance is definitely not bliss

THE DOCS CHAT ABOUT THE PELVIC ORGANS

DR. R: That's a lot of stuff to remember for body parts that don't work anymore! Tell us about prolapse of the uterus.

DR. J: Prolapse, or dropping, of the uterus is not as common as the other conditions we discussed but does occur in women of our age. You'll know it if you have it. Quite literally, the uterus sags or drops down into the vagina.

DR. R: Hmm… A fallen uterus. Is that where the term "fallen woman" came from?! What causes it?

DR. J: It's caused by weakening of the muscles and tissue that regularly support the uterus. This weakening is due to aging, childbirth, and/or a lifetime of those things that cause pressure to the abdomen, such as obesity, heavy lifting, or chronic coughing. Some women also develop prolapse of the bladder or rectum. Our old enemy, gravity, is taking its toll again.

DR. R: How do we know if we have it, and what should we do about it?

DR. J: The most common symptom is a feeling of pressure or a bulging in the vaginal area, though once it is more advanced, you can actually feel the uterus dropping down into the vagina. This is only an emergency if you have severe pain or bleeding with it; otherwise, you should make an appointment with your gynecologist as soon as possible. The only permanent cure is surgery to repair the damaged pelvic muscles and tissue; some doctors recommend a hysterectomy too. If it is a mild case, pelvic floor muscle exercises can help, as can a pessary, which is a rubber device placed inside the vagina to support the uterus (see chapter 7).

DR. R: The behavior of all those STIs sounds like a plot against women! I mean, really. We can get an infection we don't know we're getting, from someone who either doesn't tell us or doesn't know he/she has it, and this infection can lead to serious consequences. How fair is that? So what do you really recommend so that we don't worry constantly?

DR. J: I recommend taking the bull by the horns (not your partner—the problem) and being pro-active about it. Even if you're not sexually active right now, if you've had an STI or a history of multiple partners, or if you had a partner in the past who you suspect was sexually active outside your relationship or who became ill, then get tested for all the STIs.

DR. R: Hate to break up this party, but gotta run. I'm going to make *both* of our *gyn appointments* right now!

PEARLS OF WISDOM FOR THE REPRODUCTIVE TRACT

○ Get a yearly pelvic exam, and ask about a Pap smear and STI testing.

○ Know what tests are being done. If you need surgery—know exactly which organs will be removed and which will remain. Get your operative report.

○ Ask you doctor if there are alternatives to a hysterectomy for you.

○ See your clinician ASAP for any postmenopausal bleeding.

○ See your clinician ASAP for abdominal bloating that persists.

○ For sudden and severe abdominal/pelvic pain lasting over an hour, go to the ER.

○ Know the risk factors for STIs. Talk to your partner openly about them.

CHAPTER 7

The Urinary Tract: How to Stay Dry on the Outside

What is the one uncontrollable bodily occurrence that probably embarrasses us even more than hot flashes? That's right—leaking urine. It's such a common fear that Dr. J remembers the most popular skit in her medical school end-of-year Follies included a song that went like this (sung to the tune of "Chattanooga Choo Choo"): "Pardon me Doc, but I'm incontinent at parties!" But it's no laughing matter. The good news is that loss of control of urine doesn't have to happen as we age, and there are things we can do to correct, and even prevent, this problem.

THE NORMAL URINARY TRACT

The function of the *urinary tract* is to maintain the appropriate water and chemical balance in the body while getting rid of the toxins. The *kidneys* are responsible for processing the fluids, chemicals (for example, potassium and sodium), and waste products of the body. The resulting fluid is urine. Once the urine has been made, it flows out of the kidneys into the bladder through two long tubes, the *ureters*. The *bladder*, a sac covered by a membrane, holds the urine until it is pushed out of the bladder neck into a short tube, the *urethra*, that opens to the outside of the body.

The Muscles of the Urinary Tract

Control of urination is all about muscles, a few of which are under your control, and several that are not. The bladder is enclosed by a powerful muscle called the *detrusor muscle* and sits on a muscular structure known as the *pelvic floor*, which is like a sling from the pubic bone in front to the bottom of the spine in back. In addition, more muscles surround the *bladder neck* (the internal sphincter muscle) as well as the *urethra* (the external sphincter muscle). When you want to keep yourself from urinating, you control the external sphincter muscle and some of the pelvic floor muscles by consciously contracting them. The other muscles are controlled by the brain and are automatic, or involuntary, actions; they are not under your conscious control.

THE URINARY TRACT AS IT AGES

There are many factors associated with aging that can lead to the urinary tract not working well. For instance, the ability to hold one's urine depends, for one thing, on the ability to think clearly enough to contract those muscles, which is one reason that people with alcohol intoxication, or dementia, cannot hold their urine. Other factors that may lessen your ability to control urination include a history of vaginal deliveries or a history of pelvic or abdominal surgery, which may have damaged or left scar tissue in the pelvic floor muscles and surrounding tissue, which then prevents the urine from exiting out of the body.

The sensation that the bladder is full, the ability to put off voiding, and the ability of the muscles to contract all decline with age. Moreover, as we age, the muscle surrounding the bladder often doesn't work as well and may contract randomly (Resnick and Yalla 2007). In most circumstances, however, none of these age-related changes *alone* causes severe problems without another problem of the urinary tract being present. That is, just because you keep having birthdays doesn't mean you will become incontinent.

URINARY INCONTINENCE (UI)

Urinary incontinence is a symptom, not a disease. It is defined as the complaint of any involuntary loss of urine. It can be temporary, occurring only once or several times, such as in the presence of a urinary tract infection; or it can be chronic or long lasting, such as when the urinary tract muscles are damaged.

How Common Is It?

Approximately 50 percent of the adults of both genders in the U.S. report having experienced UI, the overwhelming majority being women (Nygaard, Thom, and Calho 2004). Urinary incontinence increases with age. UI is more common than most research shows because many patients will not admit to having experienced it, even when asked by their clinician.

Types of Urinary Incontinence

As mentioned, urinary incontinence may be temporary or chronic.

TEMPORARY URINARY INCONTINENCE

Some of the causes of *temporary incontinence*, or the loss of control of urine just once or over a limited period of time, include urinary tract infections, excess fluid intake, constipation with the resultant straining during bowel movements, restricted mobility, and severe depression. Certain medications also may cause this symptom, such as some of the drugs used for high blood pressure (diuretics like hydrochlorothiazide), those used for nasal congestion (like pseudoephedrine), sleeping medications, antidepressants, and, in some people, caffeine. In almost all cases of temporary UI, once the problem that causes it goes away, the UI itself resolves. For instance, if you have leakage of urine while you've had an infection, once you've taken antibiotics and the infection goes away, so should the incontinence.

Dr. R's Scare (as Told by Dr. J)

At much too early an age, Robin had a scare that she had developed urinary incontinence. This was when we were in training together, both in our thirties, and before Robin was married. She had a date with someone new, and when he came to pick her up one chilly night, she was impressed to see that he had a great new car—a Saab—which was "the" car to drive back then. When they pulled into the restaurant parking lot, to Robin's horror, she felt an unfamiliar sensation of warmth creeping from the back of her knees up the back of her thighs and to her rear end. She was frantically thinking up an excuse to explain why she needed to go back home to change clothes, when her date said, as he opened her door, "How do you like the new heated seats?"

CHRONIC URINARY INCONTINENCE

There are three main types of chronic urinary incontinence based on the symptoms of each. These include *stress, urge, and mixed urinary incontinence*. Stress incontinence is the main type in younger and middle-aged women, while urge and mixed incontinence are more common in older women. Why is it important to have at least heard of these types? Because they have different causes and thus are treated differently. It's also important to know that any urinary incontinence, no matter the symptoms or cause, is considered abnormal and must be discussed with your clinician. Most cases can be improved or corrected with treatment, which doesn't always include surgery.

Stress urinary incontinence. The main symptom of stress urinary incontinence is that of leakage of urine *only during* any activity that applies pressure to a full bladder, that is, *stresses* the bladder. Such activities include coughing, sneezing, laughing, and high impact exercises, to name a few. The leaking stops when the activity stops. Stress incontinence is due to damage to the muscles, nerves, and/or connective tissue within the pelvic floor muscles (which support the bladder), the bladder neck, and the urethra. Because of the damage to these structures, neither the urethra nor the bladder neck can close completely. Therefore, any pressure at all on the bladder neck or the urethra, such as occurs with coughing or laughing, causes urine to leak out.

Urge urinary incontinence. The primary symptom of urge incontinence is *involuntary* leakage of urine accompanied by, or immediately following, the urge to urinate. With this type of UI, you cannot stop the urge to void, even temporarily; thus, you may be surprised to find that you've already urinated. This is also called irritable bladder or overactive bladder, and can cause symptoms such as frequent urination day or night, without any leakage of urine. It may occur anytime; many women get it only at night, and it is not associated with any particular activity. This type of UI is due to random and/or frequent contractions of the detrusor muscle surrounding the bladder.

Mixed urinary incontinence. This type has symptoms of both stress and urge UI, and other symptoms not classified under either of these categories. The other, less common symptoms can include continuous leakage of urine, leakage only at night, and *unconscious UI*, in which there is leakage not accompanied by the urge to urinate or by some activity. Mixed urinary incontinence has the risk factors associated with both of the types described above.

Are You at Risk?

It is well-known that the aging process can cause a general weakening of the muscles involved in voiding, though not everyone develops incontinence at the same rate, if at all. Although it used to be thought that stress urinary incontinence was a natural consequence of going through menopause, caused by a lack of estrogen, this is no longer believed to be true. Other risk factors include prior pelvic surgery; vaginal deliveries; obesity or a large weight gain; chronic constipation; chronic respiratory problems (including smoking cigarettes) with frequent coughing; exercise; heavy lifting; medications (especially some sleeping agents); anxiety and depression; diseases such as diabetes; genetic factors; and damage to the central nervous system such as occurs with multiple sclerosis, Parkinson's disease, spinal cord injuries, and stroke. Having any one of these risk factors alone doesn't mean that you will definitely develop incontinence. However, having a combination of several of them makes it more likely.

How Do You Know if You Have It? What Can You Do About It?

If you leak urine at all, it is important to notice when, how often, and with what activities it occurs. For instance, you may have been jogging for years with no problem and then noticed UI only after a recent surgery. You do not have to figure out the type of incontinence that you have—that's your clinician's job—but it helps tremendously if you are able to give specifics. UI is not an emergency unless accompanied by another more serious condition; unless you have severe pain or bleeding along with urine leakage, you don't need to seek emergency care. UI alone is not medically serious, although it can certainly disrupt your life. Make an appointment to see your clinician about this symptom.

How Is It Diagnosed?

After your clinician has asked you the specific questions noted above, she will examine your abdomen do a pelvic exam, and obtain urine and blood samples. Diabetes, for example, which can cause you to drink and urinate more often and at night, can be diagnosed from blood tests and a urinalysis. She may want to measure what is called the "post-void residual urine volume," or the amount of urine left in your bladder after you've finished urinating. You may need to have imaging studies, such as an intravenous pyelogram, or IVP (an x-ray, with dye, of the entire urinary tract, which can show abnormalities), CT, or MRI scan. Or your doctor may want you to have urodynamic testing, which shows how you urinate. You may also need a cystoscopy, in which the doctor looks into your bladder with a lighted tube inserted into your urethra. This procedure is done in an operating room and you must be given anesthesia.

How Is It Prevented or Treated?

For temporary UI, correcting the problem that led to it will get rid of the problem of leaking urine. You may be thinking that the only way to get rid of chronic incontinence is surgery. Not so. Most women with overactive bladder/urge incontinence can benefit from a combination of medication and bladder training techniques. And while it is true that surgery is the one most effective treatment for stress incontinence, approximately 40 to 50 percent of women with this disorder can avoid surgery and still be satisfied with the outcome of more conservative therapies (Payne 2007). The important thing to understand here is that trying noninvasive methods first is always a must. After learning the options from your doctor, you have a large say in what type of therapy you want; you can still have surgery later if other therapies do not work.

COMPLEMENTARY AND ALTERNATIVE APPROACH

Acupuncture has been successful for urinary incontinence (see chapter 14).

BEHAVIORAL THERAPY

Behavioral therapy refers to a group of treatments based on the concept that a person with UI can be educated about her condition and taught strategies to get rid of, or lessen, the UI. These also include lifestyle changes.

Bladder training. Do your eyes deceive you? Just when you thought you were finished with this kind of training—"potty" for your kids and "house" for your pup—you have to go through this training yourself. At least you know it works! This training is most helpful if you have overactive bladder/ urge incontinence. You are given a fixed time schedule to void, the idea being that if you void often enough, you will urinate *before* you experience either leaking or the urge to void. The goal is for you to learn that you can wait two to three hours to void without leaking urine. This retraining of the bladder has been shown to work in 85 percent of patients initially and to still be effective in 48 percent of patients three years later (Holmes, Stone, and Barry 1983). Sometimes bladder training works best when, at the same time, you take a medication that relieves the detrusor muscle spasms, such as Ditropan (oxybutynin) or Detrol (tolterodine). Most experts tell you to first decrease and then stop that medication several months after the bladder training has been shown to be working. Bladder training may be tried in stress incontinence to lessen the actual amount of urine leaked when the stress activities occur.

Kegel exercises (pelvic floor muscle training). You've probably heard of Kegel exercises. They are the forceful contraction of the pelvic muscles originally recommended to treat and prevent UI after pregnancy. The idea behind these exercises is the same as with exercising any muscle: That multiple repetitions of a specific exercise will improve the muscle's function. However, in recent years it has been found that half of patients cannot perform Kegel exercises properly with only simple instructions, and up to one-fourth can actually *cause* incontinence by doing them wrong (Bump et al. 1991). Because of this, it is now thought that the exercises should be taught by a health professional and monitored over time; this is now known as *pelvic floor muscle training*, and it includes Kegel exercises. These exercises do work. In fact, the authors of a recent review of ninety-six randomized, controlled trials of nonsurgical treatments for UI in women, published in English from 1990 through May 2007, reached the conclusion that pelvic floor muscle training resolves nearly 50 percent of UI cases (Shamliyan et al. 2008). We recommend that you ask your doctor to have you trained properly.

Vaginal cones. These are small weights used to improve pelvic muscle control.

Biofeedback. This is a device designed for home use in which a probe, placed in your vagina or rectum, relays information about the strength of your pelvic floor muscle contractions to a monitoring device, allowing you to learn to control that muscle better.

Lifestyle changes. These include correcting or preventing constipation, cessation of cigarette smoking (to decrease or stop associated coughing), loss of weight, maintenance of a normal intake of fluids (see chapter 11), and restriction of carbonated beverages. As for the last recommendation, there is a definite link between these beverages and both types of incontinence, but not between caffeine per se and UI. Therefore, unless coffee or tea causes or increases your symptoms, there's no need to avoid either one (Payne 2007).

Bottom line: A recent opinion paper by the NIH states that pelvic floor muscle training, biofeedback, and the lifestyle changes of weight loss and exercise are effective in preventing, and may reverse, UI (Landefeld et al. 2008). We believe that these behavioral methods should be tried first, before devices, medications, or surgery.

DEVICES TO DECREASE OR STOP URINE LEAKAGE

The mechanical devices available for dealing with urine leakage include vaginal pessaries as discussed in chapter 6 (a tampon placed inside the vagina before exercise works the same way and will keep you dry); urethral occlusive devices applied directly to the opening of the urethra to create a dam effect (CapSure, FemAssist); urethral plugs (FemSoft stint) which must be removed to urinate and then reinserted; and, when all else fails, adhesive pads. (How to use the pads? It *Depends...* With *Serenity?* Sorry—couldn't resist!)

MEDICATIONS

There are several types of medication used in the treatment of UI.

Medications for urge incontinence. These medications include Ditropan XL (oxybutynin) and Detrol LA (tolterodine) orally, and a newer skin patch, Ocytrol (oxybutynin). They work by delaying the initial urge to void and inhibiting the spasms of the muscle surrounding the bladder, which increases the capacity of the bladder. They provide relief for most women, particularly when the long-acting or extended release forms are used. Because there are so many side effects, and since some of the behavioral methods, such as pelvic floor muscle training, work so well with urge incontinence/ overactive bladder, it is wise not to start with these drugs until other methods have failed.

Medications specifically for stress incontinence. This group of drugs strengthens the smooth muscle that opens and closes the internal sphincter muscle surrounding the bladder neck. This group includes ephedrine and pseudoephedrine (commonly in over-the-counter decongestants and appetite suppressants). A recent review of these drugs, however, came to the conclusion that they are not very effective (Shamliyan et al. 2008).

Sally's Story

Sally, a sixty-three-year-old patient of Dr. J's, loved traveling with her family—four kids, two dogs, and her very patient partner who always drove. Since the kids were tiny, she'd load them up into the huge SUV with a huge plastic bag of food goodies—cheese, apples, carrot sticks, doggie treats—and off they'd go. These trips continued uneventfully until she reached her fifties, and out of the blue she found she was disrupting their trips by having to make a bathroom stop at least every thirty minutes. Even then, she often wet herself before she got to the gas station toilet. Then she hit upon the idea of using those foodie plastic bags for another purpose: She peed in them! That way, she could pee (discreetly of course) when she had to, and make fewer bathroom stops. It worked! That is, until one day a dog smelled something familiar, and while she was grabbing her plastic bag filled with yellow fluid, the dog accidentally punctured it with his canine tooth. After that, Sally knew she had no choice but to admit she had a problem and pay a visit to the specialist Dr. J recommended. After a brief workup confirmed that she had an overactive bladder with urge incontinence, she successfully trained her bladder while also taking Detrol LA. Now, as she is slowly coming off her medication, she is happily back to taking her trips again.

NEUROSTIMULATION

In some people with overactive bladder/urge incontinence, stimulation of the sacral nerve, the nerve near the tailbone that influences the muscles that control the bladder, may relieve those symptoms. Available as InterStim, it is recommended only for those with overactive bladder who have not responded to behavioral or drug therapy.

INJECTION THERAPY

This type of treatment involves the injection of a substance/medication directly into the bladder or bladder muscles to help them relax. These include botulinum toxin (Botox), capsaicin, and bulking agents (GAX collagen). The first two are the most commonly used to treat overactive bladder resistant to other forms of therapy. Botulinum toxin (yes, the very same used for facial creases) has been shown to be effective in relaxing an overactive detrusor muscle surrounding the bladder (Payne 2007).

SURGERY

There are many surgical procedures for UI, and as with the other types of therapy, the procedure chosen depends on the type of UI the patient has. Generally, surgery is not recommended for women with urge incontinence, and if it is, it is usually directed at the sacral nerves, located in the tailbone, which control the bladder. The only group of women for whom surgery is considered as early therapy are those with severe stress incontinence. For women with milder stress incontinence, surgery is effective and relatively safe but only reccommended when the more conservative therapies have failed.

THE DOCS DISCUSS
THE URINARY TRACT

DR. R: What about that very common symptom of burning when urinating? Are urinary tract infections (UTIs) still common as we get older?

DR. J: Absolutely. But the issue at our age now is that urinary burning does not always mean that there's a UTI present. There are other possibilities caused by the effects of menopause and by the lack of estrogen in the vulva and urethra. Because the tissues there are so thin and dry after menopause (if not being treated with estrogen topically), they can become easily irritated and raw from day-to-day activities or even from allergic reactions to bath products. This can cause a burning sensation when urine flows over the area.

DR. R: So we shouldn't jump to the conclusion that we have a UTI every time there's burning, right?

DR. J: That's right. And do *not* take that leftover antibiotic in the medicine cabinet without making sure there is a UTI. Other things that can cause the same symptom are a vaginal infection (not necessarily sexually transmitted) that causes the area to be raw, and sexually transmitted infections (STIs) like genital herpes. If you get urinary burning, call your primary care clinician; she may want you to drop off a urine sample at the lab, and if it's negative for infection, to come in for a pelvic exam. But whatever you do, don't treat yourself! You could make it worse.

DR. R: What do we need to know about our kidneys at this age?

DR. J: The major causes of kidney disease and failure include some of the same factors that lead to heart disease and strokes: uncontrolled high blood pressure and diabetes. There are kidney diseases that are inherited as well. If we concentrate on taking care of our high blood pressure and diabetes, know our family history, continue with a healthy lifestyle, especially drinking an adequate amount of fluids daily, and adhere to our health maintenance schedule, we will be taking care of our kidneys as well.

PEARLS OF WISDOM
FOR THE URINARY TRACT

○ Leaking urine at any time is abnormal and should be evaluated for a cause.

○ Urinary incontinence does not automatically occur with aging.

○ Most cases of urinary incontinence can be resolved or improved.

○ Be sure to notice when your urine leaks—is it only with coughing or exercise?

○ Be sure to notice if your body or your lifestyle changed before the UI occurred. Did you gain weight? Increase your fluid intake? Start drinking carbonated beverages?

○ Do not restrict your daily fluids just because you have UI.

○ When you have burning on urination, notice whether there are other symptoms. Do *not* take a leftover antibiotic pill without talking to your clinician!

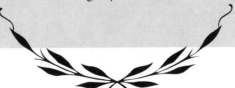

CHAPTER 8

Muscles, Joints, and Bones: How to Keep Moving and Grooving

Our bodies are made up of a framework of 206 bones that fit together in very intricate ways. These bones are arranged and held together with muscles that allow us to move, run, twist, dance, and perform an infinite number of tasks. Joints are where different bones meet: They can act as hinges (as in the knees and elbows), pivots (as in the head on the neck), and ball and sockets (hips and shoulders). The whole package is our vehicle and protector (thank goodness for that hard skull that protects our brain, and the rib cage that protects our heart and lungs) and provides us with our own unique identity, our shape. How beautiful and well organized our structural foundation is!

Like any machine, the body takes constant abuse as we age. Those who have taken care of their bodies seem to weather aging more gracefully than those who've ignored them. From the age of thirty onward, a woman's muscles begin to decline. A healthy woman in her seventies (who is not a bodybuilder) has lost about 20 percent of the muscle mass that she had at the age of thirty. When the body mass of menopausal women was studied, researchers found that the bones were the first to go, followed by shifting of body fat (more jiggle around the middle), and then muscles diminish, in that order (Morita et al. 2006).

This chapter covers common problems affecting the bones, muscles, and joints. We discuss fibromyalgia and sports injuries as well.

BONES

Bones appear to be solid, but they are made up of a matrix, or crisscrossing, of a protein called collagen, as well as calcium, phosphorous, sodium, and other minerals. This structure allows both strength and flexibility. Inside most bones is the *marrow*. This is where stem cells produce the red blood cells that carry oxygen, the white blood cells that help fight infection, and the platelets that help blood to clot.

Bones don't just stand there looking strong. They are constantly being torn down and built up again. When we are young and growing, the building up far exceeds the tearing down. Peak bone mass is reached about the time we turn thirty, and then more bone is lost than is replaced. This process increases, and can accelerate after menopause. If it continues unchecked, *osteopenia*, or mild bone loss, can develop, followed by *osteoporosis*, or excessive bone loss.

OSTEOPOROSIS

The loss of bone mass or density is known as osteoporosis. According to the National Institute of Arthritis and Musculoskeletal and Skin Diseases, 10 million people in the U.S. are estimated to have osteoporosis, and 34 million have a low bone mass, or osteopenia, putting them at risk for developing osteoporosis (2007). Here's what happens: Osteoporosis causes bones to become more porous, thus causing them to weaken and break. The bones most commonly injured are the vertebrae (or spine), the ribs, the wrists, and the hips. Spinal fractures cause loss of height and what is known as a dowager's hump, both of which can be very painful.

Hip fractures are no joke. In 2001, about 315,000 Americans over the age of forty-five were admitted to a hospital for osteoporosis-related hip fractures. Twenty-four percent of hip fracture patients over the age of fifty die of complications in the year following their fracture (National Osteoporosis Foundation 2007).

One out of every two women will experience a fracture in her lifetime due to this silent disease. That's the bad news. The good news is that with strength training exercise, the appropriate nutrients, and medication as needed, these changes can be prevented and even reversed.

Are You at Risk for Osteoporosis?

There are certain factors that can increase the chances of your developing osteoporosis, although not all women develop it, even with age. As with heart disease, some factors can't be changed, but others can. The risk factors you *cannot* change are listed below:

Gender. Women are at higher risk, especially after menopause. Women who are small with thin bones are at greater risk.

Race. Caucasian and Asian women are at a greater risk than Hispanic and African-American women.

Heredity. Osteoporosis tends to run in families.

Those risk factors you *can* change include the following:

Hormones. Early menopause and lack of hormones after menopause are associated with osteoporosis.

Anorexia. This eating disorder increases the chances of osteoporosis due to deprivation of nutrients.

Alcohol. Excessive consumption can increase bone loss.

Cigarette smoking. Cigarettes increase bone loss.

Sedentary lifestyle. Activity helps to build bones; walking (literally, pounding those bones against the pavement) and strength training are both necessary. If you aren't moving or bearing weight, then your bones won't be building. For instance, swimming is great exercise, but because your bones aren't bearing your weight while you're doing it, it is not helpful in preventing bone loss. Because they are weightless when they go into space, bone loss is a big issue for astronauts. NASA has found that astronauts on the space station lose almost 1 percent of their bone mass per month (Lang et al. 2004).

Mood. Depression has been found to increase the chances of developing osteoporosis (Eskandari et al. 2007).

Medications. Steroids, heparin, Coumadin (warfarin), medication for seizures such as Dilantin (phenytoin), and too much thyroid hormone can cause bone loss. The use of proton pump inhibitors, such as Prilosec (omeprazole) and Nexium (esomeprazole), has been associated with bone loss (Yang et al. 2006). If you are on any one of these medications, it is important to take adequate supplements of calcium and vitamin D, and your doctor will need to follow your bone density.

Calcium and vitamin D. We need these for healthy bones; most of us don't get enough of either of them. Recommended dosages are discussed later in this chapter.

How Do You Know if You Have Osteoporosis? How Is It Diagnosed?

People with osteoporosis generally have no symptoms until they fracture a bone. The best way to know if you have osteopenia or osteoporosis is to find out *before* a fracture occurs. If you are menopausal, or if you are younger but have a family history of osteoporosis or have fractured one or more bones, ask your clinician to order a baseline bone density scan. Also known as a DEXA scan, this is done using a dual-energy absorptiometry test; it is somewhat like a regular x-ray, although it uses a very low amount of radiation. It is quick, painless, and you don't even have to take your clothes off! Most doctors recommend that you have a baseline study at menopause and, depending on the results or your risks, that you repeat it periodically depending on your age, your activity level, your medications, and any changes in your health status.

How Is Osteoporosis Treated and Prevented?

Because bone loss is a gradual process that can be slowed and even reversed by lifestyle changes and diet, we will discuss treatment and prevention at the same time. The following recommendations can apply to either. Even if you are currently on medication for osteoporosis, it is important to make dietary and lifestyle changes as well.

DIET, CALCIUM, VITAMIN D, AND OTHER NUTRIENTS

Almost all the nutrients you need to keep your bones strong you can get in your diet. They are as follows.

Calcium. When the effect of dietary calcium versus supplemental calcium was studied, getting calcium through food was found to be better for bone density than calcium pill supplements (Napoli et al. 2007). Great sources of calcium include low-fat milk, yogurt, cheese, and dark green vegetables such as broccoli, chard, and spinach. Canned sardines and salmon that include the ground-up bones, tofu, and almonds are also good sources. You also can find food fortified with calcium, such as orange juice, cereals, and breads. If you don't get enough calcium in your food (although this is preferable), you may need to take a supplement. The recommended amount of calcium for women over fifty is between 1,200 and 1,500 mg per day. There is still debate on whether we actually need this much calcium (Feskanich et al. 1997). **Caution:** The ingestion of too much calcium (2,000 mg or more per day) can result in kidney stones. Calcium citrate is the form that is easiest to absorb. Since this form doesn't require stomach acid to work, it is a good choice for women taking medications, such as

Prilosec, that reduce the acid in the stomach. Calcium carbonate usually contains more calcium per pill, so you may need to take fewer pills in this form, but it does need acid to be absorbed.

We recommend staying away from the "natural" calcium products like those made from bone-meal and oyster shells. Many of these products have been found to contain heavy metals, including lead. Also, don't forget that calcium can lead to constipation, so if that is already an issue for you, then talk to your clinician about what you can do before you start taking calcium supplements. Also, avoid high-protein diets since they leach calcium from your bones.

Vitamin D. This vitamin is very important for bone strength and health. It must be present in your body for calcium to be absorbed from the gut. Vitamin D does many other very important things, discussed in chapter 13. How do we get it? It is absorbed through the skin from sunlight, then converted to its active form by the body. Unfortunately, as we age, our bodies don't do a great job of converting vitamin D to its active form. In addition, sunscreen blocks our skin from absorbing it. (This doesn't mean you should stop wearing sunscreen!)

Many people get vitamin D in a calcium supplement or from fortified foods such as orange juice and milk. It is also found in eggs and oily fish. However, that still may not be enough. Some researchers are now recommending that women have a total of at least 1,000 IU a day. Dr. R has noticed in her practice that nine out of ten patients she sees are deficient in vitamin D. Therefore, we recommend you have your vitamin D level checked with a simple blood test so your doctor can determine the appropriate dose for you. **Caution:** Too much vitamin D is toxic, and for that reason it is important to have blood levels checked periodically when you are ingesting high doses of supplements.

Vitamin K. This vitamin is found in dark green leafy vegetables such as kale, lettuce, broccoli, and Brussels sprouts. Low intake of vitamin K has been correlated to low bone density in women (Weber 2001). The key is to eat one or more green leafy vegetables a day. However, if you are taking Coumadin (warfarin) to keep your blood from clotting, vitamin K may reverse the effects. Therefore, talk to your doctor before you alter your diet.

Dr. R and Dr. J's Story (Told by Dr. R)

After checking our patients' vitamin D levels, Janet and I finally decided to check our own. (We both avoid the sun like the plague.) We weren't taking any extra supplements, and we were both shocked when we saw our levels. We had the lowest levels of all the people we had tested. Our results were marked as "severe deficiency"! Once both of us started taking vitamin D, we noticed that we had more energy and muscle strength. Neither of us would have believed this if we hadn't experienced it for ourselves.

Genistein. This supplement made from soy was recently studied in almost 400 women with low bone density. After twenty-four months, the bone density of those taking the supplement had increased significantly compared to the women taking a placebo (Marini et al. 2007). This may be a reasonable alternative to conventional medication, provided there is no history of breast cancer since soy products are not recommended for those with that history. (See chapter 12.)

LIFESTYLE CHANGES

Lifestyle changes are every bit as important as supplements and medication in preventing and treating osteoporosis.

Exercise. Weight-bearing exercise, like walking, promotes bone building and is important for the bones of the lower body. For the upper body, strength or resistance training is important. Pumping iron can help. If you don't want to lift weights, you can get very good upper body strength training from yoga or Pilates.

Cigarette smoking. If you smoke, you need to quit. See chapter 15 for help.

Alcohol. As little as two to three ounces a day of alcohol can hurt the bones. If you drink, it's important to do it in moderation.

Caffeine and soda. These products can promote calcium loss in the urine. If you like caffeine in your coffee or tea, then drink it with a milk product. If you like soda pop (now we're showing our age!), make sure you also get adequate calcium and vitamin D.

MEDICATIONS

If the preventive measures listed above haven't been effective in slowing bone loss, or if you have already been diagnosed with osteopenia or osteoporosis by a bone density scan, your doctor will want to reverse or at least slow down that process with a medication. This is especially true if you are on a drug, such as prednisone, that is known to cause bone loss. It is actually possible to improve your bone density with these medications, and to avoid, or reverse, osteoporosis to some extent.

The group of drugs known as the *bisphosphonates* includes Fosamax (alendronate), Actonel (risedronate), and Boniva (ibandronate). These medications can be taken as a pill, either daily (Fosamax, Actonel), or weekly (Actonel, Fosamax), or monthly (Boniva, Actonel). Boniva is also available as an intravenous injection given every three months, and Reclast (zoledronate), a newer bisphosphonate, is given intravenously once a year. A rare complication that has been reported with the use of high-dose intravenous bisphosphonates in cancer patients is called osteonecrosis of the jaw, or death of the jawbone. This risk appears to be very small for those taking oral bisphosphonates. For those being treated with intravenous bisphosphonates, the consequences of a fracture due to osteoporosis are likely to cause more significant pain and disability than the jaw problem (Grbic et al. 2008). Since most dentists know what to look for, you can be monitored for the early appearance of this condition and treated. If you're considering the use of intravenous bisphosphonates, see your dentist for an evaluation before you start it. Also, talk to your clinician about the proper way to take bisphosphonate pills, and the possible side effects.

Another type of medication that helps to build bones is the group known as the selective estrogen receptor modulators (SERMs). Evista (raloxifene), a member of this group, is often used for prevention of osteoporosis in women unable to tolerate the bisphosphonates.

There are four hormones available for use in women with bone loss who cannot tolerate the bisphosphonates: calcitonin, parathyroid hormone, estrogen, and progesterone. Calcitonin is available as a nasal spray and is used only in women who are at least five years past menopause. Parathyroid hormone is available in an injectable form known as teriparatide (Forteo), which must be given daily. It is used also for women with bone loss who are at high risk for developing a fracture, or those who have not responded to bisphosphonates.

Estrogen and progesterone when taken together by menopausal women are known as hormone replacement therapy (HRT). They have been found to reduce bone loss, increase bone density, and prevent fractures. You've probably heard that the Women's Health Initiative study found an increased risk of breast cancer, stroke, and heart attack in women who were taking HRT. We discuss this study, the benefits and risks of HRT, and whether HRT should be taken only for bone health in chapter 10.

Margaret's Story

Margaret is a fifty-five-year-old, tiny Asian-American bundle of energy who had her initial bone density scan right after her first visit with Dr. J, at the time of her menopause at age fifty-one. It showed severe osteopenia. She wondered how this was possible since she is "always running around," although she does no exercise, eats a "healthy" diet, except for never drinking milk, has never smoked, and prides herself on taking no vitamins (since she "eats so well"); she never took hormone replacement. When Dr. J specifically asked her about bone loss in her family, she recalled that her mother had lost an inch in height in recent years and that her grandmother has a dowager's hump. Not one to accept her diagnosis as her fate, she applied her usual energy and focus to a one hour a day walking program, three thirty-minute weight lifting sessions a week, calcium and vitamin D supplementation, and one of the bisphophonate pills. After two years of never straying from this regimen, her bone density scan had improved, and after four years, her scan was almost back to normal. She continues to keep up her bone-building regimen and now takes her mother, grandmother, and two daughters walking with her!

JOINTS

In order for our muscles and bones to work, the joints, or connectors of muscles to bones, need to be healthy as well. The slippery coating on the joints that serves as the actual connecting tissue is the *cartilage*. When joints are abused, injuries occurring from wear and tear can lead to *osteoarthritis* (inflammation of the joint). It makes sense that overuse is not the only cause of arthritis; wear and tear occurs naturally with aging. Another form, *rheumatoid arthritis*, is an autoimmune disease that causes inflammation in the entire body, resulting in the body attacking its own joints. It is far less common than osteoarthritis.

Osteoarthritis

Osteoarthritis (OA) is the most common threat to healthy joints. Before age fifty, it is most common in men. After age fifty, women take the lead (Lawrence et al. 1998). When it comes to work and disability, it has a greater impact on women as well (Theis, Helmick, and Hootman 2007). This disease commonly leads to joint surgery, for both repair and replacement.

WHAT CAUSES OSTEOARTHRITIS?

Osteoarthritis starts with the breakdown of cartilage. Normally, the slippery cartilage allows for easy motion; it also acts as a shock absorber. Over time, with wear and tear, or after injury, the cartilage breaks down and wears away. When this happens, the two bones, normally connected by the cartilage in that joint, start to rub together. This causes inflammation, leading to swelling and pain. Eventually, bone spurs may grow around the edges of the joint, and pieces of bone and cartilage fall into the joint space, causing further pain, inflammation, and occasionally fluid accumulation, which shows up as swelling of the joint. The joints most commonly affected are the hands, feet, hips, knees, low back, and neck.

ARE YOU AT RISK FOR OSTEOARTHRITIS?

Osteoarthritis for the most part is a disease of aging, and it tends to run in families. If it affects a young person, it is usually as the result of a joint injury. Other factors that can initiate and accelerate it include being overweight, having deformed joints or joints that haven't healed properly, having a genetic defect in the cartilage, or getting "overuse" injuries related to jobs that require repetitive actions or sports (professional athletes, marathon runners).

HOW DO YOU KNOW IF YOU HAVE OSTEOARTHRITIS?

If you have OA, you *will* eventually feel it. You may first notice that some of your joints are stiff, and that the stiffness tends to get worse as the day goes on. Or you might notice a swelling in a joint or pain when you press on it. You also might hear or feel a crunching. Many people with osteoarthritis of the hands will develop nontender nodules at the middle joints and/or at the joints nearest the ends of their fingers. Some people will develop bunions on their toes, although there are other causes of bunions. All of these symptoms either recur or are permanent. This is different from the temporary joint pains you may get after working too hard in the garden, which eventually will go away.

WHEN SHOULD YOU MAKE AN APPOINTMENT TO SEE YOUR CLINICIAN?

If joint pain and swelling occur overnight, especially if accompanied by a fever, call your doctor immediately. This set of symptoms usually indicates an infection of the joint and must be treated quickly. Otherwise, make an appointment within a month or so. The development of OA is not an emergency, even though the pain it causes may make you feel that it is. In and of itself, OA is not dangerous except in advanced stages when the broken-down cartilage leads to instability of the joint, and then, to a fall.

HOW IS OSTEOARTHRITIS DIAGNOSED?

There are several ways to diagnose OA. On physical examination, your clinician may notice swelling or tenderness of a joint, nodules on the fingers, or bunions on the feet. Or when she moves your knees or hips to different positions, she may notice that you cannot flex or extend them the full amount. X-rays will show the characteristic bone spurs and loss of joint space due to your loss of cartilage. If the signs on exam, or the x-rays described above, are not helpful in diagnosing your joint symptoms, your clinician may want to order further studies.

CAN OSTEOARTHRITIS BE PREVENTED?

There are several steps you can take to prevent OA. They are discussed below.

Weight loss. Maintain a healthy weight. For some women, losing just eleven pounds can cut their risk of developing osteoarthritis of the knee by 50 percent (Felson et al. 1992).

Exercise. A recent study found that midlife women who exercised for twenty minutes at least once in the last fourteen days had a higher volume of cartilage in the knee joint than those who did no exercise at all (Hanna et al. 2007). They also found that the exercise did no harm to the joint. Because preventing cartilage loss can prevent OA, the finding that exercise may protect against developing OA is of great interest and needs further study. Other benefits of exercise include maintaining the flexibility of the joints and the strength of the muscles surrounding the joints, both of which help mobility. Also, stretching exercises are important for all the joints, but especially for the hands and feet.

Avoid excess stress on your joints. Unfortunately, when we were younger we thought we were invincible, and many of us stressed our joints as well as our parents. For those of us who have OA, it's not too late to talk about stopping its progression. This means that it is important to be fit and to find exercises that do not stress the joints. Perhaps you could cut back on your jogging and try swimming instead? Mixing up your types of exercise and avoiding overuse of any one set of joints is important. (See Robin's story in the text box.)

CAN OSTEOARTHRITIS BE TREATED?

There are a variety of treatments available for the symptoms of OA.

Diet and lifestyle changes. Exercise and weight control are essential. *The best way to take pressure off of the joints, particularly the hips, knees, and feet, is to maintain a healthy weight.* Think about this: For every one pound lost there is a four-pound reduction in the load placed on the knee for each step taken (Messier et al. 2005). We recommend that weight control be achieved by eating a diet rich in fruits, vegetables, and healthy oils, known as an anti-inflammatory diet, which also can help to decrease overall inflammation in the body (see chapter 11).

Exercise is helpful both for losing weight and for treating osteoarthritis. Be aware of which activities cause pain, and then back off if pain occurs. We recommend consulting a qualified trainer or physical therapist to find out what will work best for you, and to be taught stretching and warm-up exercises to do with your regular activities.

Dr. R's Story

I remember John F. Kennedy's call to physical fitness when I was in grade school. I took it very seriously. I'm one of the chronic baby boomer exercisers. I used to run but had to give it up because my knees started to hurt. Now I walk. I did gymnastics for a while, but I hurt my neck, so I had to give that up too. Now, I work out using weights with a trainer (whom I fondly refer to as the "Torture Princess"), and I am very careful about how I do things so that I don't put further stress on my joints. PS, I also stopped stressing my parents!

Medications. For many people, mild pain relievers are all they need. Acetaminophen (Tylenol) is quite effective for pain control when the recommended dosage is taken. It has the advantage of not causing bleeding as aspirin and drugs like Advil (ibuprofen) do. Aspirin works both as an anti-inflammatory and a pain medication, but can cause bleeding and irritation in the gut. Over-the-counter non-steroidal anti-inflammatory (NSAID) medications, such as ibuprofen, Advil, or Motrin can reduce pain and inflammation, but also can cause bleeding in the gut. COX-2 inhibitors, a type of NSAID (such as Celebrex, or celocoxib), can reduce inflammation and are less irritating to the gut. However, this class of medication has been linked to an increased risk of stroke and heart attack. Cortisone injections into the joint are often used to help reduce joint inflammation. Hyaluronic acid (Synvisc) is injected into the joint and can restore the cushioning of the joint fluid for up to six months. It requires a series of three shots given weekly over a fifteen-day period. It does not work for everyone.

Which medication we recommend for symptoms depends on the individual woman and her medical condition and history. We often recommend that women on chronic anti-inflammatory medication protect their stomachs with a proton pump inhibitor medication (Prilosec, or omeprazole) as well. We usually reserve Synvisc and steroid joint injections for those with severe arthritis. Unfortunately, the medications discussed above treat only the symptoms of osteoarthritis, not the disease. Currently, there is no permanent cure for OA other than replacing the diseased joint. However, remember that you may be able to slow the progression of OA by taking good care of your joints through lifestyle changes.

Herbs and Supplements. These can be effective for some women. See chapter 13 for more information. Fish oil has anti-inflammatory properties and may help with pain. Recent studies have found that for patients with moderate to severe OA of the knee, 1,500 mg of glucosamine and 1,200 mg of chondroitin a day can help with pain relief and decrease inflammation (Clegg et al. 2006). Many people find relief with these supplements. **Caution:** Since glucosamine can thin the blood, discuss this supplement with your clinician if you are taking Coumadin (warfarin) or another blood thinner. Since glucosamine is derived from shellfish, talk to your clinician before taking it if you have an allergy to shellfish or iodine.

Herbs and spices such as holy basil, turmeric, ginger, and green tea can have an anti-inflammatory effect similar to the COX-2 inhibitors. (Dr. R recommends a supplement called Zyflamend, which contains these spices, to her patients with OA.) MSM (methylsulfonylmethane) has been touted as a good treatment for arthritis, although no good studies exist supporting these claims. SAMe, or S-adenosylmethionine, occurs naturally in the body and helps with immune support and the breakdown of serotonin; it also helps in the formation of cartilage. It may work just as well for some people as the anti-inflammatory medications.

Physical therapy. Special physical medicine doctors, called *physiatrists*, are available for consultation for musculoskeletal problems. They have extensive training in how to improve and restore joint and muscle function, and often prescribe physical therapy in addition to medications. Equally as effective for low back pain as for recovery from just about any injury, physical therapy can help strengthen the muscles surrounding arthritic joints. Physical therapists help by using treatments such as heat, electrical stimulation, and ultrasound, and low-tech methods like stretching and strengthening exercises. Although many insurance companies will not pay for massage, acupuncture, or chiropractic, almost all will pay for physical therapy prescribed by your clinician.

Surgery. When a joint is totally worn out and treatment with medications and joint injections have failed to control the pain and disability of OA, it may be necessary to have the diseased joint replaced with a prosthetic joint. According to the American Academy of Orthopaedic Surgeons, in 2004 there were 233,000 hips and 455,000 knees replaced in the U.S. (Brenn 2004). Joint replacement is a good option for getting rid of pain and improving joint function. Prosthetic joints generally last between fifteen and twenty years. We hear a lot about hips and knees, but other joints can be replaced as well, including ankle, foot, shoulder, elbow, and even finger joints. According to the American Academy of Orthopaedic Surgeons, nine out of ten people with joint replacement are satisfied.

Now, you might ask when you will know if your joints need to be replaced. If your activity is restricted to the point that you can't get out of a chair or get up from a fall, and you can't sleep due to the pain in your joints, it is time to consider joint replacement. Or if your pain is causing you to be isolated and unable to socialize and there is no pain relief from medications or other treatments, it may be the time to look at surgery. Most orthopedic surgeons, however, will not even consider doing a joint replacement until all the noninvasive therapies have been tried first. In addition, the orthopedic doctor may want you to lose weight before the surgery. The techniques for joint replacement will continue to improve, as will the prostheses used to replace them. In fact, recently, prosthetic joints made specifically for women are being used. Surgical time to do the procedure is getting shorter, and patients are recovering faster.

CAM treatments. Acupuncture has been found to be effective for treating the pain caused by osteoarthritis of the knee. When compared to those patients getting fake acupuncture or education regarding knee pain, the acupuncture group showed significant improvement in pain and function of the joint over a fourteen-week period (Berman et al. 2004). It is a very useful short-term treatment to use in addition to medication, diet, and exercise. Massage can be very effective for neck and back pain that results from osteoarthritis. Chiropractors manipulate the bones and muscles to relieve pain and to improve the overall function of the body. Which treatment works best will vary according to the individual. (See chapter 14 for discussion of chiropractors.)

MUSCLES, BONES, AND JOINTS

This last topic involves the musculoskeletal system as a whole.

Fibromyalgia

According to the American College of Rheumatology, 3 to 6 million Americans suffer with fibromyalgia, and 90 percent of them are women (NIAMS 2004). It usually affects women between the ages of twenty and sixty. No one is quite sure how many people in older age groups have it, but in a community study done in Kansas, over 7 percent of women between the ages of sixty and seventy-nine were found to have fibromyalgia (Wolfe et al. 2005). This condition is made up of a complex of symptoms that can include muscle pain, many tender points over the body, fatigue, problems sleeping, morning stiffness, headaches, and irritable bowel syndrome. Fibromyalgia patients may also have painful menstrual periods, numbness and tingling of the arms and legs, restless legs syndrome, temperature sensitivity, and "brain fog" or memory problems. Although the pain and discomfort of fibromyalgia can interfere with daily activities, it does not cause inflammation that damages the joints the way rheumatoid arthritis or osteoarthritis does.

WHAT CAUSES FIBROMYALGIA?

No one really knows what causes fibromyalgia, although it is often triggered by a traumatic or stressful event, such as a car accident.

HOW DO YOU KNOW IF YOU HAVE FIBROMYALGIA?

There is no definite blood test or imaging study that lets you know you have fibromyalgia. The diagnosis is ultimately made by the combination of your symptoms and the findings of a physical exam. There are eighteen points on the neck, shoulders, back, hips, and upper and lower extremities that can be tender on physical exam if you have fibromyalgia. If you have eleven out of the eighteen designated tender points, as well as widespread pain of your muscles and/or joints that lasts for more than three months, you may meet the definition of fibromyalgia. Remember though, there are other diseases that can cause pain and tender points lasting for over three months. Your clinician will look for these first, because unlike fibromyalgia, they may have serious or life-threatening complications that are treatable. Often, these other diseases can be diagnosed by laboratory tests. Although fibromyalgia itself doesn't lead to any serious or deforming complications, it is possible to have fibromyalgia plus another disease, such as rheumatoid arthritis, that can cause serious complications.

One of the more serious of the diseases that has symptoms like fibromyalgia is polymyalgia rheumatica (PMR). However, unlike fibromyalgia, PMR is due to inflammation in the blood vessels rather than the joints or muscles. It is most common in older women and can cause extreme pain and/or weakness in the upper arms and the upper legs. The weakness can become so severe that you cannot get up from a chair by yourself or you have trouble lifting your arm to comb your hair. PMR can be diagnosed based on your symptoms, a physical exam, and a blood test known as the sedimentation rate. Unlike fibromyalgia, PMR can be treated, and the illness can go into remission. Some patients with PMR have inflammation specifically in their temporal arteries, located on either side of the head. This is known as temporal arteritis (TA).

When TA is present, you will usually have pain in the area of the temples on either side of the head or a severe headache. In addition, either or both of the temples hurt when pressure is applied to them on exam. TA can lead to blindness if left untreated. (See the section "Headaches" in chapter 1.) We have had several patients who were told they had fibromyalgia when they actually had PMR. It is also possible to have fibromyalgia and then develop PMR. This is why your clinician needs to check for other causes that have severe complications and are treatable before diagnosing fibromyalgia.

CAN FIBROMYALGIA BE TREATED?

There are a variety of treatments for the symptoms of fibromyalgia, but not for the disease itself because the cause is unknown. It is important to treat other diseases that may be associated with the syndrome, such as an underactive thyroid, rheumatoid arthritis, or PMR. When the other diseases are adequately treated, the fibromyalgia symptoms usually improve, at least temporarily.

Education. If you have fibromyalgia, it is important to understand how far you can push yourself when you exercise and to learn how to do gentle stretching before and afterward. It is also crucial to know that fibromyalgia is a recognized syndrome. Many patients feel stigmatized by some clinicians who do not believe it is real. It is. So if you think you have it, speak up! Be your own advocate.

Lifestyle changes. One of the easiest things to do first is—you guessed it—exercise! For those with fibromyalgia this is often hard to do because they fear it may worsen their pain. However, studies looking at the effect of aerobic exercise on fibromyalgia have found that those who exercise have an increased ability to exercise more, decreased pain levels, and a higher tolerance for pain (Busch et al. 2002). It is important to consult with a certified trainer or physical therapist to develop a safe personal exercise plan.

Medications. Nonsteroidal anti-inflammatory drugs such as ibuprofen can relieve pain. Tylenol (acetaminophen) or Ultram (tramadol)—both pain relievers, not anti-inflammatory drugs—may also be helpful. Antidepressants can reduce pain by boosting the serotonin levels in the brain. Cymbalta (duloxetine), Prozac (fluoxetine), Paxil (paroxetine), and Zoloft (sertraline) have been used to treat both depression and pain. Tricyclic antidepressants such as Elavil (amitriptyline) in low doses can help with the sleep disturbance. Muscle relaxers such as Flexeril (cyclobenzaprine) can be helpful. Anticonvulsants such as Lyrica (pregabalin) may help some fibromyalgia patients. In a study of over 500 patients in whom Lyrica was compared to placebo, there was a greater than 50 percent improvement in pain, and improvements in sleep, fatigue, and overall quality of life (Crofford, Rowbotham, and Mease 2005). Drugs for Parkinson's disease such as Mirapex (pramipexole) have been found to help some fibromyalgia patients. Because they have the side effects of weight loss, anxiety, diarrhea, bloating, and morning drowsiness, many doctors will try them only when other therapies have failed. These medications may be used alone or in combination to treat the symptoms of fibromyalgia.

CAM therapies. These therapies work well when used in concert with conventional medical therapies. One or several may be helpful. Hypnotherapy and biofeedback have been found to improve the symptoms of fibromyalgia. (See chapter 14.) Cognitive behavioral therapy (CBT) is a form of psychotherapy that examines how what we think affects how we feel. It is generally a short-term therapy. It has been extraordinarily successful with fibromyalgia patients. A study using meditation and CBT found significant improvement in fibromyalgia patients over thirty months after treatment (Goldenberg, Kaplan, and Nadeau 1994). Acupuncture may be helpful to fibromyalgia patients. A study done at the Mayo Clinic divided fibromyalgia patients into two groups, one receiving six sessions of acupuncture while the other received fake acupuncture. The acupuncture group reported significant improvement with pain, fatigue, and anxiety, although after seven months without treatment, their symptoms returned (Martin 2006). Acupuncture may need to be continued on a quarterly or even a monthly basis to maintain its effect.

Herbs and supplements. SAMe has been found to improve morning stiffness and mood in fibromyalgia patients. Because magnesium (found in nuts, seeds, green leafy vegetables, whole grains, and supplements) and malic acid (found in apples) help to make energy for the cells of the body, both could theoretically be of benefit to fibromyalgia patients. 5-HTP (5-hydroxytryptophan) increases the serotonin levels in the brain and has been found to help pain, stiffness, and anxiety. 5-HTP should not be taken with selective serotonin reuptake inhibitor antidepressants.

CAN FIBROMYALGIA BE PREVENTED?

Because we don't know what causes fibromyalgia and we don't know exactly who is at risk to get it, there are no recommendations for prevention other than our usual counsel: eat well, exercise, and keep yourself in great condition.

SURVIVING FIBROMYALGIA

Fibromyalgia is a chronic problem. The key to successfully dealing with it is to adopt a positive attitude, accept support from others, exercise, and learn when to stop pushing and rest. The best approach to treatment appears to be a multidisciplinary one that uses both conventional medicines and complementary therapies. Talk with your primary care clinician to find the combination that works best for you. This is a disease in which our motto of the four A's can help immensely. Be *aware* of the disease, be *alert* to your symptoms, take *action* in seeking medical help for it, and *advocate* for yourself if you don't get good initial responses from medical practitioners.

THE DOCS CHAT ABOUT
THE MUSCULOSKELETAL SYSTEM

DR. J: I've heard that sports injuries are a big deal in our generation. Is that right?

DR. R: Yes. They sure are. In 1998, the U.S. Consumer Product Safety Commission reported that sports-related injuries in the baby boomer population was on the rise (U.S. Consumer Product Safety Commission 2000). In that year alone, there were over 1 million injuries in this group. The major injuries were from basketball and bicycling. According to this report, the many head injuries associated with bicycling were probably due to the lower use of helmets in baby boomers.

DR. J: We're still doing the extreme sports thing, but we aren't protecting ourselves?

DR. R: Sure seems that way. Whereas 69 percent of children wear helmets, only 43 percent of baby boomers wear them! Although doing these sports keeps us active and is good for us, we need to be more aware of available protection out there, especially as we get older. And we're talking more about that in chapter 11, right?

DR. J: Sure are. One other question. Finding the right doctor and hospital for surgery is so important. What do you tell your patients?

DR R: I tell patients to ask their primary care clinician for a referral to a surgeon that she would trust to operate on her or her family. When they meet with the surgeon, they need to find out how many procedures she has performed and how many complications she has had; it is important to look for a surgeon who does a lot of procedures and has very few complications. When choosing a hospital, they should find out what the infection rate is at that hospital, since one of the major complications of joint replacement is hospital-acquired infection. It is vital to find the hospital with the lowest infection rate.

PEARLS OF WISDOM FOR YOUR BONES, JOINTS, AND MUSCLES

○ Take care of your bones by getting adequate amounts of calcium, vitamin D, and weight-bearing exercise!

○ Ask your doctor to order a bone density scan if you're menopausal, if you have a family history of osteoporosis, or if you are taking prednisone long term.

○ Ask your doctor to check your blood level of vitamin D.

○ Know the ways to prevent the progression of osteoarthritis.

○ Fibromyalgia does not have to be a debilitating condition, but it may require a team of professionals and several medications to keep it under control.

○ Ask your doctor about polymyalgia rheumatica (PMR) if you have new-onset joint pain with or without severe muscle weakness.

○ Ask your doctor about temporal arteritis (TA) if you have the above symptoms and/or a new-onset severe headache or pain over your temples.

○ Wear protective gear when you exercise.

○ Protect your joints to avoid, or at least postpone, the need for their replacement.

○ Be proactive and advocate for yourself, your bones, your muscles and your joints!

CHAPTER 9

How to Keep Your Skin Moist, Smooth, and Firm

The skin is the first and most noticed body part. It is also the body part where our state of health and all those birthdays initially show up. Not only is it the largest organ of the body, but it's considered by many to be the major organ of sexual attraction, due to the all-important sense of touch related to the skin. The skin is extremely important to our health for other reasons as well. It's a major part of our body's defense system because it protects the organs from injury and keeps foreign substances, such as infectious organisms, outside the body. The skin also helps to keep us hydrated by preventing the loss of body fluids from inside the body. It has an important mechanical function in its ability to stretch when necessary, more in some locations than in others (think of your belly after weight gain or during pregnancy). It also has glands that can produce odors, reminding us, or others, that it's time to clean up.

Therefore, whether you hate your wrinkles and obsess about your skin because of them, or you love your wrinkles and never think about your body's covering, it's imperative for you to keep your skin intact and in good condition for the health of the rest of your body. In this chapter, we discuss what happens to the skin, and some of the common skin problems that occur, as it ages. We also talk about what treatments make sense for maturing skin. And most important, we discuss the ins and outs of sunblock. Skin cancers are discussed in chapter 12.

SKIN: IN YOUTH AND AS IT AGES

Most descriptions of the skin discuss the two main layers: the epidermis and the dermis. We will too. The *epidermis* is the top layer of the skin, and is made up of skin cells known as *keratinocytes*. In the top part of the epidermis, the keratinocytes are dead and are constantly being shed at the same time that new living cells are forming, in a routine cycle lasting three to six weeks. The living keratinocytes are known as *squamous cells*; they can give rise to one of the most common types of skin cancer, *squamous cell carcinoma*.

As the skin ages, the keratinocytes divide more slowly, causing the shedding of the dead cells to slow and the cycle of loss and renewal to take place less often. This leads to the piling up of dead cells that do not reflect light, causing the surface of the skin to appear dull and gray. In addition, those dead skin cells do not absorb topical medication or skin care products such as moisturizers well, and this leads us to recommend that you do regular home *exfoliation* (or microdermabrasion in a professional office) as you age.

The other main layer of the skin, the *dermis*, lies beneath the epidermis and contains many types of cells, including those making up blood vessels, nerves, and the immune system. Also in the same area are large collections of *collagen* and *elastic fibers*, which give the skin its structure and elasticity. With aging, the fibers unravel and loosen, causing sagging, furrows, and a decrease in elasticity of the skin.

The site where the epidermis meets the dermis is sometimes called the *transition layer* of the skin. The cells that form pigment, *melanocytes*, are found in this area. The brown-black skin pigment, called *melanin*, does two things: It helps to protect against the damaging rays of the sun, and it determines a person's skin coloring. With age, melanocytes may increase in number and cluster together. They are then seen on the skin surface as small, dark, flat or raised spots, known as liver spots or harmless moles. However, some of those dark skin spots that look like moles may be malignant—a sign of the deadly cancer melanoma, which is discussed in chapter 12.

Both the epidermis and the dermis become thinner with age. This leads to thinning of the skin and an increased susceptibility to trauma; this, in turn, results in areas of easily torn skin. Because of the slowed turnover of dead cells into new cells, breaks in the skin heal more slowly with age. Since the blood vessels in the dermis are closer to the surface of the skin and are more fragile themselves, we tend to bruise more easily with age. Because the oil-secreting and sweat-secreting glands within the skin decrease with age, the skin loses its ability to retain moisture and becomes scaly and dry. Now you can see why, with each birthday, our skin becomes drier, thinner, duller, saggier, more wrinkly and bruised, and has more dark spots! Skin aging differs between light-skinned women and women of color, as discussed in the next section.

What Causes the Skin to Age?

On first glance, asking what causes the skin to age may seem like a stupid question. But the answer with regard to the skin is not simply time, as it is with the other organ systems of the body. Put another way, why do some women have skin that doesn't seem to age, while other women feel that they become more prunelike by the day?

PHOTOAGING

As with the other organs of the body, aging of the skin is a natural process caused by a combination of factors including heredity, environmental exposure, and hormonal influences; the aging of the skin due to the passage of time only is known as *chronoaging*. Most of the skin changes that occur with aging, however, are due to sun exposure, known as *photoaging*. The more sun exposure you've had during your lifetime, the more photoaging you will have.

There are two types of ultraviolet radiation produced by the sun: ultraviolet A (UVA) rays and ultraviolet B (UVB) rays. Both types penetrate the top layers of the skin, attacking and damaging the DNA inside the skin cells; this leads to harmless lesions as well as to cancers. UVB usually penetrates only the outer skin layers and is the main agent causing sunburn; UVB rays are at their most intense during the midday hours and the summer months. Also, UVB is filtered through window glass while UVA is not.

UVA ray intensity is less variable than that of UVB; therefore we are exposed to it no matter how bright or dull the intensity of the sun. This is why wearing sunblock is recommended anytime that there is daylight outside, even during the hours when the sun is not at its brightest, and even on cloudy days. Because UVA is able to penetrate to the deeper layers of the skin, it tends to be more responsible for photoaging than is UVB. Knowing about these two types of ultraviolet rays is important in choosing a sunblock; many do not offer protection against both types. Tanning beds give off both types of radiation, with many machines using predominantly UVA rays, which can lead to premature aging (Boiko 2001).

Photoaging in light-skinned women. Because light-skinned women tend to have fewer melanocytes than women of color, and thus less protection against the sun, they tend to get all of the effects of photoaging mentioned above. For the same reason, a larger percentage of Caucasian women have skin cancers—including melanoma—than do women of color (Halder and Ara 2003). (See chapter 12.)

Photoaging in women of color. The large number of melanocytes that women of color have in their skin protects them from UVA and UVB rays; one study showed that five times the amount of both types of UV light penetrates the skin of white women as compared to that of women of color (Kaidbey et al. 1979). Because of this superior protection against UV light, photoaging effects are seen much less in women of color. In fact, the only photoaging effects seen are mostly fine wrinkling and splotches of darker color, known as *hyperpigmentation*; even these changes may not begin to appear until they're in their fifties (Halder and Ara 2003). For those of Asian background, photoaging tends to show up as harmless darkened and scaly lesions known as *seborrheic keratoses* and as liver spots (Griffiths 1998). There is little known about photoaging in Hispanics, although when occupationally exposed to sunlight over many years, Hispanics can develop deep wrinkles (Halder and Ara 2003).

It is important for women of color to note that, although you do have better protection against the damaging rays of the sun due to your skin color, you are not completely immune from those rays either. That protection against the sun is not complete; that is, some UV light does penetrate your skin. Therefore, the recommendations for sun protection discussed later in this chapter apply to you too.

OTHER CAUSES OF AGING SKIN

Although photoaging is responsible for the majority of skin changes with age, other factors also play a role. With the differences each of us has in our heredity and our lifetime exposures, you can see how individual women may age in different ways and at varying rates.

A portion of how much and how quickly the skin ages is related to heredity. Female hormones play a role; estrogen increases the amount of collagen in the skin, which results in thicker skin with fewer wrinkles and less sagging (Ghersetich et al. 2001). Cigarette smoking also plays a large role. In one study, female smokers had a risk for wrinkling three times greater than that of women who never smoked, and two times greater than former smokers (Castelo-Branco et al. 1998). In another study, the longer and more heavily the research participants had smoked, the more wrinkling they had (Ernster et al. 1995). Air pollution, particularly ozone, may be a problem for the skin.

COMMON BENIGN SKIN PROBLEMS OCCURRING WITH AGE

There are several commonly seen skin problems that occur more frequently as the years go by.

Excessively Dry Skin

Severely dry skin may be the most frequent skin issue in women over the age of sixty-five, affecting almost 75 percent of women (and men) in this age group (Roberts 2006). This dryness often affects the hair and nails as well.

What are the factors that cause, and increase, the dryness of skin? The factors that can worsen dryness include excessive bathing, particularly in hot water; personal cleaning products such as harsh soaps and detergents or acetone- or alcohol-based products; environmental humidity, with the lower humidity of winter causing the greatest water loss from the skin; long-term use of central heating or air-conditioning, both of which lower the humidity inside; illnesses such as an underactive thyroid; and medications such as diuretics.

How do you know if you have dry skin? Believe us, you'll know! The skin becomes very flaky and rubs off easily. It may feel rough, scaly, and uncomfortable and look red and irritated. Probably the most common symptom is itchiness all over, with no specific rash to account for that symptom. Besides being uncomfortable, dry skin tears more easily, and the resulting wound does not heal as quickly as before, which may lead to infection. Dry skin is not just a cosmetic problem.

How is dry skin treated and prevented? Avoid losing moisture from the skin, and add moisture to it. There are several ways to both treat and prevent dry skin, including avoiding hot baths or showers; limiting the amount of time you spend bathing and your bathing frequency; using a humidifier inside; and avoiding harsh soaps and detergents, such as those dispensed as foam (recommended cleansers include Dove Sensitive Essentials Non-Foaming Cleanser and Cetaphil). In addition, the use of different types of moisturizers is extremely important. You should use an occlusive moisturizer (one that acts as physical block against the elements and traps moisture in the skin) while the skin is still damp, such as lanolin-based products, petrolatum (Vaseline), or products made with almond or olive oil (our favorite is Olivella All Natural Olive Oil Moisturizer). But remember, a little bit of oil goes a long way. At other times, you should use a thick, oil-free moisturizer such as Cetaphil, which is found in drugstores. If you are having difficulty keeping your skin moist despite doing the right things, like limiting baths and showers and using moisturizer daily, discuss this with your clinician.

Rosacea

Rosacea is a common disease that occurs most frequently in fair-skinned women between the ages of thirty and sixty. Currently it affects approximately 14 million Americans (Mayo Clinic Staff 2006).

How do you know if you have rosacea? What can you do about it? Affecting the skin on the face, rosacea often begins as redness across the cheeks, nose, forehead, or chin, and may progress to small, broken blood vessels or red pimples and bumps filled with pus. It also may involve the eyelids and the white part of the eye, causing both to become inflamed. It may occur cyclically, flaring up for weeks to months then disappearing, only to reappear at a later time. Because of its appearance, rosacea may be confused with acne or eczema. Though it is not life-threatening, it does not clear up on its own and if left untreated, will progress. Therefore, an initial diagnosis is important. If you have new skin issues, see your clinician within several weeks *while* you are having the outbreak.

What worsens rosacea? Anything that increases blood flow to the surface of your skin will aggravate rosacea. This includes spicy foods, hot foods or beverages, excessive sunlight, alcohol, extremes of temperature (including hot baths or saunas), overdoing your exercise, stress, and medications that dilate blood vessels, such as some high blood pressure medications.

How is rosacea treated and prevented? Your dermatologist will start treatment with medications that may include a topical antibiotic, such as metronidazole, a topical anti-inflammatory drug known as azelaic acid, oral antibiotics such as tetracycline, or, for more severe cases, isotretinoin (Accutane). For more advanced cases of rosacea, laser and electrosurgery may be used. Since the cause of rosacea is unknown, there are no known ways to prevent the disease itself, but you can prevent its worsening by avoiding the aggravating factors and by the regular use of sunblock.

Lumps and Bumps and Other Uglies

We're sure you've had the experience of awakening one morning to find one or more weird spots on your skin that weren't there the night before. We certainly have. Most of these are harmless, benign, and just a nuisance. Unfortunately, there are many different types, including liver spots, also known as "age spots" (you know what those look like), tiny bright red spots that look almost like blood blisters beneath the skin known as cherry angiomata, scaly raised brown bumps known as seborrheic keratoses, and those huge bruises that appear out of nowhere. The only thing these have in common is that they're all ugly!

We can reassure you that many of these ugly skin things are harmless; but we cannot tell you to ignore them. The reason is that skin cancer is the most common cancer in our age group, and often skin cancer can look like one of the harmless ugly spots. So, how do you tell the difference? You make an appointment for a full skin exam with a dermatologist, even if you're having no skin problems, and let her tell you which of your skin spots may be dangerous and which are not. With that instruction, make sure to do a monthly exam of your skin to notice if there are new lesions, or if any of your old ones have changed. To know specifically what to look for, read the section on skin cancer in chapter 12.

Changes in the Face and Neck: Wrinkles, Sagging, and Dark Spots

When you look in the mirror these days, do you ever wonder when you started looking like your grandmother? Or maybe you only recently looked around your office and noticed that many of your coworkers look like they're twelve years old, and knowing the high value that our culture places on a youthful appearance, you've become worried that your current appearance may affect your job—a not-uncommon concern in women our age (Gupta and Gilchrest 2005).

If you've had any of these thoughts, you're certainly not alone; both Dr. R and Dr. J, and probably a few million other women, are feeling the exact same way. So if your current appearance upsets you or worries you as to how it will affect your job, read on. On the other hand, if you aren't bothered by this issue from either a personal or workplace perspective, you can skip most of this chapter. But please don't skip the part about prevention and sunblock, as it's important for everyone.

Mary's Story

Mary is a beautiful sixty-five-year-old African-American grandmother who is constantly told that she looks so young she could be her thirty-five-year-old daughter's sister. Her only skin issues, which she brought to Dr. J's attention during her routine exam, were all the new spots that were continually appearing on her body. One in particular, on her chest, kept catching on her bra, ripping a bit, and bleeding; this was the one she was most worried about. During the exam, Dr. J saw many lumps and bumps of aging and noted the harmless skin tag on Mary's chest that was causing the problem. It wasn't until she took off her shoes and hose that Mary thought to mention the new large, dark spot on the sole of her foot. In the classic location that it occurs in women of color, this turned out to be a melanoma, which was caught early, surgically removed, and considered cured. This story has a happy ending, but only because Mary did two things: She kept her appointments for routine exams, and she was aware of new and changing skin lesions on her body.

HOW ARE THE SIGNS OF AGING IN SKIN TREATED?

Have you read about, or seen on television or the Internet, vitamin C/grape seed products/seaweed/diamond dust/specks of gold and their "miraculous" new use in getting rid of the wrinkles/sagging/dark spots on your face? Despite heady claims of the effectiveness of any and all of these products, the claims cannot be uniformly validated because the FDA, the governmental agency regulating the safety of our foods, and the safety and effectiveness of our medications, does not regulate these products. However, many of them have been scientifically studied and do, in fact, work. Because Dr. J has been a skin care nut since her mother started her using Pond's cold cream and Noxzema at age twelve (and made her wear a hat all the time), she will take over the rest of this chapter.

Skin Care Products

There is now a large range of products and procedures that successfully treat, although usually only temporarily, many of the signs of aging skin. I'm going to make this simple. All you really need to do to care for your skin, especially your face, is to keep it clean (including removing the dead cells on top by exfoliating), moist, and protected against the sun. If you want to treat the signs of aging skin as well, then that adds another step or two. But don't get discouraged by the huge number of products out there; caring for your skin does not have to be complicated. Also remember that the signs of aging show up on your hands as quickly as on your face; so do the same steps on your hands as you do for your face.

Caution: Before you buy any products, find out what type of skin you have; your dermatologist can tell you, although you probably already know. (For instance, do you have very fair skin that burns easily and is sensitive to most products?) Also, to make sure your skin is not allergic to a new product, do a skin "patch test" first. Apply a quarter-sized amount of the product only to the side of your neck or the inner part of your arm (somewhere it won't be seen if there is an allergic reaction) the first time you use it. If there is no redness, swelling, or itching in that area the following day, go ahead and use the product as directed.

Cleansers. Keeping the face clean is essential. But plain old soap may be harmful, particularly if it is harsh and drying. There are many types of cleansers in many forms, including lotions, gels, foams, and even the good old bar of soap. If you have particularly dry skin, use the form that moisturizes the best, a lotion cleanser; some of these are just tissued off and don't even require water. Avoid products that foam or contain alcohol, which are drying. I have normal to dry, very sensitive skin and have had great success with Cetaphil cleanser, which may be purchased in any drugstore. Dove, Olay, and Neutrogena also make good cleansers.

Exfoliants. The reason for exfoliating your skin, including your face and your entire body, makes sense: it gets rid of the dead cells piled up on the outer surface of your skin. You'll definitely look better after you do this. But there's another important reason to exfoliate: It removes those dead skin cells that act as a barrier to the absorption of other treatment products. After all, what good are the best antiwrinkle creams or simple moisturizers if they cannot get into the deep layers of your skin, where they need to be?

There are two types of exfoliant products readily available without prescriptions: the fruit acids (alpha and beta hydroxy acid, also called AHA and BHA), which chemically dissolve and lift off the dead skin cells when used in high concentrations, and the exfoliants that physically scrape off the dead cells. The latter group includes products with tiny rough beads, or sugar or salt crystals, or even your own bath towel! How often should you exfoliate? It depends on how your skin reacts, but you can exfoliate with a strong product at least once a week and with milder products more often. The instructions on the bottle will tell you how often is best with that particular product. But be aware, you can definitely overdo this. Aggressively exfoliating can lead to severe skin irritation (Gordon 2005).

I have used several different exfoliants. As a mild facial and body exfoliant in the shower, I use Peter Thomas Roth Botanical Buffing Beads. For less frequent, heavy duty facial exfoliation, I like Dr. Brandt Microdermabrasion (in a jar), or Philosophy Microdelivery Exfoliating Wash. Also, Dove makes a good exfoliant.

Toners and facial water. Most toners contain alcohol, although this will be indicated on the label. Avoid these if your skin is dry, and instead spray plain facial water after cleansing and follow it with your treatment products and moisturizer. I skip this step entirely, mainly because, for me, the simpler the routine, the better.

Moisturizers. Although we know that moisturizers make our skin look and feel better and improve mild inflammation of the face in the winter (Kikuchi et al. 2003), there is disagreement in the dermatologic community concerning any long-term benefit that accrues to the skin with moisturizing it regularly (Gordon 2005). Definitely use a moisturizer if you have dry skin. Hyaluronic acid is a component of many antiaging products and is also available as the pure substance. I've used SkinCeuticals B_5 Moisturizing Gel, which contains hyaluronic acid and vitamin B_5, for years and love it. In the summer, I try to combine the steps in my regimen and use a sunblock that is moisturizing. (See the discussion of sunblocks later in this chapter.)

Antiwrinkle products. There are so many products out there that lay claim to getting rid of wrinkles and sagging that I don't know where to start. The first thing I'll tell you is that, often, lines and wrinkles on your face are partially the result of dryness, and you can look much better just by using a moisturizer and assuring its absorption by first exfoliating. Another important thing to remember with all of these products, including sunscreens, is that their active ingredients may become inactive over time; so always check the expiration date on your skin care products.

Of all the ingredients that make claims of antiaging effects, the only one that is FDA-approved (which means that it has been scientifically shown to do what it says it does) are the antioxidants known as the retinoids, or retinol (vitamin A) (Gordon 2005). The two products in this group that are available by prescription are tretinoin (Retin-A, Renova) and tazarotene (Tazorac, Avage). Both of these improve fine wrinkles, the skin's texture, and the areas that are darker due to photoaging (Kligman et al. 1986). Although many over-the-counter (OTC) products contain this type of ingredient as retinol, it is present in lower concentrations than in the prescription products. Therefore, the OTC products containing retinol may help, but they are not as effective as prescription products.

The other popular antioxidants also work by offering protection from damaging free radicals produced when skin is exposed to UVA and UVB, and can promote collagen synthesis, lighten hyperpigmented areas, and improve areas of inflammation. The list of these products is seemingly endless and includes ascorbic acid (vitamin C), vitamin E, lipoic acid, idebenone, green tea, pomegranate juice, copper, grape and grape seed products, and on and on.

Of these, I will mention only a couple. There is reasonable scientific evidence that topical vitamin C is effective (Farris 2005). However, it too must be absorbed by the skin in order to work, so it must be contained in a product that is easily absorbed. Vitamin C in some forms is highly unstable; make sure when you're using it that you check the expiration date, which will be on the bottle. It can be quite irritating when first used, so you might want to mix it with your moisturizer initially. Another antioxidant that is effective is idebenone (McDaniel et al. 2005), which is an ingredient in the commercially available products Prevage and Kinerase. Alpha lipoic acid has been shown to have significant antioxidative effects, as well as anti-inflammatory properties, and is recommended especially for the skin of African-American women (Jackson 2003); this ingredient is contained in many of the Dr. Perricone line of skin care products.

I've been using the retinoid Tazorac (0.5%) several times a week for a year or so, and I love it. On the other days of the week I use *one* of the other antioxidant products, such as vitamin C (I love SkinCeuticals C E ferulic), Prevage, or Kinerase. (I use one of these products until it is gone, and then I switch; but I always use the Tazorac two or three days a week.)

Skin-lightening products. Because the darkened (hyperpigmented) areas on the skin caused by aging are common and distressing, skin-lightening products are an important part of your antiaging regimen. The safety and effectiveness of these products is especially important for women of color, in whom hyperpigmentation is common (Holloway 2003). Of the various substances, only one is covered under the FDA's review of over-the-counter preparations, hydroquinone 1.5 percent to 2 percent. Higher concentrations may be obtained by prescription.

Nonsurgical Cosmetic Procedures

To go through the myriad of nonsurgical procedures now available would require us to scrap the rest of this book! So, here is the best advice we can offer you about when, how, and how often to get Botox, cosmetic fillers, Thermage, microdermabrasion, and/or laser therapy: Find either a board-certified dermatologist or plastic surgeon with whom you are comfortable and whom you trust. How can you find such a doctor? Through recommendations from patients who have been satisfied, and by asking your primary care provider and other clinicians for recommendations. We cannot advise you to go to a mall "spa" that does cosmetic procedures unless it is under the direction of a qualified physician who is easily accesible at all times.

Want more advice? Let your dermatologist or surgeon know if you plan to lose weight. Loss of weight can affect the shape of your face, and therefore can also affect how many, and what type of, procedures are needed. Also, be sure to ask your dermatologist or surgeon before the procedure about the possible complications and how frequently they been reported to occur. Many women are surprised to discover that such seemingly "simple" procedures can cause problems. Most importantly, make sure your primary clinician knows you are planning to have these procedures done and has given you an okay from a medical standpoint, even though such clearance may not required. Getting that okay is a smart thing to do because your primary care provider knows the most about your total health. That's just good medicine.

Cosmetic Surgery

Since we didn't go through all of the nonsurgical cosmetic procedures, you know we're not going to discuss all the types of plastic surgery here as well. Nevertheless, we still have several things to say. If you're considering plastic surgery, the same advice applies: Find the best doctor for yourself. This physician should be board certified, and preferably a plastic surgeon. If you're unsure about what you've been told, take the time to meet with, and get opinions from, several physicians in this field, particularly to see if the same procedures are recommended. Most of these surgeons have available computerized simulations of how you'll look after various procedures. Also ask to see photos of other patients after their surgery.

It is very important to think about the reasons you want to have the surgery done and what your expectations are. If you want to look as if you're twenty again, think again, as that is unrealistic. If, however, you want to look more rested or like a better version of yourself, go for it! If you're just recovering from a bitter divorce or another traumatic life experience, consider postponing the decision until you're completely back to yourself. Also, remember that as we age, the skin does not heal as quickly. Be sure to discuss this and any other of your health concerns with your primary care provider before you make your final plans for the surgery. Remember also that there is risk associated with any type of surgery. For a discussion of these risks, read the "Hysterectomy" section in chapter 6.

Cosmetics

A word about makeup. The newer foundations, powders, blush, and eye makeup available today can actually transform your face—if used correctly. If you'd really like to look better but are unsure about having a cosmetic procedure, then first try changing your makeup. Go where your favorite makeup line is sold and have a makeover. You may look so good that you decide to put off the procedure for a while. We both like the new makeup lines made from minerals. (I use the Bare Escentuals powders.) Remember, though, not to keep your makeup forever, particularly eye makeup; when you buy it, ask how long it stays good. One rule of thumb: When it develops a bad odor, toss it. We include an excellent book in the Resources section about how to best use makeup on our more seasoned faces.

How Are the Effects of Aging and Skin Cancer Prevented?

You can already guess what I'm going to talk about here: sun protection.

SUNSCREEN PRODUCTS

I have an admission to make here. I love sunblock. It is probably my favorite of all skin care products. Why? Because it works; it absolutely does what it says it's going to do. And how many things can you say that about these days? When enough is used in an appropriate way, sunblock actually prevents (most of) those UV rays from penetrating into the skin. How do I personally know this? Because I have that sensitive type of skin that never tanned and always burned to a crisp, causing me to get sick with a high fever ("sun poisoning") whenever I was exposed to the sun for even a short period of time. Since I started using certain sunblocks all the time, I have never burned. Nor have I gotten a lot of those brown aging spots. In addition, certain sunblocks definitely prevent some types of skin cancer and are thought to prevent other types (see chapter 12). So if you use no other product on your exposed skin, please use this one. This goes for women of color and light-skinned women.

What does it protect against? The first and most important thing to know about sunblocks is that not all of them protect against both UVA and UVB rays. Therefore, with certain products, you may not get any protection at all against UVA rays, which cause most of the photoaging and contribute to skin cancers. Sunblock products are regulated by the FDA. In the summer of 2007, they changed their recommendations as to the labeling, formulation, and testing of these products based on suggestions made by the American Academy of Dermatology (FDA 2007b). The new regulations now require that the amount of UVA protection be shown on the label; thus, if the product does not contain enough UVA-blocking agent, the label will say that there is no UVA protection. Therefore, you will be able to tell, based on the labeling, if your sunscreen protects you from both types of UV light, as it should.

What are the categories of active ingredients? There are two categories of active ingredients in sunscreen, which work in different ways. The type with broader UV coverage is said to be a *physical blocker* because it literally physically blocks the absorption of the sun's rays; it is like wearing a shield. Remember that thick white cream you used to use on your nose—zinc oxide? The modern version of this is titanium dioxide. The other types are *chemical blockers*, which actually chemically react with your skin to prevent absorption of UV light. The majority of these, like PABA, protect only against UVB rays and may cause irritation or allergic skin reactions. The one chemical blocker that protects against both types of UV rays is Mexoryl. It is now available at drugstores in the U.S. in the Anthelios line of products, as well in department stores as Lancôme's UV expert 20 with Mexoryl.

How is it formulated? The active ingredients mentioned above are available in many products, including moisturizers and makeup. Which you use is up to you and depends on the state of your skin.

What is the best way to use it? You must apply *at least two tablespoons to each area* of the body that will be exposed to the sun at least half an hour before exposure, *reapply at least every two hours*, or sooner after swimming or excessive sweating, and use a product with an SPF (sun protection factor) of at least 15. Don't forget about using a sunscreen on your lips. Use sunblock with any sun exposure, which includes riding in your car, walking outside even briefly, or sitting inside if you are next to a window. Wear it during the winter months as well as the other seasons. That's basically every day of the year!

Also, keep in mind that various areas of the country receive different amounts of UV radiation depending on factors such as elevation of the land and amount of air pollution. A recent study showed that there is a higher incidence of certain skin cancers in locations receiving the highest amount of UV radiation, such as in the southern U.S. (Qureshi et al. 2008). In those places receiving high amounts of UV radiation, you should be even more careful about protecting yourself, especially if you have had skin cancer in the past or have a family history of it. To find out about the amount of UV exposure you will receive in any location in the U.S. on any given day, go to the Environmental Protection Agency's website at www.epa.gov/sunwise.uvindex.htm/#map.

Don't allow yourself to burn, and avoid tanning. Avoid sun exposure between 10 a.m. and 4 p.m. (Don't forget to factor in daylight savings time.) Drink plenty of fluids. Don't forget to wear a hat and the appropriate sunglasses (see chapter 2), and consider specially treated sun protective clothing (see below). Moreover, since all of the recommendations above are designed to limit your sun exposure, don't forget to ask your clinician to check your vitamin D level. That's because sunlight is necessary to metabolize vitamin D in the body, and many people become deficient in this important vitamin just by following sunblock recommendations. (See chapter 8 for further discussion of vitamin D.)

You may be wondering if I use sunblock every day all year as I've recommended. Yes, I really do. I don't walk out of the house without rubbing some on my face and my exposed arms or hands. What specifically do I use? I've tried many sunscreens over the years but keep coming back to two old favorites and one new one: Neutrogena for Sensitive Skin and Skinceuticals Physical UV Defense SPF30, both of which contain titanium dioxide; and a newer one, Anthelios with SPF50+. Blistex makes a lip product with a high SPF that can be found at most drugstores.

PROTECTIVE CLOTHING

Not all clothing is equally protective against the sun. Although some dermatologists think that densely woven fabrics, such as denim, wool, or polyester materials, especially in dark colors, are protective (Lautenschlager, Wulf, and Pittelkow 2007), there now exists specially manufactured clothing that is treated to give high UV protection. This is important for you to consider if you've had skin cancer, have a family history of it, or have fair and sensitive skin. My favorite is made by the Solumbra company. I wear one of their hats all the time and their tracksuit for long summertime walks. They do work, even after many washings.

THE DOCS CHAT ABOUT
HAIR AND SKIN

DR. R: I'm curious about how hair changes as we age.

DR. J: There are two main issues with our hair as the years pass: not enough in some places, and too much in others. Like real estate, it's about location, location, location! Seriously, a natural effect of aging is the thinning of hair on our scalps. This may be as subtle as the part that you make in your hair appearing wider than it used to be; this would indicate hair loss around the part. The important thing to know is that there are many causes for hair loss other than aging. For any type of hair concern, I would advise a woman to see her primary care clinician or dermatologist and be checked for illnesses such as an underactive thyroid. If there isn't another illness, it's still important to be seen because there are many options for treatment.

DR. R: Anything else we need to know about how our hair changes as we get older?

DR. J: Yes. Just as our skin does with the passing years, our hair becomes drier and more brittle. I never used a conditioner in my younger years, or paid much attention to the type of shampoo or other hair products I used. When I noticed in recent years that my hair was in worse condition than it used to be, I started washing it less often to help prevent it from being so dry, and using a conditioner after every wash. And when I do wash my hair, I try to limit the time I use the hair dryer to the least amount possible, since hair dryers can cause damage too.

DR. R: Doesn't your hair get greasy if you don't wash it often?

DR. J: Sometimes. But then I use what we all used in the old days—one of those "dry sham-poos." Most hair care lines have just started making them again. And blondes can use baby powder. Also, I've started paying attention to the shampoos and other hair care products I use now. For the past few years, I've used only Schwartzkopf products; at this point in time, they are sold in the U.S. mostly in certain hair salons. (Thanks, Jill!) There are other hair product lines available in drugstores that are very moisturizing as well. Now, I have a questions for you. Are there any CAM therapies that might help with the effects of aging on our skin?

DR. R: Yes, acupuncture has been used successfully in some people to diminish the appearance of wrinkles. And, of course, we all look better (and smoother) when we relax and stop worry-ing; so try meditating or getting a massage. Another one for you. Do exercises for the facial muscles help get rid of wrinkles and sagging?

DR. J: There's no scientific evidence that they do, but some women swear by them. But don't you dare tell me to add them to my daily routine; I barely have time to exercise the rest of my body! I'm curious, though, how do you take care of your skin?

DR. R: I have to admit, I don't do as much as you do, but I have a special cleanser that I use for dry skin called True. I also use Retin-A three times a week, and in the morning I used to use Total Effects by Olay, and have now switched to Regenerist with sunscreen, which was recommended by my dermatologist. I also use a mineral makeup that is a natural sunscreen. And I have a microdermabrasion treatment every month—it's great!

DR. J: Not to worry about not doing as much as I do. You'll catch up and pass me when we compare our exercise regimens!

Pearls of Wisdom
about Skin

○ Know that the main culprits responsible for the aging of the face and skin cancer are the UV rays of the sun.

○ Smoking cigarettes can cause wrinkling of the skin, so stop smoking!

○ Wear a sunscreen that gives protection against both UVA and UVB rays; this goes for women of color as well as light-skinned women.

○ Examine your skin regularly. Don't ignore new or changing skin lesions.

○ See your dermatologist regularly.

○ Smile lots and often. It does wonders for facial drooping or sagging!

CHAPTER 10

Menopause and Hormones: How to Stay Cool if You Are One Hot Mama

Let's start this discussion by stating unequivocally that menopause is *not* a disease. It is a natural process that occurs when we outlive our ovaries. This is a relatively new phase of life for women to have to deal with because our average life span has increased from forty-eight years to eighty since 1900 (Arias 2006).

MENOPAUSE

Menopause is a normal part of the aging process. Just as puberty is one of life's natural and healthy transitions, so is menopause.

Definitions and Terms

As we enter our late thirties or early forties, our ovaries gradually slow down, and then stop functioning. It is as if they step on the brakes and say, "No more, I am done!" The process is usually gradual and can last years. Most women experience their last period in their late forties or early fifties; the average age for periods to end is fifty-one.

Menopause itself is defined as the absence of a menstrual period for one year. The period of time before actual menopause is completed is termed *perimenopause*. *Surgical menopause* refers to the removal of the ovaries, called *oophorectomy*. If the ovaries are gone, menopause occurs immediately due to the loss of hormones. If only the uterus is removed (*hysterectomy*), although you won't have a period, you will still go through menopause at your destined time. Factors that are associated with earlier menopause include smoking, a history of osteoporosis, heart disease, and race. Hispanic and African-American women are more likely, and Chinese and Japanese women are less likely, to have early menopause (Gold et al. 2001).

What Are the Symptoms of Menopause?

Some women experience only a few symptoms, while others are "lucky" enough to experience them all. These are discussed below.

Irregular periods. You may notice that your periods are occurring more often or getting heavier or longer. Or you may spot between periods, or even skip several periods. If you've always had irregular periods, you might not even notice that you are experiencing perimenopause.

Joint aches. In a study of over 400 women who were going through menopause, the symptoms that correlated best with menopause were joint aches and stiffness (Freeman et al. 2007). The good news was that after the women had transitioned through menopause and their hormone levels had stabilized, the joint aches and pains improved.

Dr. R's Story

When I started perimenopause, there were three months when I had no period. I felt pretty good with minimal symptoms, and I thought I was done, no sweat! I bragged to a friend of mine who is a gynecologist about how easy menopause was, and she laughed. She told me my ovaries were just recharging their batteries and getting ready to throw out a few more eggs. Although I scoffed and told her she was wrong, sure enough, a week later my periods were baaaaack!

Hot flashes. No one is quite sure of the exact cause of a hot flash. However, the sudden drop in estrogen triggers a reaction that can be as mild as a flush, or that is intense enough to cause red blotches, sweats, a sense of intense heat over the entire body, and the feeling that you've been ignited from the inside out. At night, it can wake you from a sound sleep with the feeling that the sheets have been heated or set on fire. Hot flashes can come out of the blue without warning or can be triggered by spicy food, caffeine, alcohol, smoking, and stress.

Approximately, two-thirds of women will experience hot flashes; one-third of those will have them for up to five years and 10 to 20 percent will find them very distressing (Stearns et al. 2002). (They needn't have done any research studies for that last one—they could've just asked us!) In the Study of Women's Health across the Nation (SWAN), Japanese and Chinese women reported fewer hot flash symptoms and African-American women reported more symptoms when both groups were compared to Caucasian women (Gold et al. 2000).

Dr. R's Story

I remember watching an episode of the TV show Cybil *many years ago. Cybil was in a restaurant and got a hot flash. She took the ice from her water glass and stuffed it down her shirt. At the time, I thought she was being a bit melodramatic. After I started having my own hot flashes, I wonder why she didn't pour the whole glass of water and ice down her shirt!*

Vaginal and bladder problems. As we lose estrogen, our vaginal tissue dries out and becomes thinner and less elastic. This can make sex painful and also make us more prone to bladder symptoms and infections. (See chapter 7.)

Sex and libido. Some women lose interest in sex around the time of menopause, possibly due to a decrease in testosterone levels. Others have an increased interest in sex with the newfound freedom of not worrying about getting pregnant. However, as discussed in chapter 6, you can never be free of worry about contracting sexually transmitted infections. It is important to be careful no matter what age you are!

Sleep problems. Many women in our practices have listed lack of sleep as their number one problem related to menopause. The problems can run the gamut: trouble falling or staying asleep, or not sleeping altogether.

Memory lapses, or mental-pause. During menopause, many women feel like they are losing their minds. They forget names, dates, and all sorts of simple things. However, although we think our memories are declining, studies have found that this is not the case (Thompson 2003). One study followed 800 women over six years postmenopause. Their memories were tested over that time period and not only did their memories not decline, they got better (Henderson et al. 2003). See chapter 1 for more on memory problems at this age.

Body changes. After menopause, we lose lean body mass and many of us gain weight, especially around the middle (see chapter 11). During this time, we are at increased risk for osteoporosis (see chapter 8) and our risk for heart disease starts escalating (see chapter 3).

Can the Symptoms of Menopause Be Treated or Prevented?

Although menopause is a natural process, there are many things we can do to improve and, in some cases, prevent the symptoms.

IRREGULAR PERIODS

Don't ignore extremely heavy or frequent periods, as you may be losing a lot of blood. Also, don't write off these symptoms as "just part of menopause." There could be another cause, such as an underactive thyroid, which often occurs along with menopause, and which also can cause the weight gain, fatigue, joint aches, and sleeping problems that may be attributed to menopause.

HOT FLASHES

The most effective way to stop hot flashes (and joint pains) is with estrogen. But for women who would prefer to avoid hormone replacement, there are some alternatives as discussed below.

Lifestyle changes. A diet rich in soy protein may decrease hot flashes. A recent study found that eating half a cup of soy nuts divided into three or four portions throughout the day, along with a healthy diet, can cut hot flashes by half (Welty et al. 2007b). Avoiding dietary triggers such as caffeine, alcohol, and spicy foods can reduce hot flashes. Another interesting study found that eating in general suppressed hot flashes for about ninety minutes; the resurgence of the hot flash correlated with the drop in blood sugar (Dormier and Howham 2007). That doesn't mean you should eat all day, but try stretching your daily calories over five small meals throughout the day.

Exercise, too, is important. Because women who are overweight are more likely to have hot flashes, exercise can reduce their body mass index and potentially decrease the number of flashes (Whiteman et al. 2003). Using cooling devices can also be helpful. Dr. J always has a portable handheld fan from Sharper Image in her purse (although paper fans will do in a pinch). It is also important to layer your clothes for the quick on and off (and back on again) that has to be done, and *never* wear wool!

Dr. J's Story.

A few years ago when I had just started to have hot flashes, I bought myself the little portable fan mentioned earlier and carried it everywhere. One evening at a large dinner party, all was going well until the end of the meal, when I started having hot flashes big time. No hiding it. I could just feel my hair sticking in clumps to my head, and sweat dripping into my eyes. So I did what I had always done in that situation. I took out my trusty little fan and starting using it. The woman sitting next to me was about my age, had never seen one, was fascinated, and just had to try the fan. Then several other women from the other end of the table came over to look at it. The low buzz of the excited voices of these pre- peri-, and postmenopausal women was suddenly interrupted by the displeased voice of our hostess, a lovely eighty-year-old, directed right at me. "Frankly, Dr. Horn, I'm shocked. I've always liked you so much, until you brought out that…thing. We do not discuss those issues in public." She had barely gotten the words out when another voice piped up and said, "Oh don't be such a stuffy gussie." And who was this speaking in my defense? The hostess's ninety-eight-year-old mother!

I sure learned about the difference in attitudes toward menopause that night. But do you think I gave up my fan after that? No way! I was just more careful about where I went to dinner until my menopause was over!

Medications. The groups of antidepressants known as the SSRIs (selective serotonin reuptake inhibitors), such as Paxil (paroxetine) and Prozac (fluoxetine), and the SNRIs (serotonin-norepinephrine reuptake inhibitors), such as Cymbalta (duloxetine) and Effexor (venlafaxine), have been found to reduce the number of hot flashes when compared to a placebo (Nelson et al. 2006). Tibolone, a synthetic steroid not yet available in the U.S., has been used successfully in Europe and Asia for the past twenty years to treat hot flashes, night sweats, vaginal dryness, and bone loss.

Herbs and supplements. The three main types of natural estrogens found in plant foods (phytoestrogens) are the isoflavones, the coumestans, and the lignans. Studies of the foods that contain these have shown they are of no help in relieving hot flashes. Black cohosh is the most popular supplement used to treat hot flashes, although the studies looking at its effectiveness have been conflicting. However, Dr. R found that Remifemin (a popular black cohosh preparation) helped with her hot flashes. (See chapter 13 for further discussion of black cohosh.)

CAM therapies. Acupuncture may be of benefit in reducing the severity of hot flashes (Nir et al. 2007). Since it is relatively safe, it is worth trying. It is also helpful for joint aches. There is also a study showing that meditation can be helpful in reducing the number of hot flashes (Freedman and Woodward 1992).

VAGINAL PROBLEMS

Vaginal lubricants, such as Replens, can be used on a regular basis to relieve vaginal dryness. Others, such as K-Y personal lubricant, K-Y Liquibeads, and Astroglide, can provide lubrication during sexual intercourse. None of these creams contain estrogen. Estrogen cream or tablets inserted into the vagina are also helpful; these are only minimally absorbed into the bloodstream. A ring, Estring, that is inserted every three months, delivers tiny amounts of estrogen on a daily basis.

SEX AND LIBIDO

Other common menopausal complaints have to do with almost all aspects of sex, including new-onset pain during intercourse, decreased enjoyment of sex or a diminished sexual response, and complete loss of interest in having sex.

Pain or discomfort during sex. Correcting vaginal dryness, as discussed above, can help ease the discomfort that may occur with menopause caused by the thrusting during sex. If, however, you feel pelvic pain with sex, that most likely is due to another problem. (See the section "Pain: Abdominal or Pelvic" in chapter 6.)

Decreased libido or sexual responsiveness. If your interest in sex is low or has decreased due to menopause, get your testosterone level checked; if it's low, adding a little testosterone may make a difference. In the form of a cream that is applied to the inner thigh or pubic area in small doses, it can also help restore the intensity of orgasms and sexual response. Your clinician should monitor your testosterone level before you grow a beard from taking too much! Several other sexual enhancement creams are available over-the-counter, such as Zestra, Excite, and O'My, all of which contain an amino acid called L-arginine, which improves blood flow to the genital areas. Although there are no large studies, many women find these creams help to increase the sensation of, and the ease of reaching, orgasm. Some contain menthol and peppermint to produce sensations of heat and tingling, but some women find these ingredients irritating.

A supplement called ArginMax, containing L-arginine, ginseng, ginkgo, damiana, vitamins, and minerals, improved both desire and the level of satisfaction with sex, especially in those who were postmenopausal, in a study of over 100 women (Ito et al. 2006). This supplement can cause genital herpes infections to flare, and shouldn't be used if you have this infection. The recommended dosage is six tabs per day, and it takes two to four weeks to work. If there is no improvement after six weeks, it isn't going to work. The use of Viagra and medications like it is currently being studied. If you want to try ArginMax or Viagra, talk to your doctor first to make sure it is safe to take with the other medications you're on.

In addition to the creams and supplements described above, the devices commonly known as vibrators (sometimes called "intimate massagers") are designed to increase the blood flow to the genital area, and thus assist in achieving orgasm. In fact, all of these aids are easily found these days, which shows how common the problem is and how popular a treatment these have become.

One of the major factors affecting sexual response and desire is what goes on in our brains. If we are stressed, upset, tired, and cranky, sex is the farthest thing from our minds. You need to explain that to your significant other. Try to have regular date nights when you can relax, be pampered, and get in the mood. If you've lost interest in sex since your menopause started, talk to your clinician. Don't be embarrassed or just write it off. There may well be another medical reason for it that can be easily treated. Sex is a good thing. It helps us to connect with our loved ones or ourselves, as the case may be. Having an orgasm releases endorphins into our system, boosts the immune system, and provides a sense of well-being. Please note: These effects result whether we achieve orgasm with a partner or by ourselves.

SLEEP

Avoid caffeine and alcohol at least several hours before bedtime. Keep your bedroom cool. Use several layers of blankets, so that you can remove or add one at a time depending on your fluctuating body temperature. See chapter 14 for meditation and relaxation techniques.

MENTAL-PAUSE

First, make sure that there is not another reason, besides menopause, for your brain fog, such as an underactive thyroid. If there is no other reason, several things can help, including stress reduction techniques, exercise, and talk therapy. Learning how to nurture yourself is also very important. (See chapter 1 for more ideas on improving brain fog.)

BODY CHANGES

The best way to slow down or stop the body changes associated with menopause, from weight gain to bone loss, is... exercise! See chapter 11 for specifics on exercise.

HORMONE REPLACEMENT THERAPY: FRIEND OR FOE?

Before we talk about the benefits and risks of hormones, let's first talk about the players. What are these hormones we are talking about?

Estrogen. Actually made up of a group of hormones—estradiol, estriol, and estrone—much of the body's estrogen is made in the ovaries by developing egg follicles. It is the main sex hormone for women and is responsible for regulating our menstrual cycles and for developing our secondary sex characteristics (breasts and pubic hair). It also can cause fluid retention, increase the risk of breast cancer, raise HDL cholesterol and triglyceride levels, and lower LDL cholesterol levels.

Progesterone. Produced by the ovaries (and the placenta during pregnancy), progesterone also helps to regulate our menstrual cycle and works to make our body fertile. Birth control pills use a synthetic form of progesterone called progestin to trick the body into thinking it's pregnant and thus prevent ovulation. Progesterone (not progestin) boosts the immune system, reduces swelling, prevents inflammation of blood vessels, stimulates the thyroid and keeps bones strong and nerves functioning normally.

Testosterone. Although considered a "male" hormone, testosterone is produced in the ovaries in small amounts. In men and women it prompts the growth of body hair. The drop in the testosterone level that occurs with aging can result in mood swings, loss of sex drive, fatigue, and muscle loss; replacement to premenopausal levels can reverse all of these.

Dehydroepiandrosterone (DHEA). Made in the adrenal glands, DHEA can be converted into estrogen, progesterone, and testosterone. It is suggested that DHEA may have beneficial effects on the changes of aging; however no long-term studies have been done.

The Controversy: The Women's Health Initiative Study

Since the release of the results from the Women's Health Initiative (WHI) study, there has been much confusion regarding the safety of hormone replacement therapy.

THE PURPOSE OF THE STUDY

The purpose of the study, begun in 1997, was to look at the overall health benefits and risks of hormone therapy in postmenopausal women in the U.S., with special attention given to coronary artery disease, breast cancer, colon cancer, and fractures.

THE PARTICIPANTS AND DESIGN OF THE STUDY

In this study, the average age of the participants was sixty-three. Although healthy overall, many of the women were being treated for high blood pressure and high cholesterol. More than 16,000 women with intact uteri were given either daily doses of 0.625 mg of Premarin (equine estrogen) and 2.5 mg of Provera (progestin) or daily placebo pills (sugar pills containing no medication). Over 10,000 women who'd had a hysterectomy were given 0.625 mg of Premarin alone or a placebo.

THE RESULTS

+ In 2002, the study was stopped early when researchers found an increase in breast cancer, heart attacks, and strokes in the women who were taking combination hormones compared to the women taking placebo pills.

+ The finding that the women who were given hormones and were over sixty-five had twice the rate of dementia as those receiving placebo pills was worrisome as well.

+ Interestingly, the women who were on Premarin alone (those who'd had a hysterectomy prior to the study) had no increase in breast cancer or heart disease. They did, however, have an increased risk of benign proliferative breast disease, which can cause the breasts to become more dense and lumpy, making mammograms and breast exams more difficult to interpret. In addition, this type of breast disease may put one at increased risk for breast cancer. Also of note, this part of the study was stopped early (in 2004) due to an increased risk of stroke in these women.

+ Also interesting was the finding that the younger women, ages fifty to fifty-nine, who were placed on hormones within ten years of their menopause, had no increased risk of heart attack; in fact, these women had less evidence of heart disease than women in the same age group who did not take hormones (Manson, Allison, and Rossouw 2007).

Bottom line: After the results came out, the medical and research communities had many concerns about the design of the study. Here's what we do know from this research: The study was done in older women to see if hormone therapy could prevent heart disease and dementia, and we now know that it did not prevent either. But it did show that hormone therapy was safe, in terms of heart disease, for younger women if taken within ten years of menopause.

Other Issues of Hormone Replacement Therapy

As mentioned above, the WHI study raised important practical questions.

Synthetic versus natural hormones. Most doctors and studies do not distinguish between Provera (medroxyprogesterone acetate, or MPA), which is synthetic, and natural progesterone. They are not the same; one is man-made and the other is found in nature. Studies show there are differences. The risk of breast cancer is lessened with natural progesterone when compared to MPA (Greendale et al. 1999). The risk of developing a blood clot goes up with MPA and not with natural progesterone. Natural progesterone has a positive effect on good and bad cholesterol; MPA does not (Writing Group from the PEPI Trial 1995). In a study of nearly 100,000 women in France, those on estrogen alone had a 30 percent increased risk of developing breast cancer. When natural progesterone was used in combination, there was no increased risk of developing breast cancer; when synthetic progestin (such as MPA) was used along with estrogen, the breast cancer risk went up by almost 50 percent (Wood et al. 2007). **Bottom line:** Natural progesterone is safer overall than synthetic progesterone.

Pill versus the patch or gel. The French study mentioned above also found that transdermal estrogen, delivered by patch or gel through the skin, did not increase the development of blood clots in postmenopausal women, while estrogen in pill form did. Natural or micronized progesterone used in association with this was also safe (Scarabin, Oger, and Plu-Bureau 2003). Therefore, the transdermal form, rather than the pill, may be a better alternative for women who are at risk for heart problems, blood clot, or stroke.

Your Choices for Hormone Replacement Therapy

Most physicians agree now that hormone replacement therapy can be safely used at the time of menopause, for a period of five years or less, to treat severe symptoms of menopause in women who have no risk factors for breast cancer or stroke. If you are bothered by hot flashes, vaginal dryness, insomnia, or moodiness, or you are at risk for bone loss, you might want to talk to your doctor about hormone treatment. If your uterus has not been removed, you need to be on both estrogen and progesterone to prevent the buildup of the uterine lining, which increases the risk of getting uterine cancer. It is important to carefully discuss with your clinician the benefits versus the risks to *you*.

Forms of estrogen. This hormone comes in several forms; the most commonly used are Premarin and bioidentical estrogen. The standard dose of Premarin pills is 0.625 mg/day by mouth. The body sees bioidentical hormones as a match to your hormones. The pill form is estradiol; the standard dose is 1 mg/day. Another way to get this type of estrogen is to have a pharmacist compound it for you in the dose and form that you and your doctor prefer. Compounded medication is not regulated; however, it is available from registered pharmacists who are regulated. It can be compounded in pill, patch, cream, gel and drop forms, and as troches (these go under your tongue). One of the pharmaceutical brands is Vivelle-Dot patch.

Types of progesterone. The pharmaceutical brand of natural progesterone is Prometrium, which is taken at 100 to 200 mg per day. If you don't want to take estrogen, you can try this hormone alone for possible relief of hot flashes and sleeping disturbances. Compounded progesterone can be made in cream, capsule, lozenge, or drop form.

Testosterone. This is usually prescribed in a low-dose cream that is relatively safe.

DHEA. This can be found as an OTC supplement. It is relatively safe, *but you need to let your doctor know you are taking it.* High doses lead to liver problems and acne.

When to Start Hormones and How Long to Take Them

It is now thought to be a safe option for a woman within ten years of her menopause and not at high risk for breast cancer or stroke to take estrogen and progesterone replacement therapy for relief of severe menopausal symptoms for no longer than five years. If you decide that you are going to take hormones, it is mandatory that you optimize all of your risk factors for heart disease and breast cancer by not smoking, maintaining a normal blood pressure, and getting yearly mammograms (Rossouw et al. 2007), and that you see your clinician every year for your routine screening exams, including a breast and pelvic exam. There are no recommendations regarding how long to take testosterone and DHEA.

FURTHER THOUGHTS

As unique individuals, we experience changes in our own way, and we deal with these changes in our own way. Our recommendation is to find what works for you in consultation with your clinician. For Dr. R, hormones work great. Because of her medical history, Dr. J used other methods to help her through menopause and is not a fan of hormones (although she is a fan of fans!). It is important to find a doctor who will work with you and help you in your own "adventure" through menopause. Also, please bear in mind that we wrote the recommendations above in early 2008; by the time you read this book, they may have changed yet again.

THE DOCS CHAT ABOUT MENOPAUSE

DR. J: I know you take hormones. Why did you decide to take them?

DR. R: I was having so many hot flashes a day, I thought I was personally responsible for global warming, and I couldn't sleep. That was rough! My family gently suggested that I needed something for my moodiness. What a difference a few days on hormones made. I decided to use the Vivelle-Dot patch (I love my patch) and the natural progesterone tablets under my tongue. I feel like a new woman.

DR. J: You had a hysterectomy, so why do you take progesterone?

DR. R: Although it is usually recommended only along with the estrogen when the uterus is intact (to protect against endometrial cancer), I thought that it might be helpful to take it after looking at what natural progesterone can do. It is the "feel good" hormone of pregnancy, so it helps my mood and it also helps me to sleep. Since I have a family history of osteoporosis, it also helps my bones. I know you don't take hormones. Why not?

DR: J: Never did, never will. With my particular physical makeup, hormones and I just don't get along. I have migraines, which got much worse when I took birth control pills many moons ago. So I don't want to chance that. I have a family history of breast cancer, and whether or not the study discussed in this chapter was flawed, I'm not willing to take the risk. There is no osteoporosis in my family, and my baseline bone density scan was normal, so I didn't feel I needed hormones for that reason. Though my menopausal symptoms were fairly severe, especially the hot flashes and insomnia, the symptoms were not disruptive enough to me to chance taking the hormones. The broader issue for me is that I still don't think we know as much as we should about the long-term effects of hormones. I don't have a problem, though, with others who have the appropriate physical makeup and family history—like you!—taking them for a limited period of time, provided that they have discussed all the risks and benefits with a knowledgeable clinician and are regularly followed medically.

Pearls of Wisdom for Dealing with Menopause

○ Menopause is not a disease.

○ If you are tired, gaining weight, and achy, make sure you have your thyroid checked.

○ Don't blame any new symptoms you have on menopause; get them checked out.

○ Find out what combination of medications works best for you.

○ If you want to take hormones, discuss the benefits and risks for your particular physical makeup, as well as the best form for you (natural or synthetic; pill or patch) with your clinician; and then reevaluate your decision every year.

CHAPTER 11

Fitness and Food: Keep Your BMI Fine, Learn to Dine, and Avoid the Jiggle in Your Waistline

Have you ever been so involved in a story, watching a film or reading a book, that you wondered why the heroine was making the decisions that she was? Why, for instance, didn't she realize that she was doing things that were not good for her? That's exactly how we've both felt about our own bad habits in recent years, and how we've often felt about those of our patients in our age group and older. From the title of this chapter, you already know what we're talking about—the complex and related issues of body weight, physical activity, and eating.

We know how difficult these issues are to manage; if they weren't, there wouldn't be an obesity epidemic today. We also know that there seem to be millions of opinions and recommendations out there, all of which make these subjects even more confusing. We want to simplify them for you. Besides discussing physical activity, eating, and body weight, in this chapter we tell you about our own eating and exercise plans (some successful, some not so), as well as giving you simple ways to approach these all-important health issues. In addition, we discuss the common problems of type 2 diabetes, metabolic syndrome, and thyroid disease, and how they relate to your weight.

PHYSICAL ACTIVITY AND YOUR MATURING BODY

For many of us the word "exercise" has negative associations. For Dr. J, it brings to mind all those years of gym class in school, and how she dreaded it. Besides hating gym itself, she was terrified of getting hit in the face (she didn't want her coke-bottle-thick eyeglasses to break) with a ball—be it a tennis ball, football, basketball, or volleyball. She either hid in the locker room hoping all the teams would be picked or tried to come up with an excuse to miss gym that day. (Despite that, she is proud to say that she never got lower than a B, because she always scored high on the "Tries Hard" part of the evaluation.) And unlike Dr. R, who was inspired by President Kennedy's program for physical fitness in the early 1960s, which spurred her on to doing regular physical activities for the rest of her life, all that Dr. J remembers of that program is the government-endorsed song produced to accompany children while they did the approved workout routines in class, the "Chicken Fat Song." (Remember "Go, you chicken fat, go"?)

So we won't call it exercise here. Neither are we going to refer to it by any of those other clinical-sounding names, like "workout" or "physical activity." We'll just call it "moving." Simple and to the point.

Why Moving Is So Important to Your Health

Movement and mobility are so important to the quality of life. We've already told you about studies that have shown how important physical activity is to retaining memory (chapter 1), maintaining balance (chapter 2), the health of your heart (chapter 3), and your musculoskeletal system (chapter 8). You already know the relationship between moving and your weight. However (and this may surprise you, just as it surprised us), a recent study that followed more than 2,500 people over the age of sixty for an average period of twelve years found that those who were fit, whether they were overweight or not, had a significantly lower death rate than those who were not fit (Sui et al. 2007). So, being fit is every bit as important as being at a healthy weight. Also, regular physical activity has been shown to help psychological health and well-being, increase longevity, increase your basal metabolic rate, suppress your appetite, help you sleep better, decrease the risk of common chronic diseases that tend to occur more often with aging, lessen many of the physiologic bodily changes that occur with aging, and help to prevent and treat disability (Singh 2004). Does it sound like a magic bullet? It is. If we were to tell you that there was a pill that could do all these things, wouldn't you take it (and buy stock in the company that makes it) without hesitation?

Why Doesn't Everyone Do It?

If you happen to be one of those women who either loves to do regular physical activity or doesn't like it but is still disciplined about doing it, accept our congratulations. The following does not apply to you. But if you have trouble doing regular exercise, you are not alone. In recent years, surveys have shown that nearly one-third of American adults do not do any regular exercise, and that almost half do not meet the activity levels recommended by government agencies (Bonow and Gheorghiade 2004).

Given all the positive and lifesaving effects of regular physical activity, why doesn't everyone do it? Both of us have observed that many of our very smart patients do not, in fact, exercise regularly, even though they're concerned about their health. And although she hates to admit it, Dr. J falls into that category. Because this is the case for her, she will take over this section.

Many of my patients have told me that the recommendations for exercise or for eating properly are so complicated that they just don't have the desire to wade through them. Add to that the fact that many people don't enjoy being active physically, or *think* that they don't enjoy it (me included), so they either don't make it a priority or cannot sustain a routine of regular physical activity, despite knowing on some level that it's good for them.

I think the reasons for this are complicated; at least they are for me. One is that during the twentieth century, we became spoiled about instant gratification; in other words, we like to do things for which we see results quickly. We like, and have become used to, instantly prepared food from microwaves and instant communication through the use of cell phones and e-mail. We have no patience or time (so we think) for a long, drawn-out program, particularly if it's not enjoyable. Also, we like to tackle a problem, find the solution, and be done with it—not to have to keep working at it forever so it is incorporated into our daily lives, which is the way a fitness program should be.

Another reason is that in our younger years, keeping fit used to be a "nice" thing to do; good for our health, yes, but not crucial. In recent years, the knowledge about the beneficial effects of physical activity for our health has mushroomed. It's no longer a "nice to do"; it has become a "must do." If we don't keep reminding ourselves how beneficial and necessary physical activity is to our health, we forget; instead we see it as just one more chore and make it our lowest priority, so that the first thing to go when we get busy is our exercise routine.

The final reason is what Robin and I mentioned in the introduction of this book. Virtually all the women we know, ourselves included, have always been so busy taking care of others that we neglect ourselves. This may be due to lack of time or it may just be habit. Whatever the reason, most of us have not done a great job of taking care of ourselves.

All of these reasons are true for me. My life, like yours, is very busy and crowded with things I have to do to keep it humming along. I don't have the desire or discipline to do things that don't immediately affect my life, especially if they aren't fun to do. Therefore, in the past when I was given recommendations for a fitness regimen by my doctor or a colleague, I either filed it in my brain, thinking I would get to it eventually, or I put it into action immediately—but quickly stopped doing it. I did this despite the fact that I've always told every one of my patients how important it is. Simply put, I know the reasons why exercise is so important, I just don't keep thinking about them in terms of my own health. If I did, then I wouldn't stop doing it.

Regularly moving is crucial to our long-term health, especially now that we're older. Like breathing, we need to move regularly to live. Unlike breathing, we won't die quickly if we stop exercising, which makes it easier to stop doing it after a while. Another example is wearing seat belts. Don't you automatically put them on when you get into the car, even though it can be a pain? (If you don't, you should.) Perhaps an even better analogy is that of brushing your teeth. Aren't you fairly regular about doing that? Have you ever stopped to think why? It's either because this habit was drummed into your head since you were little, or because you know on some level that if you don't, you will eventually have gum disease and lose your teeth. We must learn to think the same way about physical activity (not that you'll lose your teeth if you don't do it, but that there will be health consequences).

Robin and I believe that you'll be most successful at keeping yourself healthy as the years pass if you understand the reasons for our recommendations, and if those recommendations are simple and easy to understand. So now I will tell you what finally worked for me.

First, I found several physical activities that I actually like to do, like dancing to old disco tunes, walking the hills of my neighborhood, and riding my exercise bike while reading gossip magazines. Second, I remind myself regularly of the positive benefits of physical activity for my health. Third, when the idea of maintaining my own good health isn't enough to keep me moving regularly, I think about my loved ones, an event coming up, or all the books I still want to read, and how I would like to be around and in good health for a long time to enjoy all these good things. Fourth, I make a conscious effort everytime I finish a session, to note how good I feel afterward. Do I do regular physical activity without fail? No, but I now do much more in any given week than I used to do.

So we're back to the four A's we've discussed throughout this book. We need to be *aware* of how important regularly moving our bodies is to our health, be *alert* to our own boredom or desire to stop the exercising, take *action* to keep moving, and *advocate* for ourselves when other life activities compete for our time.

TYPES OF PHYSICAL ACTIVITY

Thus far, we've talked about moving in generalized terms. But there are actually four different types of physical activity that you need to be doing at this age.

Aerobic exercise. When we refer to "exercise," what we all usually think of is the aerobic, cardio, or endurance type of physical activity—the type of exercise that gets your heart pumping and your pulse climbing in the short term, in order to get the heart muscles stronger and the pulse slower in the long term. This type of activity can reduce high blood pressure, improve your lipid profile, decrease your risk of heart disease, keep your brain active, and improve function in the various types of arthritis, among other benefits. Examples of this type of exercise are jogging, walking, swimming, and bicycle riding. If you have pain or osteoarthritis in your knees or hips but like walking, try Nordic walking. This is walking for fitness with the use of specifically designed long poles similar to the ski poles used for cross-country skiing (though shorter in length). Many people have found that their knee or hip pain is relieved through use of these poles, which work by shifting part of the body weight from the joints of the walker's legs to the upper body. The poles are available at sporting goods stores. (Thanks Annie!)

Strength training. This type of exercise is also known as resistance training. It builds muscle strength, helps to build bone, reduces disability, improves the daily functioning of our bodies, increases metabolism, and more recently has been shown to aid in keeping the heart healthy. The most common example of this type is weight lifting. This type of exercise also firms your body.

Balance training. The third type of exercise is balance training. It is known to greatly reduce the risk of falls (Tinetti et al. 1994), improve thigh muscle strength, and improve overall functionality. An example of this type of exercise is tai chi. Another way to improve your balance is to do your weight training while standing on a BOSU trainer. Also known as a BOSU ball, it is a rubber device that looks like a huge beach ball cut in half. One side is inflated, just like a ball, and the other side is flat and rigid. When you stand on either side, it provides an unstable surface that forces you to maintain your balance, and while doing so, strengthens the lower half of your body. Dr. J loves the BOSU ball thanks to her excellent trainer (thanks, Jessica!), but Dr. R hates it.

Flexibility training. The last type of exercise, which is also the least studied, is flexibility training. The more flexible we are, the less likely we are to be injured. The classic example of this type of exercise is stretching, although yoga and Pilates are helpful too. These last two practices also help to strengthen our core, or the middle section of our bodies, which helps both balance and flexibility.

RECOMMENDATIONS FOR REGULAR PHYSICAL ACTIVITY

The official recommendations by the American Heart Association and the American College of Sports Medicine for the amount of physical activity necessary to improve and maintain our health include both aerobic activity and muscle-strengthening activity (Nelson et al. 2007).

Recommendations for aerobic activity. These recommendations advise aerobic activity of moderate intensity for thirty minutes daily, five days a week. Alternatively, one can do aerobic activity of vigorous intensity for twenty minutes a day, three days a week. How are "moderate" and "vigorous" intensity defined? Vigorous intensity is when you are pushing yourself as hard and as fast as you can; moderate is somewhat less than that. Here is a useful tip: With moderate intensity exercise, you should be able to talk and exercise at the same time. It is acceptable to break up your exercise sessions into three ten-minute intervals throughout the day to reach a total of thirty minutes a day of moderate-intensity activity.

What should you do specifically? Climb up those steps at work for ten minutes at a time; take the dog for a thirty-minute walk up a nearby hill; take your grandchild (or borrow your neighbor's) in her stroller and jog in an empty parking lot for ten to twenty minutes. You're clever and inventive—mix it up! Make it a priority.

Recommendations for muscle-strengthening activity. Recommendations for this type of activity include doing eight to ten exercises involving the major muscle groups, with eight to twelve repetitions each, at least twice a week. You can use free weights, a barbell, a machine that simulates weight lifting by resistance, or elastic resistance bands.

Recommendations for flexibility and balance. Recommendations for balance and flexibility type exercises include at least two days a week for those at risk for falls. Here, we disagree with the official recommendations. We would have everyone incorporate balance, flexibility, and core exercises into their regular routine at least two days a week, because we all are at risk for falls.

A FINAL THOUGHT ABOUT REGULAR PHYSICAL ACTIVITY

We've often heard comments from our patients that go something like this: "I'm too old to change my lifestyle, and what good will it do me at this age anyway?" Or, "I've never been athletic, or a jock, like my friends; I can't start now." We have an answer to these comments. A recent study was done with more than 15,000 middle-aged adults who were divided into two groups: One group adopted four healthier habits, including eating five or more servings of fruits and vegetables each day, regular exercise, maintaining their weight within a reasonable range, and not smoking; the other group did not adopt any new behaviors for a healthier lifestyle. Over the next four years, total deaths and heart attacks were much lower for the group that engaged in healthier habits (King 2007). This study shows that it's never too late to begin a program of eating healthy and engaging in physical activity, to receive health and longevity benefits from these changes.

EATING WELL

Are we really supposed to tell you, in this one section in this one chapter, *all* you need to know about eating and nutrition and calories and carbs as you keep having birthdays? Of course not. And are the recommendations for eating well to stay healthy at this age really that different from those we've seen

Dr. J and Dr. R's Eating Habits, Part 1

In school and in training, we didn't always eat as well as we do now. When Janet was in training and on call every other, or every third, night in the hospital, she ate what she fondly referred to as the "VM diet." Can you guess what that stands for? The vending machine diet!

Robin's eating habits were not quite as bad as Janet's because she bought her food from the grocery store, so at least she knew how fresh it was. Her regular and favorite meal? A bowl of popcorn! Although sometimes she would supplement that with a Caesar salad (heavy on the croutons). Read on to learn about the effects of these diets.

in the past? To answer that, we can tell you that the official dietary guidelines put out by the government in 2005 recognized Americans over fifty as a specific group that needed specific nutritional recommendations for the first time (USDHHS 2005).

We hope to simplify this subject by having you understand your body's changing nutritional needs as you get older. We feel fairly confident that we can do this because in recent years we've each been through some radical changes in our own eating patterns.

What Happens to Our Nutritional Needs as We Age?

Remember when you were asked out on a date for the following weekend and you could lose five pounds the week before? No more. Our bodies change both in composition and needs as we grow older. Not only does the percentage of body fat increase with age, but the distribution of that body fat shifts, with most of it being deposited in the trunk.

To add insult to injury, there is a natural decline in muscle and fluid mass as we age (that is, if you do not do regular strengthening exercises). And even worse, our *metabolic rate* (the rate at which we metabolize the nutrients in foods into the energy our body uses) decreases as the years pass. This means that we don't need as much food to function as we used to, and that if we continue to eat the same amount as when we were younger, we will gain weight. Moreover, there are changes in other parts of the body that affect our food intake, including a decrease in the motility of the GI tract, an increased likelihood of constipation, and a possible decrease in our sense of smell, taste, or appetite, to name a few. These can lead to our avoiding certain foods that are nutritious and eating those that are not.

Bottom line: Gaining weight is easier to do now than it used to be, and losing it is tougher. And because many of us are usually too busy to think about what we put in our mouths, we've been able to get in enough calories, just not enough *nutritious* calories (Noel and Reddy 2005).

Calories. Because there is a decrease in our metabolic rate as we grow older, as mentioned above, there must also be a decrease in the number of calories we need to take in. If not, any calories not used by our body as energy will be stored as fat. It is estimated that for each decade of life, there is a decrease in the needed number of calories of 2 to 5 percent (Andres 1995). Counting calories may be the simplest way to figure out how much you can eat each day without gaining weight.

Remember, when you're calculating the calories you need, you also should factor in how much physical activity you will be doing. The more active you are, the more calories you can take in over your baseline needs. One quick way to estimate the *baseline calories* you need (that is, the number you need if you do no physical activity) is to multiply your body weight in pounds by ten. So, if you weigh 145 pounds, you can eat approximately 1,450 calories a day. Please remember though, this is a rough estimate as each person's metabolic rate varies. The lowest number of daily calories you can safely eat is the product of your body weight in pounds times eight. So if you weigh 145 pounds and you need to lose weight, the number of calories you need daily is 1,160, a difference of only 270 calories. To lose one pound a week, you need to decrease your calories by 500 a day. You can easily do that by cutting out 250 calories in food a day and working off another 250 calories a day with exercise.

Carbohydrates. What exactly is a carbohydrate? Simple—it's a sugar. *Complex carbohydrates*, also known as starches, are those foods, such as grains, in which many sugars are bonded together so that the body has to work harder to digest them; it takes a while for the sugars to get into the bloodstream and then to be used by the body as energy. *Simple carbs* are either smaller molecules of one sugar, or smaller sugars that are easily and quickly absorbed in large amounts into the bloodstream. Because our cells don't usually need the amount of energy that simple sugars provide, simple carbs are more likely to be converted into fat than complex carbs are. Sugar, in its simple carb form, has become such a common part of eating only in recent centuries. Think back to cavewomen. No pure sugar was available then; they got their carbs for energy through fruits and grains they collected. Today, the amount of pure sugar and simple carbs we eat is responsible in large part for the epidemics of diabetes and obesity.

As we age, based on the changes in our body composition, we also need to *decrease* the amounts, and change the type of, carbohydrates we eat. This often comes as a surprise to our patients because the emphasis in this country for years has been on low-fat diets, mainly due to the association of certain types of fat with heart disease. During this same time period, not much has been said about limiting carbohydrates except to those with diabetes. Recently, a study of over 15,000 women confirmed prior studies and showed that a diet with too many carbs is also associated with increased cardiovascular risk, including heart disease and strokes (Hu 2007). So, eating that entire tray of brownies or a package of Tollhouse chocolate chip cookie dough (Dr. J's former favorite) is not benign, for either your heart or your arteries, or your waistline.

We advise avoiding refined sugars or simple carbohydrates, and eating complex carbs. Specifically, stay away from baked goods, white bread, candy, and ice cream; take care of that sweet tooth with fruits high in fiber, such as apples or pears. How do you know which are high in fiber? Simple—just think, the crunchier, the better.

Dr. J and Dr. R's Eating Habits, Part 2

For a long time after our training, we each were suffering with what we thought was an unusual degree of fatigue. Interestingly, neither of us discussed it with the other until recently. Although Robin was good about exercising and keeping her weight stable, she wasn't at all conscious of the nutritional value of the food she was eating. She knew exactly how many calories she needed each day to keep her weight stable, but she would eat French fries or popcorn as a meal, just as long as what she ate did not go over her daily calorie restrictions. However, after she completed her fellowship training with Dr Andrew Weil, in which she learned the importance of eating nutritious food, she decided she had better start taking the advice she gave to her patients and completely changed her way of eating. She was shocked at the unexpected benefit of eating nutritiously; her fatigue completely disappeared.

Although Janet had stopped eating from vending machines (only because there weren't any in her office building), she still didn't think about what she ate. She had her own solo practice by this time, so eating was simply something she had to do from one day to the next, and she neither counted calories nor thought about nutrition. Neither was she was exercising regularly. No time! Intermittently, she would try to lose the weight that, inevitably, she had gained by eating so poorly by going on the Atkins diet (high in protein, very low in carbs). During this phase, she got into the habit of considering all carbs as bad and staying away from fruits. You can probably guess the results of this: A weight that kept going up and down, increasing fatigue, and poor nutritional intake. This went on until one day after a routine physical, her blood tests returned showing almost all of the values as abnormal. She got scared, sought the advice of her physician, started exercising regularly, and, most importantly, began to think about every bite of food she put into her mouth. To her amazement, she lost weight—even while eating fruit, which astonished her. After maintaining this healthy regimen for several months, her fatigue also lessened.

Fats. Since the composition of the body changes with age to contain more fat, we need to eat less fat in our food. But remember, just as with carbohydrates, there are good and bad fats. Saturated and trans fats are the bad fats. In fact, trans fats have proven to be so bad for our hearts that the New York City Board of Health considers them a bona fide health hazard and has passed a mandate limiting their use in the restaurants of the city, as of July 1, 2007. Bakers and makers of deep-fried doughnuts have until July 1, 2008, to stop using trans fats and find an alternative (Okie 2007).

Here's an easy way to remember which are which. The good fats are usually from plant or vegetable sources. Examples of good fats are olive oil, flaxseed oil, and almond oil. Fish oil is also a good fat. Saturated fats are mostly from animal sources, such as meat and full-fat dairy products. Trans fats are usually made when hydrogen is added to vegetable oil by manufacturers in order to increase the stability of the flavor and the shelf life of the foods containing these fats. Trans fats can be found in many snack foods, margarines, vegetable shortenings, and some fried foods. Naturally occurring trans fat may be found in some animal-based foods, though in very small amounts.

Proteins. The good news about protein is that our needs change very little as we grow older. This means you can still enjoy protein in your diet, the recommended daily amount being approximately 1 gram of protein per kilogram (kg) of your body weight (to find your weight in kilograms, divide your weight in pounds by 2.2).

Recommendations: What and How to Eat

We are not going to give you a specific diet plan here, but will tell you the principles that can make eating at this age simple, easy, and nutritious. You pick the individual foods according to your own likes and dislikes. Make your daily eating plan fresh, colorful, and varied. Eat small portions spread out over the day, and include only good carbs and fats. Make sure you drink between eight and eleven eight-ounce glasses of fluid a day (this includes water and tea, and some coffee), and specifically avoid processed food and sweets (simple carbs), and cut back on animal fats. These principles are a simplified version of the key recommendations from the 2005 governmental report on eating (USDHHS 2005).

One example of a specific eating plan that meets these criteria is the Mediterranean diet. Traditionally, dietary patterns of the Mediterranean cultures, such as Greece, Crete, parts of Italy, and southern France, usually include an abundance of natural whole foods, especially fruits, vegetables, and nuts, as well as olive oil, fish, and moderate amounts of wine, while not including an overabundance of simple carbs. We both love this way of eating. It is so good for keeping your heart healthy that the American Heart Association endorsed it in 2001 (Kris-Etherton et al. 2001). A recent study that followed nearly 160,000 women over the age of fifty for ten years found that those who ate according to a Mediterranean-type diet plan had a 20 percent decreased risk of dying at a young age compared to those who did not eat this way (Mitrou et al. 2007). In addition, we were both pleased to see the results of an Italian study that showed that this diet improved sexual function in women with metabolic syndrome (Esposito et al. 2007). Since this was a small study, further work is needed to confirm it, but we certainly applaud the researchers for looking into this!

THE IMPORTANCE OF BODY MASS INDEX (BMI)

Losing pounds and maintaining an appropriate body weight is not about being a size 0 and looking like a supermodel; it's about staying healthy and functional and enjoying a good quality of life as those birthdays keep coming. Staying physically active and eating the right amount of nutritious foods is important to your health no matter what you look like. The consequences of not doing it can be deadly.

There are several simple measures used to assess body fat, including the measurement of abdominal girth, the waist-to-hip ratio measurement, and the easily calculated body mass index (BMI), which is a measure of your weight in relation to your height. Traditionally, BMI is the most commonly used, both in clinical practice and in research studies (to calculate your BMI, see below). By definition, you are *overweight* if your BMI is between 25 kg/m2 and 29.9 kg/m2. You are considered *obese* if your BMI is equal to or greater than 30 kg/m2. You are considered underweight if your BMI is less than 18.5 kg. Simply put, being overweight or obese refers to the fact that there is an excess amount of body fat, and being underweight means that there is too little body fat.

Calculating Your BMI

Here's how to calculate your BMI: your weight (in pounds) x 703/your height (in inches) squared. *Example:* Let's say you weigh 150 pounds and your height is 5 feet 4 inches, or 64 inches. 150 x 703 = 105,450, and 64 squared = 64 x 64= 4,096. Your BMI = 105,450/4096 = 25.7; you are slightly overweight.

A Word About Being Underweight

Being overweight or obese is far more common in women in our age group than being underweight. But having a low BMI can be just as dangerous. In a recent study in adults over the age of twenty-five, it was shown that those who were underweight (BMI less than 18.5 kg) had a significantly increased risk of dying from noncancer, noncardiovascular diseases (such as lung disease) than were those of normal weight (Flegal et al. 2007). Women who are small boned and underweight also have an increased risk of osteoporosis, which can lead to hip fractures and being bedridden. In addition, being underweight makes it more likely that you are not getting the nutrients you need, and thus that you will become undernourished. Those of you ladies who live by the saying that "you can never be too thin," think again. You definitely can.

How Common Is Obesity? Who Gets It?

There has been a dramatic increase in the number of overweight and obese adults in the U.S. over the past twenty years or so; approximately 60 percent of American adults are either overweight or obese. Specifically, 40 percent of Americans between the ages of sixty and sixty-nine are obese, as are 30 percent of those between the ages of seventy and seventy-nine. Equally as concerning is the fact that while more men are overweight than women, more women are obese than men (Jensen 2008). In addition, there is now considered to be an obesity epidemic worldwide.

What Causes Obesity?

Obesity is caused by an increase in body fat which then results in an increase in body weight. Simply put, we gain body fat by taking in more calories than we use up with physical activity. The components of those calories—whether from carbs, fats, or protein—matter as well, since eating more carbs and fats than protein leads to obesity.

You've probably heard that an increase in the size of your muscles can also cause an increase in your body weight. This occurs through an increase in physical activity, including lots of muscle-building exercises, such as lifting weights, and eating more protein, fewer carbs, and less fat. But weight gain due to an increase in muscle mass is obviously not the same as weight gain due to fat, especially in terms of the danger to your health that each type of body weight increase poses. The increase in body fat, or obesity, can be deadly; an increase in muscle mass most often is not.

A recent medical-sociological study observed that, in fact, one may be able to "catch" obesity from another person, much like one catches a cold. This clever research showed that if your close friend becomes obese, then your risk of becoming obese increases by 57 percent, greater even than if your partner or your sibling becomes obese (Christakis and Fowler 2007). This study demonstrates how important the social environment is to us, especially in our perceptions of body size, and our health habits, including eating and exercising (Barabasi 2007). What we think it also says is that we women are so in tune with our friends that when they eat, we eat. And when they gain weight, we do too. Therefore, the flip side should work as well; if you're having trouble eating well or staying physically active, ask a friend or two for help and support.

Why Is Being Overweight or Obese Bad for Your Health?

Being overweight or obese leads to many complications that can significantly impact your health in the following two ways: The first is that the actual mass of fat in your body can have physical effects on nearby body parts. One good example of this is *sleep apnea*, which is caused by an increase in the size of the fat deposits on either side of your pharynx, or throat. This can lead to the narrowing of that opening which can cause you to snore and, occasionally, can lead to its closing, which causes you to intermittently stop breathing. Another physical effect of increased weight is osteoarthritis. Greater wear and tear of the joints, especially the knee joints, occurs from carrying around an increased amount of fat (Bray 2004).

The second way that obesity leads to medical complications is this: The enlarged fat cells actually produce substances that cause changes throughout the body. Some of these changes include increased fat or sugar stored in the liver or muscle, leading to poor functionality; increased inflammation throughout the body (this plays a role in high blood pressure, stroke, and heart disease); increased production of estrogens by the fat mass (this may increase the risk of breast cancer); and shortened life expectancy (Bray 2004). In a British study of more than 1 million women aged fifty to sixty-four, researchers found a significant increase in cancer risk in those women with a higher BMI (Reeves et al. 2007). Two other important complications caused by being overweight are type 2 diabetes and metabolic syndrome.

TYPE 2 DIABETES

Just as there is an obesity epidemic in the U.S., so too is there an epidemic of type 2 diabetes. It is currently estimated that approximately 15 to 17 million Americans have diabetes, with almost a third of them unaware they have the disease. Among those Americans aged forty-five years or older, the number of cases of diabetes increased 170 percent between 1960 and 1990 (Bonow and Gheorghiade 2004).

What is diabetes? This chronic and incurable disease occurs when there is a total lack, or a decreased amount, of the hormone insulin in the body. Insulin, produced by the pancreas, is required to help glucose, or the sugar from food, get into the cells so that energy can be produced from the glucose. When insulin is decreased or absent, glucose can't get into the cells to produce energy, so it builds up in the bloodstream. Many short-term complications (dehydration, thirst, weight loss, fatigue) and long-term complications (see below) result. There are two types of diabetes: type 1, previously known as juvenile-onset diabetes, which occurs mostly in children and young adults and is caused by the body's failure to produce insulin, thought to be due to a viral infection of the pancreas, and type 2, caused by the body's inability to use the insulin, also known as insulin resistance.

How are obesity and type 2 diabetes related? There is a strong association between increased body fat and type 2 diabetes; the risk of type 2 diabetes increases as the body weight goes up—the higher the BMI, the greater the risk. This results from the body's resistance to insulin that occurs with excess weight. When this occurs, the body cannot use the insulin it has, which results in high blood sugar because the glucose cannot get into the cells. By the same token, weight loss reduces the risk of type 2 diabetes, and in many people, actually causes their blood sugar to return to normal.

Furthermore, the location of that extra body fat also matters; the more fat that is concentrated in the trunk of the body, the greater the risk. This is why people with an apple shape (fat concentrated more at the waist and abdomen than the hips and buttocks) are at greater risk for diabetes and heart disease than those with a pear shape (fat concentrated more in the buttocks and thighs than the abdomen). There is some thought that stress puts us women at increased risk of developing that dangerous extra abdominal fat (Epel et al. 2000). Stress causes high levels of the hormone cortisol to be produced from our adrenal glands, which then causes an increased amount of fat to accumulate in the abdominal area. This is under continued investigation.

Who gets type 2 diabetes? Are you at risk for it? Hispanic-Americans and African-Americans get diabetes at twice the rate of Caucasian-Americans. Native Americans are also experiencing an increase in the number of cases of diabetes (Bonow and Gheorghiade 2004). Risk factors for type 2 diabetes include a family history of diabetes, age over forty-five, long-term physical inactivity, poor diet (particularly a diet high in simple carbs), excess weight, high blood pressure, an abnormal lipid profile, polycystic ovary syndrome, and race and ethnicity. Also, if you had diabetes while you were pregnant, then you are at risk for developing it permanently at a later time.

A diet high in simple carbs has been shown to increase the risk of diabetes in African-American women independent of body weight or age (Krishnan et al. 2007). In this study, the specific foods eaten by approximately 40,000 African-American women were studied over eight years; those whose diet was high in simple carbs, regardless of their weight or age, had an increased risk for diabetes compared to women who ate a diet lower in carbs. A similar study in 64,000 Asian-American women over a five-year period found the same thing (Villegas et al. 2007).

How will you know if you have it? How is it diagnosed? Common symptoms of diabetes include increased thirst, increased need to urinate, and unintentional weight loss. Another frequent symptom is unexplained and severe fatigue. Some women get recurrent vaginal yeast infections. However, you can have this disease and have absolutely *no* symptoms. Very often, the fact that you have diabetes may be picked up when you get routine blood tests. When your blood sugar is unusually high, your symptoms can occur abruptly, and may even include passing out or becoming comatose; however, type 2 diabetes doesn't usually make itself known in this way. For the milder symptoms, make an appointment to see your health care provider as soon as possible. If you've had an episode of passing out, call your provider immediately or go to the emergency room. (See chapter 2 for further discussion on loss of consciousness.)

Diabetes is easily diagnosed by one of two blood tests: a fasting blood sugar (glucose) test, using blood drawn when you have had nothing to eat or drink for at least eight hours, and the glycated hemoglobin (A1c) test, which may be drawn at any time, and which provides information about how your body has handled sugar during the prior three months. A fasting blood sugar of 126 mg/dL or higher on two separate occasions indicates that you have diabetes; a fasting blood sugar level from 100mg/dL to 125 mg/dL is considered *prediabetes*, which means you have a high risk of developing diabetes. The normal level for the A1c is 7 percent or less.

What are the complications of type 2 diabetes? As mentioned in chapter 3, diabetes is one of the major risk factors for coronary artery disease. Other complications include kidney disease and failure, decrease in eyesight, blindness, damage to the peripheral nerves causing chronic numbness and tingling in the legs, damage to blood vessels that can lead to amputations of the lower extremities, and liver disease. A recent study found that life expectancy is seven to eight years shorter for people who have diabetes at age fifty or older than for those of the same age who don't have the disease (Franco 2007).

A similar study also found a shortened life span in people who were prediabetic; that is, they had mildly elevated levels of blood glucose, without meeting the definition of diabetes, when compared to people who had normal levels of blood glucose (Barr et al. 2007). Yet another study found that although the number of men who died from diabetes and its complications decreased from 1988 to 2000, the number of women dying from diabetic complications increased during the same time span (Gregg 2007). This disease seems to take a heavier toll on women.

Prevention and treatment of type 2 diabetes. You can control many of the risk factors for type 2 diabetes, including high blood pressure, abnormal blood lipids, physical inactivity, and excess body weight, simply by exercising, cutting back on the carbohydrates in your diet, losing weight, and possibly keeping your stress level low.

There are medications to treat type 2 diabetes that keep the blood sugar within the normal range, including many types of pills, as well as insulin. Remember, though, these medications do not *cure* the disease; the only cure is to prevent it in the first place. Even though the medications help to keep your blood sugar at a normal level, you still have the disease and you are at risk for the long-term complications. Since, in some people, losing weight causes the blood sugar to return to normal without medications, it is much better to try to bring the blood sugar level down by losing weight (through exercise and a proper diet), rather than to rely on medications to keep the blood sugar normal.

METABOLIC SYNDROME

Another complication of being overweight or obese is metabolic syndrome, the name given to a group of risk factors that occur together. Although specialists in different medical fields disagree about the exact definition of this syndrome, they do agree that having it increases the chances of developing coronary heart disease and stroke (Mensah et al. 2004).

Definition and diagnosis. You must have three or more of the following risk factors in order to be diagnosed with metabolic syndrome (Mensah et al. 2004):

- Abdominal obesity: Waist circumference of at least thirty-five inches in a woman

- High blood triglycerides (TG; one of the blood fats): TG of at least 150 mg/dL

- Low HDL ("good") cholesterol: HDL below 50 mg/dL in a woman

- High blood pressure: Blood pressure of at least 130/85 mm Hg or greater

- High fasting blood glucose (FBS): FBS of at least 110 mg/dL

Who gets metabolic syndrome? Are you at risk? Approximately 47 million Americans have this syndrome (Ford, Giles, and Dietz 2002). Advancing age is a major risk factor, as is being overweight or having impaired glucose metabolism or diabetes. Men and women seem to get it equally, except in the African-American and Mexican-American populations, in which women get the syndrome more often.

Prevention and treatment. The preventive and initial treatment methods of metabolic syndrome are the same: exercise, eat a proper diet, and lose weight to keep your BMI below 25. Because obesity leads to all of the above-named complications, we've come full circle and are back to discussing how to treat and prevent obesity.

TREATMENT OF OBESITY

It goes without saying how difficult it is to lose weight and maintain your BMI below 25. Nevertheless, no matter how difficult it is, it is worth the struggle.

Weight loss through decreased calories and increased physical activity. Whether you count calories or carbs, eat only grapefruits or bananas, take in only liquids, or even fast, the bigger problem is not so much the loss of weight, but maintaining that weight loss. Staying aware of what you're eating and how much you are moving is crucial for maintaining any weight loss. And remember, as each birthday passes, you need fewer calories to be healthy. Talk to your primary clinician, or ask to see a nutritionist, to work out a weight-loss diet that meets your individual needs and tastes.

Medications for weight loss. You probably can guess what we're going to say here. We're not in favor of taking drugs to help you lose weight for two reasons: The first is that many people use these drugs as a crutch, and never really think about their poor eating or exercise habits. Then, once they've lost the weight and stopped the pills, their poor habits continue and the weight comes right back. The second reason is that most of the weight-loss drugs out there have unpleasant side effects or long-term effects. The National Heart Lung and Blood Institute has created obesity guidelines that recommend losing 10 percent of body weight within six months by making lifestyle changes, such as diet, exercise, and behavior modification. The guidelines also say that if patients fail to reach this goal, they then may be considered for therapy with medications, especially if they have other diseases such as diabetes, high blood pressure, or high blood fats (NHLBI 1998). We agree with this approach.

The most well-known of the traditional weight-loss drugs are in the amphetamine class. Two examples are phentermine (Adipex P and many other trade names) and sibutramine (Meridia), both available by prescription only. They are recommended only if your BMI is greater than 30, in addition to a low-calorie diet and increased exercise. They have many side effects and should not be used if you have severe high blood pressure or heart disease, seizures, glaucoma, or a history of drug abuse. The newest weight-loss drug is orlistat (Xenical). Now available without a prescription (Alli), it is used for both weight loss and maintenance, along with diet and exercise. Because it prevents the absorption of fat in the GI tract, the major side effect is diarrhea with frequent oily stools. It should not be used if you have gallbladder or gastrointestinal problems. A form of Korean pine nut oil is sometimes used for weight loss. If you take it about an hour before a meal, it will make you feel full (see chapter 13).

Surgery for weight loss. There are strict criteria that patients must meet to be allowed to have surgery for weight loss, also known as *bariatric surgery.* The most common types are *gastric bypass* and *lap band* surgeries. The number of patients undergoing these types of surgery has increased dramatically in recent years (Livingston 2005). Although traditionally reserved for morbidly obese patients, those with a BMI of 40 or greater, this criterion is being reassessed since recent studies have demonstrated that this surgery and its resultant weight loss definitely increased the life span of those who have had it (Sjostrom et al. 2007; Bray 2007). As with any type of surgery, there are risks involved with bariatric surgery.

Thyroid Disease and Changes in Body Weight

Thyroid disease is very common, particularly in women. Because information about thyroid disease is so readily available, we mention it here only briefly because it often causes a change in body weight, among other symptoms.

Hypothyroidism. An underactive thyroid, or *hypothyroidism*, causes a decreased output of thyroid hormone. Since this hormone has major effects on many different functions and organ systems, including the heart, the GI tract, the bones, the brain, and the metabolism, the overall effect of a decrease in thyroid hormone is a slowing down of the body, and the symptoms reflect that. The most common symptoms are constipation (a sluggish GI tract), slowed pulse and extra heartbeats, fatigue, sluggish thinking, hair loss, increased sensitivity to cold (or feeling cold all the time), and weight gain. Hypothyroidism is easily treated by taking a pill that replaces the body's thyroid hormone; this medication must be taken for the rest of your life.

Hyperthyroidism. When the thyroid gland makes too much thyroid hormone, or becomes overactive, this is known as *hyperthyroidism*. An overactive thyroid has the opposite effect on the body as an underactive thyroid: everything speeds up. This can lead to the following: faster pulse rate, palpitations, diarrhea, hair loss or other hair changes, increased sensitivity to heat (or feeling hot and sweaty all the time), uncontrollable trembling, feeling hyper or anxious, or loss of weight without trying. One common type of hyperthyroidism is known as Graves' disease, which can cause eye problems and skin changes, with or without the symptoms just named. Hyperthyroidism is treated by different methods, including oral medication, radioactive iodine, or surgery.

Bottom line: If you've gained weight over a relatively short period of time without changing your eating habits, or are having more difficulty than usual losing weight, or if you are losing weight without trying, with or without the other symptoms above, ask your clinician to check your thyroid; this is done by a simple blood test.

THE DOCS CHAT ABOUT MOVING AND EATING

DR. R: I've been wondering something. If having too much fat in the abdominal area of the body puts us at risk for so many bad diseases, why doesn't everyone with that problem just have liposuction there?

DR. J: Great question! That's actually been studied. The reason that having excess fat in the abdominal area is so dangerous to our health is that it is always associated with increased fat *inside* the abdominal cavity, where we can't see or feel it. Simply sucking out the fat from under our skin doesn't get rid of the dangerous fat deeper inside. When you lose weight, you actually lose the fat in the abdominal cavity, and then you decrease your risk for the diseases that come with excess fat in that area.

DR. R: We promised to tell our readers about our own regimens of eating and staying active. So, I'll go first. I walk my dogs twice a day, and then do my own walk up and down the hills in my neighborhood for at least forty-five minutes, five days a week. I work out with a trainer twice a week, doing a weight-training system called *kinesis*, which is a series of strengthening exercises using weights on pulleys. To mix it up, I ski in the winter and swim in the summer. Sometimes I go to the gym to use their elliptical machine for a change in my cardio routine.

DR. J: You're not human, you're an exercise machine! You expect me to tell my exercise regimen after that? I know I promised our readers, so here goes: I love strength, balance, and flexibility training, so I'm fairly good about doing at least one hour, twice a week, of exercises with free weights, which I often do while standing on the BOSU ball. I mix up the activities in those sessions a lot and include some yoga positions and lots of core-strengthening movements like crunches done on the large rubber ball. I have a wonderful trainer at the gym who keeps me laughing while I'm getting strong. I plan to get into Pilates next.

DR. R: Sounds great, but didn't you forget something?

DR. J: I was hoping you'd forget! As for aerobic or cardio activity, I've been just okay at keeping to a schedule of thirty minutes, two or three times a week, of exercise of moderate intensity, which I know isn't enough. I either walk outside, ride my exercise bike inside, or dance to Donna Summers, Cher, Stevie Nicks, Madonna, or Blondie. I plan to increase that to five or six days per week as soon as we finish writing this book! Now, tell our readers about your eating regimen.

DR. R: No more popcorn! Or rather, only occasionally. As mentioned in this chapter, I love the type of food that's a part of the Mediterranean diet, so I pretty much stick with that. But the one additional thing I do is called the "cheater's diet." After being very careful about what I eat for two weeks, I splurge, and for one day I eat whatever I want. The next day I go right back to my regular eating routine. It works to keep me from cheating all the time or feeling deprived. I've noticed I usually don't feel too good on the day after the splurge, so I've stopped eating as much or as badly on my "cheat" days.

DR. J: I eat similarly with the addition of drinking oodles of green tea, which keeps me full. I drink it hot and cold, made from scratch (my favorite is made by Stash). I supplement the tea with Poland Springs Sparkling Water with lime essence. The other food I get in daily is ground flaxseed, which I love sprinkled on yogurt, my favorite being Dannon Light & Fit Yogurt (carb and sugar control). I adore salmon and could eat it daily, too. Lastly, although I love sweets, I realize that they are worthless in terms of nutritional value, and I constantly remind myself of this. I don't have a regular "cheating day" like you, but occasionally I do have ice cream or a cookie, and I no longer let the fact that I've "cheated" demoralize me or destroy my new way of eating. Also, I do one thing that sometimes stops me from eating that piece of cheesecake, which is right up your complementary medicine alley! I actually visualize the cheesecake being made with several cups of refined sugar being poured into the batter. That's enough to stop me from eating it!

PEARLS OF WISDOM ABOUT MOVING AND EATING

○ Get moving now and keep moving!

○ Do all four types of physical activity regularly: aerobics, strength training, balance, and flexibility exercises.

○ Wear seat belts! (If you read the chapter, you'll see how this fits in.)

○ Be aware of everything you eat.

○ Try the Mediterranean way of eating.

○ Remember that those extra pounds you may be carrying are dangerous to your health.

○ Get your blood sugar and thyroid hormone checked with regular blood tests.

CHAPTER 12

Common Cancers in Women over Fifty: How to Survive and Thrive

The diagnosis of cancer is often equated with a death sentence, which might have been valid 100 years ago. Even fifty years ago, cancer was a taboo topic; family members didn't speak to one another about it or even mention the "Big C." No longer. In November 2007, America's leading cancer organizations issued a report showing the cancer death rate decline *doubled* in the past several years (Espey et al. 2007). In women, death rates from both breast cancer and colorectal cancer decreased, and the rate of increase for lung cancer greatly slowed; in addition, the number of new cases diagnosed with breast (Ravdin et al. 2007) and colorectal cancers (Howe et al. 2006), among other cancers, decreased. This significant decrease in cancer death rates shows the progress achieved through screening, early detection, improved treatments, and effective tobacco control.

In this chapter we focus on the most common cancer in women, skin cancer, and the top four killers in women: breast, lung, colorectal, and ovarian cancers. We also discuss uterine and cervical cancer. Because cancer treatments change so often, and because our emphasis in this chapter is on prevention and early detection of the most common cancers in women, specific therapies are not discussed.

WHAT IS CANCER?

Cancer is a group of related diseases that can affect virtually every organ in the body. No phrase better explains what happens with cancer than a take-off on the old cliché "girls and boys gone wild"; cancer is literally cells gone wild. Normally, in our bodies, there is a regular breakdown of cells followed by an orderly process of replacement and repair. When cancer develops, that orderly repair and replacement process is gone. Cancer cells grow out of control, eventually developing into tumors. Several factors can start this uncontrolled growth, such as exposure to toxins like cigarette smoke or chemicals, or an individual's genetic susceptibility to developing certain cancers. Unfortunately, because there are so many different types of cancer, all of the causes are not known. However, research continues to discover information that will help to unravel the mysteries of why certain people develop cancer and how to prevent it.

SKIN CANCER

Skin cancers may be divided into two types: the nonmelanoma cancers and melanoma. In Caucasian women, the most common is nonmelanoma skin cancer.

Nonmelanoma Skin Cancer: Squamous Cell and Basal Cell Carcinoma

Each year over 1 million cases of nonmelanoma skin cancer are diagnosed (ACS 2007a). The most frequent are *basal cell* and *squamous cell tumors*; both are easily treated if detected early. These cancers are most commonly found in areas of the body that have been exposed to the sun: the scalp, face, neck, arms, and hands. Basal cell rarely spreads from where it originates to other parts of the body, but if left untreated, it can grow and disfigure the area where it is located. On the other hand, squamous cell cancers can travel to the lymph nodes and spread to other parts of the body if not detected and treated early.

Are you at risk for nonmelanoma skin cancer? These skin cancers are of particular concern to women over fifty. Remember when we went to the beach (or roof if you're a city girl) loaded with bottles of iodine and baby oil and homemade sun reflectors made of record album covers wrapped in aluminum foil, and then sat out in the bright sun and fried our skin? We had no idea then that turning ourselves into crispy critters could increase our chances of getting skin cancer; all we wanted was a gorgeous tan.

Now we know better. Those of us who have a light complexion, have a history of sunburn and scarring, had excessive sun exposure before the age of eighteen, have skin diseases like albinism that increase sensitivity to the sun, or have a personal or family history of skin cancer are at increased risk for developing any form of skin cancer. However, the above risk factors do not exclude women of color from getting skin cancers; these cancers just don't occur as frequently in women with dark skin as in women with light skin. In African-American women, squamous cell cancers are more common than basal cell cancers (Halder and Ara 2003).

How do you know if you have skin cancer? What can you do about it? It is *essential* to check your skin on a regular basis, just as you routinely check your breasts. Although it may be difficult for you to tell the difference between a benign skin bump that occurs just with aging and a skin cancer, there are general things to look for. Any *new* or *old* skin lesions or moles that you discover need to be watched over time; if they grow, change shape, change color, ooze fluid, or bleed, have them checked out. Or if you think the new skin lesion just doesn't "look right"—for instance, it's very dark or irregularly shaped—see your clinician. This is one of those times that we believe your intuition is excellent—don't ignore it!

It may be helpful to keep a record of your own skin exams by actually drawing the lesions you see and writing down the date of your exam. Measuring the diameter of the lesions is also useful. That way, you will know for certain whether they have grown the next time you examine them. We strongly recommend that you have a baseline dermatological examination at your current age. In other words, make an appointment now, or just as soon as you finish reading this. Specify that you want a "full skin exam," which is exactly what the dermatologist will do. After this, you need to be seen yearly, or as often as the doctor thinks it necessary to see you.

How is nonmelanoma skin cancer prevented and treated? Both types of nonmelanoma skin cancer, if detected early, are treated with surgical removal. If squamous cell cancer spreads, it may require radiation therapy and topical chemotherapy; whereas if basal cell cancer is allowed to grow unchecked, it may require multiple surgeries, which, ultimately, can be disfiguring.

Bottom line: Catch it early! Trust your instincts! Further methods of prevention, the most important being to avoid sun exposure, are discussed in the next section.

Melanoma: The Deadliest Form of Skin Cancer

Melanoma is the sixth most common skin cancer in men and women (ACS 2007a). It was estimated that there would be 26,000 women diagnosed with the invasive form of this cancer in 2007.

The incidence of melanoma has increased 690 percent from 1950 to 2001; the number of people dying from this disease has increased 165 percent (AADA/SID 2005). This cancer originates in the pigment-producing cells of the skin. (See chapter 9.) In women, melanoma is most frequently found on the back and on the legs, although it can be found anywhere, including such unlikely places as the bottom of the foot or inside the earlobe. Melanoma is considered deadly because it can spread to other organs if not detected and treated early.

Are you at risk for melanoma? Melanoma is more common in Caucasian women than in women of color, occurring in 11 out of 100,000 Caucasians. In African-American women, it occurs in 1 out of 100,000, and in Hispanic women, in 4 out of 100,000; it is the most common form of skin cancer in Hispanic women. In all women of color, including Asian and Native American women, the most common sites for melanoma to occur are the palms, the soles of the feet, and unusual places such as under the tongue (Halder and Ara 2003).

Although melanoma is less likely to occur in women of color, it is detected, unfortunately, more often after it has spread (Hu et al. 2006). For that reason survival rates for melanoma are lower for women of color. Early on, it is often mistakenly diagnosed as a wart or a fungal infection.

Therefore, no matter what your skin color is, it is important to know your risks. These include a history of sunburn before age eighteen; excessive ultraviolet radiation exposure from the sun or tanning beds; exposure to compounds such as coal tar, creosote, and arsenic-containing compounds such as pesticides and radium; the presence of an abnormal, or dysplastic, mole (not cancer yet, but precancerous); and having a family history of melanoma.

How do you know if you have melanoma? What can you do about it? Melanoma is detected by a careful skin examination of a darkened spot or lesion, no matter how small, and if suspicious, by a biopsy of that lesion, followed by microscopic examination by a pathologist. Again, doing regular skin exams on yourself is crucial. Don't forget to look everywhere that you can, even in those areas where the sun doesn't usually shine, like the palms of your hands and the soles of your feet! In looking for a melanoma, dermatologists recommend looking for the "ABCDE warning signs":

- *Asymmetry.* The mole is not symmetrical. The two halves of the mole look different.

- *Borders.* The perimeter of the mole is irregular and not smooth.

- *Color.* The pigment is not the same throughout. It can be shades of brown, black, blue, or red.

- *Diameter.* The size of the mole is greater than the eraser tip of a pencil.

- *Expanding.* It is growing and changing in size and/or shape.

If you notice any of these changes or you are worried about the look of a certain mole, get it checked immediately. Trust your instincts! Many women have told us that they are afraid of finding out if the skin lesion is a melanoma, so they try to simply ignore it. If you feel this way, think of it like this: If it is not melanoma, you will be reassured. If it is melanoma, the earlier it is caught, the better your prognosis and survival. The five-year survival rate for people with *early* detection whose melanoma has not spread is 99 percent (ACS 2007a).

How is melanoma treated? If melanoma is detected early, treatment will involve surgery. If it is advanced, chemotherapy, interferon, and a variety of experimental therapies may be used.

How is melanoma prevented? *The best way to prevent all skin cancers is to avoid sun exposure.* Those rays may feel good, but they are damaging. A thorough discussion of ways to avoid the sun and the best products to use is found in chapter 9. Remember: Be vigilant about observing your skin and seeing a dermatologist regularly, especially if you have a lot of moles and/or freckles that make it difficult to observe each skin lesion. It is possible to catch early mole changes before they become cancerous. Be *aware* of your risk factors and *alert* to your how your skin changes, take *action* to see a dermatologist, and *advocate* for yourself if you're told that "everything looks fine" and your instincts tell you differently.

BREAST CANCER

The most common cancer in women over fifty is breast cancer. Over our lifetimes, each of us has a one in eight chance of developing breast cancer, and a one in thirty-three chance of dying from it. Although there is still no cure for breast cancer, the good news is that we are getting better at detecting it early, and survival rates are improving (ACS 2007).

Are you at risk for breast cancer? We now know there are many factors that increase the chances of a woman developing breast cancer. Just as with the risk factors for heart disease, some can be modified, others cannot. Read on.

- *Age.* The older a woman gets, the greater the chance she will develop breast cancer.

- *Race.* The chance of getting breast cancer is greatest in Caucasian women, with African-American women a close second. Asian-American and Hispanic women are next in line, and Native American women have the lowest chance of developing breast cancer. Although African-American women may have a lower incidence of breast cancer than Caucasian women do, their mortality rate is higher due to the fact that their breast cancer is caught more often at a late stage. Another reason for the higher death rate may be a recent discovery that African-American women are more often diagnosed with an aggressive type of breast cancer that is not responsive to some of the standard treatments (Amend, Hicks, and Ambrosone 2006).

· *Family history.* If her first-degree relative (mother, daughter, or sister) has had breast cancer, especially before the age of fifty, the risk of a woman getting breast cancer increases by about fifty percent. If she has two first-degree relatives with breast cancer, a woman has five times the risk.

· *Personal history of breast cancer.* If you have a history of breast cancer in one breast, the chances of getting it in the other breast are increased.

· *Menstrual and reproductive history.* The younger a woman is at the time of her first child the less likely she is to get breast cancer. Women who had their first period before the age of twelve, who went through menopause after age fifty-five, who never had children, and/or who took combined hormone treatments with Premarin and Provera (see chapter 10) are all more likely to develop breast cancer. Women who have had abortions or miscarriages are not more likely to have breast cancer. Those women who breastfed their children for fourteen months or longer have a decreased risk of developing breast cancer (Shantakurar et al. 2007).

· *Breast changes.* Oftentimes women undergo a biopsy after an abnormality is picked up on mammogram. Those who have been found to have the breast tissue changes known as atypical hyperplasia or lobular carcinoma in situ (LCIS) have an increased risk of breast cancer.

· *Genetic mutations.* Women who have many family members with a history of breast cancer are often urged to be checked for BRCA1 and BRCA2 mutations by having a blood test. These mutations increase the likelihood that a woman will develop breast cancer. What are BRCA1 and BRCA2 mutations? We all have the genes known as BRCA1 and BRCA2; they help to keep cell growth in check. When there are changes to these genes, known as mutations, they do not perform their job properly, and cells are more likely to grow wildly. Women with mutations to these genes are more susceptible to both breast and ovarian cancers. Although this is frightening, these mutations account for only about 10 percent of all breast and ovarian cancers. Your doctor can help you decide if you would benefit by being checked with a simple blood test.

· *Breast density.* Breasts are made up of fatty and glandular tissue; the latter makes and secretes milk and is surrounded by the fatty tissue. Women who have more dense glandular tissue than fat in their breasts are at greater risk of developing breast cancer. For these women, digital mammography may be a better screening test than plain mammography. (See below for further discussion on digital mammography.) Women who have more fat than glandular tissue in their breasts are not at greater risk for breast cancer.

- *Exposure to DES (diethylstilbestrol)*. DES is a hormone that some pregnant women were given between 1940 and 1971 to prevent miscarriage. Women who took it, and their daughters, may be at increased risk (Palmer 2006).

- *Exposure to alcohol*. Some studies show that the more alcohol a woman drinks, the greater her risk of breast cancer. For women who drink between two and five alcoholic drinks a day, there is a 40 percent increase in the risk of developing breast cancer (Smith-Warner et al. 1998). The risk is the same no matter what type of alcohol you drink (Li et al. 2007).

- *Radiation exposures*. Women who have had radiation to the chest for diseases such as Hodgkin's disease before the age of thirty are at increased risk. There is concern that radiation exposure from imaging procedures such as coronary calcium screening of the heart (mentioned in chapter 3), or other CT scans of the chest, may cause breast cancer due to increased radiation exposure.

- *Environmental exposures*. There are many theories that xenoestrogens (chemicals that mimic estrogen) found in some plastic bottles may be picked up by the breast tissue and cause cancers.

- *Obesity*. Women with a BMI over 25 are one and a half to two times more likely to die from breast cancer as women of normal weight (Calle et al. 2003). Estrogen is stored in fat, and the more fat a woman has, the more her breasts are exposed to estrogen.

- *Sedentary lifestyle*. Regular physical activity decreases the risk of breast cancer in postmenopausal women (Reeves et al. 2007). It does not even have to be a lot of exercise. Women in one study who did vigorous walking just one and a quarter to two and a half hours per week had an 18 percent decreased risk of breast cancer compared to the women who did no exercise at all (McTiernan et al. 2003).

How do you know if you have breast cancer? The answer to how you can find out if you have breast cancer is simple: screening and early detection. *Screening* refers to having regular exams (both physical exams and mammograms) when you have no symptoms; how often depends on your risk factors. *Early detection* refers to the timing of when the cancer is found; the earlier the better. Screening usually leads to early detection and is done in ways that vary depending on your underlying risk factors.

Clinical and self-examinations of your breasts are both extremely important. Your doctor should perform a clinical exam at least once a year, or more often depending on your risk factors. A breast self-exam is done by you. Every month, check your breasts and feel for any new lumps or changes. Since there is less friction with soap and water, which makes the exam easier to do, try doing it in the shower. Ask your clinician to show you the best way to do the exam. Many clinicians have realistic models of breasts, both normal and with lumps, on which you can practice. If you find a breast lump during your self-exam, an enlarged lymph node under your arm, bleeding from your nipple, or any other change, call your clinician for an appointment immediately. According to the National Institutes of Health, 80 to 85 percent of lumps are benign, so the odds are that even if you find one, it will be okay (NLM 2008).

Mammography is the cornerstone for screening and early detection of breast cancer. The mammogram is an x-ray study of the breasts that uses a very small amount of radiation. It is recommended that a woman in her forties have a mammogram every one to two years, depending on her risk factors. Women fifty and older should have one yearly. Some doctors recommend that a woman have a baseline mammogram at thirty-five, especially if she has a family history of breast cancer. Often, mammograms can show a breast tumor before it can be felt. For breast cancer, early detection is the key.

Some women may need further tests to take a closer look at suspicious findings, such as an ultrasound, which is good at distinguishing cysts (usually benign) from a solid mass. On the other hand, mammograms may miss some tumors, especially in women with dense breasts. For these women, a digital mammogram may be recommended. This is done the same way as a regular mammogram; however, the pictures are sent to a computer rather than developed on film. With the computer images, doctors can get a better view of different areas of the breast.

Susan's Story

Susan, a fifty-one-year-old college professor, came to Dr. R concerned about a lump in her breast that she had just found during her self-exam. After examining her, Dr. R immediately ordered a mammogram; the results were negative. Susan was still very concerned and told Dr. R she had a "gut instinct" that something was wrong with her breast despite the mammogram being negative. Because Dr. R strongly believes not only in listening to her patients, but also that women have good instincts about their own bodies, she arranged for Susan to see a surgeon and have the lump removed. Susan was right; she had early breast cancer. She had picked it up herself and remained concerned that it was cancerous in spite of the mammogram. Susan had appropriate treatment and is now cancer free. If you feel something and you are worried, insist on having it evaluated. Mammograms can miss cancers. Never ignore your gut feelings.

Magnetic resonance imaging (MRI) is a technique that uses a powerful magnet to create detailed computer images of the breast; there is no radiation involved with this test, and thus no radiation exposure to you at all. The American Cancer Society has specific recommendations regarding who should have this test based on risk factors. Your doctor can help you decide whether you need an MRI.

How is breast cancer diagnosed? Ultimately, breast cancer is diagnosed with a breast biopsy. A mammogram or clinical breast exam raises the suspicion that there is cancer, but only a biopsy can confirm it. This is important for you to know. Once a breast abnormality has been found, the radiologist or surgeon will remove a piece of the breast lump, or the surgeon will remove the entire lump.

What are the types of breast cancer? After noting the size of the lump and examining it under a microscope, the pathologist can determine whether it is *benign* (not cancerous) or *malignant* (cancerous). If malignant, she can then determine the type or classification of the cancer based on cellular type, location, and receptor status. The *cellular type* is determined by the location where the tumor originated. If it originated within a milk duct of the breast, this is known as a *ductal* tumor; if it originated within a lobule of the breast, it is known as a *lobular* tumor. The original location of the tumor is one of the most important issues, in addition to whether the cancer has spread outside of its place of origin within the breast.

Carcinoma in situ, in which the cells have not left their place of origin in the milk ducts or the breast lobules, is the very earliest stage of cancer (stage 0). It is usually considered a precancerous condition because it has not yet developed into an invasive cancer. Nonetheless, it still must be treated.

Invasive breast cancer is cancer that has spread outside the milk ducts or breast lobules into the surrounding breast tissue, and possibly into the lymph nodes and other organs. With this finding from a biopsy, more imaging studies and surgical procedures will be needed to see if the cancer has spread. Depending on how far it has spread, it is then labeled as to its stage, such as stage 1, 2, or 3. Having an invasive cancer does not mean the same thing as having *metastasis*; the latter occurs only when the tumor has broken off from its original site and spread to a distant organ through the bloodstream or lymphatic system.

Receptor status also helps to identify the characteristics of the tumor. Whether a tumor has receptors or not determines how aggressive it will be and how it will respond to treatment. These receptors include estrogen, progesterone, and HER2 receptors. Your doctors will make their treatment recommendations based on which receptors are present.

What are the special forms of breast cancer? Although not specific types of tumor, there are two conditions that are special forms of breast cancer. They are inflammatory breast cancer and Paget's disease of the nipple. *Inflammatory breast cancer* is a rare form of breast cancer. It occurs when the cancer has spread into the skin and lymph nodes. The breast becomes red and swollen due to the blocked lymph vessels in the skin of the breast. Note that this appearance may be mistaken for a simple infection of the breast.

Paget's disease of the nipple is another rare form of breast cancer, accounting for less than 5 percent of all breast cancers. Over 95 percent of women diagnosed with this have an underlying tumor. It may start as redness or flaking of the nipple. It can cause itching and burning and may cause flattening and distortion of the nipple. This is why it is important to examine your nipples when you do a breast self-exam, including squeezing the nipple to look for fluid (Kaelin 2004).

How is breast cancer treated? Treatment varies depending on the size, type, receptor status, and stage of the tumor, as well as on patient preferences. There are many options and combinations of therapies available; discuss these, and which are best for you, with your doctors. This brings up an important point. When pursuing treatment, for cancer or any other type of illness, it is important to find a doctor whom you trust and who can be your partner in healing. If you are uncomfortable with your doctor or with what you are being told, or you simply want another viewpoint, trust your instincts and get another opinion (or doctor). Second opinions are always a good idea.

How is breast cancer prevented? Healthy lifestyle choices are the main focus of prevention. You need to look at your risk for breast cancer and make certain choices. For instance, if you have a strong family history of breast cancer, hormone replacement therapy may not be the best choice for you. Also, you should consider restricting your alcohol intake.

What are the methods to prevent breast cancer for all women, regardless of risk? Lifestyle changes are important. A healthy diet, regular exercise, a monthly breast self-exam, and a yearly mammogram and breast exam by your doctor are all important for prevention and early detection. There are also certain foods and supplements that may help to prevent breast cancer. *Lignans* are found in ground flaxseed, fruits, vegetables, and whole grains. A study, over a seven-year period, of more than 100,000 women in France found that women who had the highest intake of lignans had significantly lower rates of hormone receptor positive breast cancer when compared to those with the lowest intake of lignans (Touillaud et al. 2007).

Cruciferous vegetables such as broccoli, Brussels sprouts, cauliflower, and bok choy may help to prevent breast cancer. They contain indole-3-carbinol, which may reduce the effect of estrogen on the cells (Steinmetz and Potter 1991). Soy is a phytoestrogen (a plant estrogen) that also may lessen any negative effect of estrogen on the cells of the breast (Messina and Barnes 1991). Because soy is a form of estrogen, albeit from a plant, there is still controversy as to whether patients who have had breast cancer should avoid it. However, as a food (not as a supplement) it has been found to be protective and preventive for women without breast cancer (Trock, Hilakivi-Clarke, and Clarke 2006).

Green tea may help protect against breast cancer. In one study of Asian-American women, those who drank green tea had significantly less breast cancer than those who did not drink it (Wu et al. 2003). How much to drink to get the full protective effect is unknown. Green tea is a healthy drink in general (see chapter 13), so drink up. Calcium and vitamin D are important for cancer prevention. A recent clinical trial found that supplementing women's diets with daily calcium (1,400 to 1,500 mg) and vitamin D (1,000 IU) reduced their overall cancer rate by 60 percent (Lappe et al. 2007).

What are the methods for preventing breast cancer for women at high risk? Women who are at very high risk for breast cancer, such as those with many first-degree relatives with the disease or those who have BRCA1 and BRCA2 mutations, might want to consider preventive treatment. The medications tamoxifen and raloxifene have been found to reduce the risk of invasive breast cancer by about 50 percent in high-risk women (Vogel et al. 2006) and are now recommended to some women at high risk for breast cancer. These drugs are not without side effects. They both can increase the chances of developing blood clots and hot flashes, and tamoxifen can increase the chance of developing cancer of the uterus. The risks and benefits must be carefully weighed by you and your doctor. Though useful for some women, this treatment may not be right for you.

Prophylactic (preventive) surgery is another option if you are at high risk for breast cancer. Talk with your doctor about *prophylactic mastectomies*, or removal of the breasts before cancer develops. Obviously, this will be a very serious discussion, so again make sure you trust and are comfortable with your doctor. Also consider getting several professional opinions.

LUNG CANCER

Lung cancer is the leading cause of cancer deaths in women. It kills more women than breast, ovarian, uterine, and cervical cancers combined. Deaths from lung cancer have risen 600 percent between 1930 and 1997 (Patel, Bach, and Kris 2004), although they have stabilized in women over the past several years (Espey et al. 2007). There are two main types of lung cancer, small cell and non-small cell cancers, differentiated by their appearance under a microscope. The non-small cell type of cancer tragically killed Dana Reeve, actress, activist, and wife of the beloved actor and director Christopher Reeve. The fact that she didn't smoke surprised many people. Unfortunately, that's the case more and more today; 20 percent of women who get lung cancer have never smoked (Subramanian and Govindan 2007).

Are you at risk for lung cancer? Caucasian and African-American women have the greatest risk for developing lung cancer, followed by Native American women. Asian-American and Hispanic women have the lowest chance of developing lung cancer (ACS 2007a).

Several other factors increase a woman's risk of developing lung cancer, especially *cigarette smoking*. Eighty-seven percent of lung cancers are tobacco-smoking related. When a person smokes, cancer-creating substances known as *carcinogens* are released from the cigarettes into the lungs. The chances you will develop lung cancer increase depending on the number of cigarettes smoked regularly and the number of years the habit has continued (Fu et al. 2005). In a large study of smokers, women were found to be far more susceptible to the cancer-causing effects of cigarette smoke than men. Although women were twice as likely to be diagnosed with lung cancer, they were more likely to survive than the men who developed lung cancer during the study (IELCAPI 2006). You should also know that smoking cigars and pipes can increase the risk of lung cancer when compared to nonsmokers. Even if you don't inhale, they can increase the risk of head and neck cancers.

The important thing to know is that when a woman stops smoking, her risk for lung cancer starts to decrease immediately. For help with quitting, see chapter 15.

Unfortunately, the smoke from someone else's cigarette can also produce carcinogens that are released into the air, and can be just as harmful (Reardon 2007). *Secondhand smoke* (that smoke produced by someone else smoking) can be deadly. As stated earlier, many women diagnosed with lung cancer never smoked—but their husbands did. This is a major risk factor that you should avoid. If your partner or children or others living with you are smoking cigarettes, you must get them to quit. This is one of those times when you must advocate for yourself.

Another factor that can increase your chances of developing lung cancer is exposure to *radon*, an odorless gas that occurs in soil and rocks. By damaging the lungs, it increases the risk of lung cancer, especially in smokers. In some parts of the country it can be found in houses. However, radon is very easy to detect using a kit that can be found at hardware stores. If you have high radon levels in your house, some relatively simple venting procedures can get rid of it.

Asbestos is a mineral fiber that was widely used in construction when we were growing up. When they are inhaled, the fibers break down and stick to the lungs. Workers exposed to large amounts of asbestos have three to four times the risk of lung cancer as those who have not been exposed. Unfortunately, exposure to *pollution* also increases our risk of developing lung cancer. *Tuberculosis* infection increases the chance of getting lung cancer, especially in the scarred areas of the lung. *A previous history of lung cancer* increases the chances of getting a second lung cancer, especially if the person continues to smoke or is exposed to secondhand smoke.

Remember, just because you don't smoke or never have doesn't mean that you can't get lung cancer. Be *aware* of this fact and your risk factors; be *alert* to any new chest symptoms you get; take *action* to see your clinician as soon as you can if you have any new symptoms; and *advocate* against secondhand smoke, especially in your home and workplace.

How do you know if you have lung cancer? What can you do about it? Initially, there may be no symptoms, which is why it is so hard to detect lung cancer early. Common symptoms seen in patients with lung cancer include coughing up blood, swelling of the face and neck, chest pain that doesn't improve, progressive worsening of shortness of breath and wheezing, a chronic cough that continues to worsen, repeated bronchial infections, weight loss, and fatigue. Go to the emergency room immediately if you have any of the first four symptoms mentioned above, and particularly if your shortness of breath is not allowing you to breathe comfortably at rest. If you have any of the other symptoms, see your clinician as soon as possible.

How is lung cancer diagnosed? Lung cancer is diagnosed several ways. The first test is usually a chest x-ray or a chest CT (computed tomography) scan. Chest CT scans are better at picking up tumors than are chest x-rays; so if your chest x-ray is negative and you have risk factors for lung cancer, request a chest CT scan. If there is a suspicious mass seen, then a sputum (spit) sample may be collected and examined for abnormal cells under a microscope. A bronchoscopy may be recommended next. This is an examination using a scope with a light and camera at the end (similar to a colonoscope) that is threaded down into the lung from the mouth or nose, using local anesthetic while you are sedated, in order to collect tissue and cells. Depending on the individual and the locations of the suspected tumor, other methods may be used to obtain a sample of the tissue and examine it microscopically. Remember, the x-ray or CT scan alone cannot make the diagnosis of lung cancer; a piece of the suspected tumor or of the lung must be obtained.

For years, doctors have been trying to find a way to detect lung cancer early, before those at risk (for instance, smokers) have any symptoms. Unlike mammograms or Pap smears, which have proven to be very useful for this purpose, there are currently no screening studies that alter the rates of death from lung cancer. Research is currently ongoing to determine if low-dose CT scans might be useful for screening (Bach et al. 2007). If you are at high risk for lung cancer and have no symptoms but are concerned, talk to your clinician.

How is lung cancer treated and prevented? Treatment for lung cancer may involve surgery, radiation and laser therapy, and/or chemotherapy. The choice of treatment depends on the stage and type of the cancer. As with breast and other cancers, it is important to find a doctor who will be your partner in care.

The best way to prevent lung cancer is to never smoke, or if you do, to quit! You should also make sure that those around you do not smoke either. What about supplements or medications to prevent lung cancer? For years, it was thought that beta-carotene supplements could help prevent it. However, a large clinical trial found that these supplements actually increase the chance of developing lung cancers in smokers (Goodman et al. 2004). Therefore, smokers especially need to avoid these supplements. It is better to eat a healthy diet rich in fruits and vegetables that contain beta-carotene, since food sources of this nutrient have not been found to increase the risk of cancer.

COLORECTAL CANCER

Colorectal cancer is the third most common cancer killer of women in the U.S., after lung and breast cancer, causing an estimated 26,000 deaths in women in 2007 (ACS 2007b).

Are you at risk for colorectal cancer? There are many factors that play a role in the development of colorectal cancer. Age is a risk factor, as the majority of patients diagnosed with colorectal cancer are fifty or older. A history of colorectal cancer in a first-degree relative (mother, father, sister, brother, or child) increases the risk of developing colorectal cancer. The risk is further increased if more than one relative had colon cancer. This cancer affects men and women equally. African-American women have the greatest chance of developing colon cancer, followed by Caucasian women, Native American, and Asian-American women, and then by Hispanic women, who have the lowest incidence of colon cancer (ACS 2007b).

Colorectal polyps are growths that are found in the colon or rectum. Most are benign or harmless. However, some, known as *adenomatous polyps*, can turn into cancer. When these are removed, cancer is prevented. *Hereditary nonpolyposis colon cancer* is an inherited form of colorectal cancer. On average, those with this genetic abnormality are diagnosed at forty-four years of age. Between 2 and 5 percent of colon cancers result from this condition. *Familial adenomatous polyposis* is a rare genetic abnormality that results in hundreds of polyps forming in the colon and rectum. Those with this disorder are at high risk for colorectal cancer, and it usually occurs by the age of forty. Anyone with a family history of either of these genetic disorders needs to have genetic testing. Those who test positive for the abnormal gene will be advised to have routine screening and in some cases may require surgery to remove part of the colon or rectum in order to prevent any of the polyps from becoming cancerous.

A history of having colorectal cancer increases the risk of having another tumor in the colon. Women with a history of breast, uterine, and ovarian cancers are also at higher risk of developing colorectal cancer. A history of having ulcerative colitis or Crohn's disease is a risk factor, since these diseases cause inflammation in the colon that can increase the risk of colorectal cancer. And, of course, smoking increases the risk of developing polyps and colorectal cancer.

How do you know if you have colorectal cancer? Most people have no symptoms, which is why screening is *so* important. Common symptoms of colon cancer include change in bowel habits (if you are normally constipated and now are having diarrhea, and vice versa), chronic diarrhea or constipation, or both alternating with one another, cramps and bloating, fatigue, pencil-shaped or narrow stools, blood in the stool, nausea or vomiting, or unexplained weight loss (this occurs late). Also, your clinician may find on routine blood studies an unexplained anemia, or low red blood cell count.

Because colorectal cancer can be found and cured even before it develops by removing colon polyps, which have the potential to become cancerous, screening tests for this cancer are very important. These screening tests are recommended for all women at age fifty unless you have a family history of colon cancer. In that case, it is recommended that you have your first screening ten years before you reach the age that your first-degree relative was diagnosed with colon cancer. (In other words, if your father was diagnosed at age fifty, you would want to get your first colonoscopy done at age forty.) If you have a family history of familial polyposis or hereditary nonpolyposis, your screenings would need to be started at an earlier age as suggested by your doctor.

Colonoscopy is the gold standard when it comes to cancer screening; however, your doctor may use other tests as well, including fecal occult blood testing, digital rectal exam, double-contrast barium enema, sigmoidoscopy, virtual colonoscopy, immunochemical testing, and stool-based DNA testing. The important thing to remember is that *any* screening is better than *no* screening.

Colonoscopy is *the* screening test that is recommended. It is done with a scope that reaches all the way around the entire colon. Polyps can be removed at the same time if they are not too large. Because this procedure is generally done in an outpatient procedure room with sedative medication, it is fairly comfortable. Most people sleep through the whole thing and say that the worst part of the test is the extensive preparation beforehand. The preparation includes a diet of clear liquids the day before, followed by a very salty liquid preparation or pills that induce heavy diarrhea to clean out your colon. You will probably not need another colonoscopy for ten years unless an abnormality is found or unless you have risk factors, in which case you need to be tested more often.

Virtual colonoscopy, now available in many medical communities, shows a two- to three-dimensional view of the colon using either a CT scanner or an MRI machine. The preparation for this test is similar to the colonoscopy prep, although this test takes only about ten minutes, needs no sedation, is painless, and no scope is used. A small tube is inserted into the rectum only to pump in some air, and then images are taken. The downside to this test is that if there is a polyp, colonoscopy will ultimately have to be done to remove it, and the prep will have to be repeated at a later date. When experienced radiologists do this study, it is considered to be a reliable test.

How is colon cancer diagnosed? Just as with all other forms of cancer, the ultimate diagnosis is made only by microscopic examination of tissue obtained by biopsy. In this case, the diagnosis is made after a polyp is either removed or biopsied, or an abnormal area of colon tissue is biopsied during colonoscopy. When the pathologist looks at the biopsy material, she can tell if the entire cancer has been removed or if it has spread.

How is colon cancer treated and prevented? Treatment may involve surgery, chemotherapy, or biologic or radiation therapies. It is important, as with any cancer, that you find doctors who will be your partners in healing. As with all cancers, a healthy diet and exercise program are important for preventing colon cancer. A study of over 1,000 colorectal cancer survivors found that those who ate a typical Western high-fat diet were three times more likely to have a recurrence of their cancers when compared to those who ate a prudent diet that consisted of fruits, vegetables, whole grains, fish, and poultry (Meyerhardt et al. 2007). There is still controversy whether dietary fiber can protect against colon cancer (Baron 2005).

Although some studies have found an association between low-fat diets and lower rates of colorectal cancer, the Women's Health Initiative (WHI) study did not find any such association (Beresford et al. 2006). However, a diet rich in fruits and vegetables and low in saturated fat is a healthy diet, and one that we recommend regardless. To prevent colon cancer, be screened and have polyps removed before they become cancerous. Be *aware* of your risk factors and when you need to be screened; be *alert* to any symptoms of colon cancer you may have; take *action* and see your doctor if you have symptoms, and if you don't have symptoms, remember to get regularly screened; and *advocate* for yourself if necessary.

Dr. R and Dr. J's Tips for the Least Distressing Colonoscopy Experience

1. *Don't put it off. Just schedule it. It is not nearly as bad as you think—it couldn't be!*

2. *Dr. J changes her diet to only clear liquids two days before the colonoscopy to make sure she won't have to prepare again. Make sure, though, that you drink more liquids than you usually do if you decide to do this; Dr. J tries to get in twice as much fluid as usual. Note that taking in only liquids for two days is not a good idea if you have chronic illnesses, especially diabetes or heart disease.*

3. *Don't cheat on drinking the full preparation liquid; swallow every last drop. If you're not completely cleaned out when you go in for your procedure, you will have to repeat the entire prep again to have your colonoscopy.*

4. *Dr. R suggests that on the day of your preparation you substitute baby wipes for toilet paper. Definitely more soothing!*

5. *We both suggest that whatever drink you put your laxative preparation in (GoLightly or MiraLax), use a flavor that you'll never want to taste again (until your next colonoscopy, that is). For this reason, Dr. R hates anything watermelon flavored, and Dr. J can't stand the taste of pineapple.*

    Dr. J remembers the sleep she had during her colonoscopies as being the most restful ever because of the sedative. So, when you get there, relax and enjoy the rest! Be sure not to schedule any other activities, including work, for the rest of that day and to have someone available to drive you home after the test.

OVARIAN CANCER

Although ovarian cancer accounts for only 3 percent of cancers in women, it is ranked as the fourth deadliest cancer. African-American women are less likely to develop ovarian cancer than white women. However, black women are more likely to die from the disease than white women because they receive less aggressive treatment (Parham and Hicks 2005).

Are you at risk for ovarian cancer? The risk for ovarian cancer increases as we age and peaks in our late seventies. The following factors put women at risk:

+   The current use of hormone replacement therapy (Narod 2007)

+   Being overweight (body mass index over 25)

+   A history of breast, uterus, colon, or rectal cancers

- A family history of breast and ovarian cancer (mother, sister, or daughter)

- Having BRCA1 and BRCA2 mutations

- A history of hereditary nonpolyposis colon cancer

- Living in a Western industrialized country

The following *decrease* the risk:

- Having taken birth control pills and/or having been pregnant. The risk for ovarian cancer goes down 29 percent after use of birth control pills for every five-year interval used, and the protection lasts for thirty years after they are stopped (Collaborative Group on Epidemiological Studies of Ovarian Cancer 2008).

- A history of at least one completed pregnancy decreases the risk for ovarian cancer by 45 percent (Holschneider and Berek 2000).

- A history of breastfeeding for eighteen months or longer (Danforth et al. 2007)

How do you know if you have ovarian cancer? What can you do about it? The signs of ovarian cancer are often very subtle or may mimic those of other illnesses. They include a bloated abdomen not relieved by a bowel movement; chronic pressure or pain in the abdomen, back, or pelvis; feeling full quickly or having difficulty eating; frequent urination that is not due to infection or irritation; fatigue that never seems to ease up; chronic nausea or indigestion; vaginal bleeding; and shortness of breath. If you have any of the first four symptoms almost every day for longer than two to three weeks, the Gynecologic Cancer Foundation recommends that you see your gynecologist as soon as possible (Gynecologic Cancer Foundation 2007).

How is ovarian cancer diagnosed? Ovarian cancer may be found by a pelvic exam. For tumors too small to be detected by a pelvic exam, a pelvic ultrasound or CT scan is done. A blood test, called CA125, is often used to follow the progress of ovarian cancer after it has been diagnosed in the later stages; however, it is not useful as a screening test.

How is ovarian cancer treated? Treatment depends on how far the cancer has spread. It usually involves surgery, and may involve radiation and chemotherapy as well. Again, it is extremely important to find a doctor who is going to be your partner in healing and your advocate.

How is it prevented? There is no known way to prevent ovarian cancer; however, it possibly can be detected early by having yearly pelvic examinations plus yearly, or more frequent, pelvic sonograms as recommended by your doctor. This is especially the case if you are at high risk. Pelvic sonograms, however, may miss a cancer just as mammograms sometimes do, so this screening is not foolproof. If you have known mutations of the BRCA1 and BRCA2 genes, you may be advised to have your ovaries removed before cancer can develop. In the future, there may be a blood test that can detect ovarian cancer in the early stages. For now, our mantra of being *aware* of your risks and *alert* to your symptoms, taking *action* to see your clinician immediately, and *advocating* for yourself applies to this disease too.

UTERINE CANCER (ENDOMETRIAL CANCER)

Cancer of the uterus, the most common cancer of the reproductive tract, is a highly curable tumor. It makes up 6 percent of all cancers of women in the U.S. and occurs mostly after menopause. The good news is that the number of new cases, as well as deaths from this disease, is decreasing.

Are you at risk for uterine cancer? Age and race are risk factors, with the risk of this cancer increasing as each year passes, and with Caucasian women being more at risk than African-American women. Having been on hormone replacement therapy with estrogen alone (without progesterone) increases the risk of getting this cancer, as does the diagnosis of endometrial hyperplasia made on tissue obtained from the inside of the uterus. Women who have not taken oral contraceptives (OCPs) earlier in their lives have a greater risk for this disease than women who took OCPs. Taking the medication tamoxifen for the prevention or treatment of breast cancer, having had the inherited form of colorectal cancer, or the disease known as polycystic ovarian syndrome all increase the risk for this cancer.

Several risk factors for uterine cancer are the same as those for breast cancer. These include obesity, because of the increased levels of estrogen stored in fat; diabetes and hypertension (also common in obese women); never having children; and starting menstrual periods at a young age or going through menopause at an older age.

How do you know if you have uterine cancer? What can you do about it? The major symptoms of uterine cancer include postmenopausal bleeding or unusual vaginal discharge, pelvic pain, painful or difficult urination, and pain during intercourse. How to recognize these and what to do about them are discussed in detail in chapter 6.

How is it diagnosed? How is it treated? As with all cancers, the diagnosis is made with a biopsy of the tissue, this time of the uterine lining. Known as an endometrial biopsy, this can be done in the office of your gynecologist. Before she does the biopsy, she will do a pelvic exam and may want to do a pelvic ultrasound. In order to see what stage the cancer is, you may need to have other imaging tests of the rest of your body (x-rays, MRI scans) and a colonoscopy.

Treatment includes a hysterectomy most of the time. Other treatment options are based on the stage of the cancer.

Can uterine cancer be prevented? If you choose to take hormone replacement therapy (HRT) for your menopausal symptoms, then you will be advised to take progesterone with the estrogen in order to avoid uterine cancer. Because tamoxifen increases the risk for uterine cancer, if you need this type of medication to treat or prevent breast cancer, you should talk to your doctor about taking instead the similar drug raloxifene, which has not been shown to increase the risk of uterine cancer. If you've had the inherited form of colorectal cancer, see your gynecologist regularly to be screened for endometrial cancer with a biopsy. If you are obese, lose weight; eat a diet low in saturated fats and high in fruits, vegetables, and soy, and exercise regularly.

CERVICAL CANCER

Cancer of the cervix used to be the leading cause of cancer death for American women. Due to the widespread use of the Pap smear for screening over the past four decades, this is no longer the case. The use of Pap smears is a true medical success story demonstrating how screening and early detection can truly impact cancer, and cancer death, rates. When this cancer is found early, it is highly curable.

Who gets cervical cancer? Are you at risk? Cervical cancer most often develops in women over forty; almost half of women diagnosed in the U.S. have never had a Pap smear, and an additional 10 percent have not had one within the past five years (CDC 2007a). Any woman with an intact cervix can get cervical cancer, but the risk is greatly increased if she has had a high number of sex partners or a history of sexually transmitted infections (STIs) at any time in the past. This is because having had multiple sex partners or STIs increases the likelihood that she is infected with certain types of human papillomavirus (HPV) known to cause cervical cancer (see chapter 6); obviously, infection with these types of HPV is a major risk factor for cervical cancer. Other risk factors include many full-term pregnancies, use of oral contraceptives, smoking cigarettes, having had cervical cancer in the past and still having your cervix, a diet low in fruits and vegetables, and infrequent or no screening with Pap smears.

How do you know if you have cervical cancer? Early in the disease, there are no symptoms. As it progresses, symptoms include abnormal bleeding or discharge from the vagina, painful intercourse, urinary symptoms, and pelvic pain. What to do about these symptoms is discussed in detail in chapter 6.

How is cervical cancer diagnosed and treated? It may be diagnosed by a Pap smear, but even if you have an abnormal Pap smear, you still may need a biopsy of your cervix. In addition, at the same time that the Pap smear is taken, a swab test for HPV can be done; if you have certain types of HPV, even if your Pap smear and exam are normal, you will need a biopsy of your cervix to make sure that early cancer is not present. Just as mammograms can miss breast tumors, Pap smears can miss cervical cancer. This means that even if your Pap smear is negative, you could still have cervical cancer, and you should ask your clinician to do further studies if you have continued symptoms like vaginal bleeding. Also, it's very important to let your clinician know if you have a history of STIs or multiple sex partners, which put you at risk for cervical cancer. As with uterine cancer, depending on the results of your biopsy and exam, you may need other imaging tests to see if the cancer has spread.

Treatment depends on the stage of the cancer. In the earliest stages, it can be easily treated and may not even require a hysterectomy.

Can cervical cancer be prevented? The best prevention is to have regular screening with Pap smears and the HPV test. You've no doubt heard of the new vaccine against certain types of HPV, Gardasil, which is recommended for girls and young adult women ages nine to twenty-six. Currently, it is not recommended for women older than this, based on the idea that because HPV is the most common sexually transmitted infection in the U.S., women older than twenty-six would have already been exposed to it, and thus would gain no benefit from the vaccine. Discussions are ongoing as to whether women older than twenty-six should be recommended to have this vaccine if they are planning to become sexually active for the first time. You should discuss this with your clinician when you discuss your sexual history. Other methods to help prevent cervical cancer include stopping smoking cigarettes, limiting the number of sex partners, and eating a diet low in saturated fats and high in fruits and vegetables.

What if you've had cervical cancer. A recent study has shown that even if you've been cured of cervical cancer, and still have your cervix, you are at increased risk for a recurrence and for vaginal cancers as long as twenty-five years later (Strander et al. 2007). So you must be monitored with a regular pelvic exam and Pap smears and practice the preventive methods discussed above. Chapter 6 discusses the continued need for regular pelvic exams at our current age.

PREVENTING CANCER IN GENERAL

In late 2007, the World Cancer Research Fund and the American Institute for Cancer Research released an extensive report with recommendations on preventing cancer through diet and exercise. These are their recommendations (WCRF/AICR 2007). They may sound familiar!

- ✦ Achieve and maintain a BMI within the normal range.

- ✦ Exercise thirty to sixty minutes a day.

- ✦ Eat no more than eighteen ounces of red meat each week, with little processed meat.

- ✦ Limit alcoholic drinks to one a day for women (and two a day for men).

- ✦ Consume less than 6 grams of sodium daily.

MAKING IT THROUGH THE TREATMENT IF YOU ARE DIAGNOSED WITH CANCER

Treatment for cancer can be stressful and frightening. Therapies exist that may make it easier for you and improve the outcome. Please note: Although the studies described in this section were done mostly with breast cancer patients, we are recommending you try them with the treatment for any type of cancer, as long as you discuss this with your doctor. See chapters 13 and 14 for definitions and full discussions of the CAM therapies, and herb and supplement therapies, mentioned below.

CAM Therapies

Many of the CAM therapies have been studied in cancer patients.

Acupuncture. This has been found to reduce the nausea of chemotherapy and improve energy (Ezzo et al. 2005) and has been endorsed by the National Institutes of Health (NIH) for this purpose.

Guided imagery. The use of guided imagery can improve the quality and length of life and ease the discomfort of chemotherapy for breast cancer patients (Walker et al. 1999).

Hypnosis and support groups. Both of these may be very helpful. In a study reported in 1989, eighty-six patients with metastatic breast cancer were studied. Half of the group participated in a weekly support group and used self-hypnosis for pain. The other half received routine care. Those in the support group lived almost twice as long as those without the support group (Spiegel et al. 1989).

Yoga. One study showed remarkable results among women undergoing treatment for breast cancer who practiced daily yoga. They had better general health, energy, social functioning, better sleep, and less fatigue than women who did not practice yoga (Cohen, Gerner, and Baile 2000).

Lifestyle changes. Women with cancer who exercise during treatment have been found to have greater mobility, better moods, and fewer complications than those women who don't exercise (Mutrie et al. 2007). A study that followed more than 1,400 breast cancer survivors over six years found that those with estrogen receptor positive breast cancer, regardless of their weight, who exercised thirty minutes per day and ate the equivalent of five servings of fruits and vegetables per day had a significantly improved survival rate compared to those women who did not (Pierce et al. 2007).

Herbs and supplements. There is a concern among most oncologists that herbs and supplements may counteract the effects of chemotherapy and radiation treatment. Therefore, most patients are advised to avoid them during treatment. However, the medical establishment does not object to patients getting healthy antioxidants and nutrients *from food*. Therefore, we advise eating as nutritiously as you can during your cancer treatment with a diet of organic food, rich in fruits, vegetables, and ground flaxseeds.

Diet. Flaxseeds are rich in omega-3 fatty acids as well as lignans. Ground flaxseeds (not the oil) may help to prevent or treat breast cancer. A small but dramatic study of women with newly diagnosed breast cancer found that those who were given a flaxseed muffin (containing 25 grams of flax) daily for a month had a drop in the activity of their breast cancer cells by over 30 percent (Thompson et al. 2005). Whole flaxseeds must be ground to get the full benefits (a regular coffee grinder will do), and then kept in the freezer or refrigerator to prevent them from going bad, which they can quickly do. They can be eaten on cereal and salads, in smoothies, or even in yogurt, and taste a bit like walnuts. Best of all, they're cheap.

SURVIVING CANCER

We have entered a new era when it comes to cancer and cancer care. Today, the majority of cancer patients survive their cancers and live a normal life span. Nevertheless, once someone has had cancer, it changes her outlook and her sense of identity. Many people see it as a wake-up call and are able to change their priorities and lifestyles. Others change for a while and then go back to their old ways. However, it is important to maintain healthy habits after surviving cancer and to attend to the spirit—as well as the mind and body.

Support from others—be they friends, family, other cancer survivors, or even your favorite pet—and mind-body therapies have been found to improve the quality as well as the length of life.

A diet rich in fruits, vegetables, and healthy fats is also important. Organic produce is always preferable. Exercise on a regular basis is important.

Finally, it's also important to laugh and to laugh often. There is a new discipline in medicine, called psychoneuroimmunology that studies the impact of our emotions on our body. Professionals in this field have found that laughter boosts our immune system and cancer-fighting cells.

A Survivor's Story
by Lori Taft Sours, Ph.D.

I received a breast cancer diagnosis on February 3, 2000. My world changed on that date. It became filled with doctor's appointments, questions, research, decisions, and more questions. Should I have a lumpectomy or mastectomy? Is the suggested treatment protocol the best one? What are the short-term and long-term effects of surgery, chemotherapy, and radiation? Has the cancer spread? How will I know?

Now a seven-year survivor, I know that there are few questions with definitive answers and that uncertainty is my "new normal." I have learned to live with that uncertainty. As I move through menopause and firmly into middle age, juggling the demands of family and career, the questions are confounded. Is my fuzzy thinking a vestige of "chemo-brain" or menopause? Are the aches in my joints metastasized cancer or arthritis? Are my headaches due to cancer or a stressful job? For me, the best lesson of cancer was that I must be an active member of my health care team. I must continue to ask the questions, do the research, and make the decisions. The one question that does have an answer is "How do I feel?" In the end, that is the most important question.

THE DOCS DISCUSS CANCERS COMMON IN WOMEN OVER FIFTY

DR. J: When patients come to the office or the emergency room, they are often worried that they have cancer. What is the likelihood of finding it?

DR. R: There are certain things that alarm people, such as blood in the urine, blood in the stool, bronchitis or a cough that doesn't go away, trouble swallowing, and weight loss. I look for causes of all of these symptoms. How often is it cancer? A recent study has found that if alarming symptoms have been present for less than three months in people over sixty-five, cancer is more likely than in people who have had these alarming symptoms for more than three years (Jones et al. 2007). Again, this shows the importance of our age group taking symptoms that we might have ignored when we were younger much more seriously and getting medical attention immediately. And, of course, not feeling silly about seeking medical help for what might seem to be a minor symptom.

DR. J: Are hair relaxers and hair dyes associated with cancer?

DR. R: A recent study of hair relaxers and cancer found no correlation, so they are safe (Rosenberg et al. 2007). Another recent study found a very small association between lymphoma and the use of hair dyes. This was mostly for women who used hair dyes before 1980 (Takkouche, Etminan, and Montes-Martinez 2005). The safety of hair dyes has improved since then. But this small increased risk isn't enough to stop me from coloring my hair!

DR. J: Many of my patients who have had cancer diagnosed in one organ of the body are surprised to find out that by their having this particular cancer—for instance, breast cancer—they are now at increased risk for developing a cancer in an entirely different organ, such as colon cancer. Have you had patients surprised by this also?

DR. R.: Yes. To have one cancer and to know that even after a full course of recommended treatment(s) for that cancer, they may still be at risk for it to recur is certainly enough to deal with. So, the knowledge that they are at increased risk for a second cancer is difficult. But there is an up side to this knowledge and that, of course, is that they will know to screen for the other cancers and possible catch them at a very early stage when they can be cured.

SR. J.: So, once again, knowledge is power, right?

DR. R.: Absoultely.

PEARLS OF WISDOM
FOR SURVIVING AND THRIVING

○ Know that early detection and screening are crucial for the prevention of many types of cancer.

○ Follow the recommended schedule for all screening procedures in chapter 15.

○ Know that many cancers are survivable.

○ If one of your screening tests is negative but you continue to have symptoms, ask for further tests. Trust your gut instincts and advocate for yourself.

○ When in doubt, check it out! Don't be embarrassed to seek medical attention for what may seem to be minor symptoms.

○ Don't be afraid to find out whether you have cancer; the earlier it is found, the better.

○ Attitude is everything. Having a positive attitude can help the quality and length of your life.

○ Make sure you are comfortable with your clinicians and doctors, and that they are your advocates. If they are not, find new ones, or at least get a second opinion.

○ And—all together now, in unison: Be *aware* of your risk factors, *alert* to your symptoms, *active* in getting regularly screened and in seeking help immediately if you have symptoms, and *advocate* for yourself!

CHAPTER 13

Vitamins and Nutrients:
How to Supplement Wisely

When you first saw the title of this chapter, it was likely that you had one of two reactions: either you were pleased to finally be able to learn about the huge number of supplements currently available so you will know which to buy, or you planned to skip this chapter because you think the topic isn't important. To those of you in the first group, we're hoping that you'll have a better idea of what supplements to consider taking after reading this; to those of you in the second group, please read the next few sentences before you skip the rest of this chapter.

This topic is definitely important, and here's the reason why: Some of the standard medications used successfully over the years to treat serious conditions were originally just like the substances discussed in this chapter: They were made from plants or other natural products. One example is the drug digitalis (digoxin), which is a widely used medication for several diseases of the heart and originally came from the foxglove plant. So, although the supplements that we mention may not be part of mainstream medicine *yet*, why not get the possible benefit from them, as long as they are safe?

WHAT IS A SUPPLEMENT?

Authors' note: Because Dr. R has completed a fellowship in this discipline and is currently practicing in this field, she has written this chapter.

A dietary or nutritional *supplement* is exactly what it sounds like: It is an additional vitamin, mineral, herb, amino acid, fatty acid, or protein used to supply nutritional value beyond what's available in the diet; in other words, a supplement enhances the nutritional benefits of your diet.

What Do You Need to Know About Supplements in General?

There are hundreds (and that's no exaggeration) of herbs, vitamins, and other dietary supplements out there—so many, in fact, that you could spend your family's entire savings on them. But just because they are "natural" doesn't mean they're safe.

If you eat a healthy, well-balanced diet, you may not need supplements. There are, nevertheless, some nutrients that you may not get enough of in your diet.

Buyer beware. You can never be 100 percent certain that you are getting pure products, or that the dosage of the vitamin or herb is both safe and effective.

You should always tell your clinician what supplements you take. The majority of people who take supplements don't tell their clinician or include them in the list of medications they take. This can be dangerous because many supplements can have significant interactions with medications, including causing a medication not to be effective.

Supplements currently are not overseen by the FDA. Within the next three years, the FDA will begin testing to ensure that the ingredients listed on the supplement packaging are really contained in the product, and that the products themselves are free from contamination (FDA 2007a).

Quality standards. There are organizations that monitor the quality of supplements. The United States Pharmacopoeia (USP) provides manufacturing standards for certain medicines and dietary supplements, and the National Nutritional Foods Association provides its assurance that good manufacturing practices (GMP) have been met. Many supplements will have these letters on the bottle to let you know they have passed inspection. If you don't see the letters, the supplements have not been evaluated by these organizations. But even if the bottle has these initials on it, that still doesn't mean that the supplement contained in it is either effective or safe.

That All-Important Multivitamin

Although you may try to eat a well-balanced diet all the time, that may not be realistic. Stuff happens! You get busy with your job, children, husband and/or partner, grandchildren, and life. We'll start with the basics. Because it is difficult for your diet to contain all the nutrients that you need, most adults need a good multivitamin. How do you choose a good one? These are the things you need to look for:

+ A multivitamin without preformed vitamin A; it should have a mix of carotenoids, and not just beta-carotene (which is a form of vitamin A).

+ A multivitamin with vitamin E as a mix of natural tocopherols (the components of vitamin E).

+ A multivitamin that contains 50 mg of most of the B vitamins, with the exception of folic acid. It should have at least 400 mcg of folic acid. If it doesn't, you will need to take additional folic acid as a separate supplement. See below.

+ Most multivitamins contain 400 IU of vitamin D. This isn't enough. The current recommendation for vitamin D is between 400 and 1,000 IU a day. Therefore, you may need to take additional vitamin D as a separate supplement. See below.

+ A multivitamin that contains calcium. Please note: Most multivitamins do not have enough calcium for your entire daily requirement, so you will need to get in more through your diet, or take additional calcium as a supplement, in order to meet the daily requirements. See below.

+ A multivitamin without iron, unless you are menstruating or you have iron deficiency. Getting too much iron can be dangerous.

+ A multivitamin that contains 200 mcg of selenium, an important antioxidant. It has been found to reduce the risk of secondary cancers in some patients with a previous diagnosis of skin cancer (Clark et al. 1997).

You Need More of Some Vitamins and Minerals Than Are in a Multivitamin

Folic acid. You should be taking between 400 and 800 mcg a day of folic acid. Please see the information on strokes and folic acid in chapter 1 for the reasons why.

Calcium. The current recommendations for the total calcium that you need are between 1,000 mg and 1,500 mg a day. This includes the amount that you obtain through dairy foods and milk. See the information on osteoporosis in chapter 8 for further information, especially about the different types of calcium supplements available.

Vitamin D. Since the current recommendation for how much vitamin D you need is between 400 and 1,000 IU a day, you may have to get the additional amount that you need in a supplement if your multivitamin doesn't provide enough. You may need more based on your blood level. Vitamin D3, or cholecalciferol, is the preferred form of this supplement; this should be noted on the bottle. Besides being necessary for calcium to be absorbed (see chapter 8), vitamin D has been found to do many things: It improves muscle function and balance, boosts the immune system, reduces the weight gain that can occur with menopause, and improves high blood pressure. In chapter 12, we discussed the important role vitamin D may play in cancer prevention. Finally, adequate levels of vitamin D correlate with lower mortality rates in general (Autier and Gandini 2007).

THE SUPPLEMENTS

Now that you have some ideas about how to choose a multivitamin and the additional vitamins and minerals you need, let's discuss specific supplements. First consider this: When you walk through the aisles of a health food store, it is tempting to buy almost every supplement you see. Who wouldn't want to stop the aging process, be more beautiful, have the energy of a ten-year-old, the sex drive of a teenager, the metabolism of a supermodel, and the brainpower of Einstein? When you look around at all the supplements, these are the promises that are implied or stated. But are they realistic or valid? No, because life is never that simple. Those promised results cannot be found in a bottle. (Although we can always hope.) There are far too many unsubstantiated claims out there, which is why it is important to become an educated consumer.

I'll tell you next the pros, cons, and bottom line on the most frequently used supplements; then you can decide for yourself which you want to try, based on your individual medical concerns and the state of your current health. And, again, always check with your primary care clinician to find out if there is any reason you should not take a particular supplement. Also remember that the following discussions aren't meant to be comprehensive for each supplement; I will tell you the main points about each. There are several websites on the Recommended Reading list devoted to this topic.

Ginkgo Biloba

Ginkgo Biloba is the most widely used herbal extract in Germany. A survey done in 2001 in the U.S. found that over 4.5 million Americans were currently using this herb at the time (Richman and Witkowski 2001).

For which conditions has ginkgo been used? Ginkgo extracts have been used since 2800 B.C. to combat age-related symptoms. It works as a potent antioxidant that improves blood flow. Numerous studies have shown small improvements in claudication (pain in the legs that occurs with exercise and is caused by poor circulation) when ginkgo is taken by mouth (Pittler and Ernst 2000). However, it probably is not as helpful as prescription medication (such as Trental, or pentoxifylline) or exercise therapy, and should not be taken for that problem without discussing it with a doctor. Ginkgo may help with improving memory and in dementia treatment (not prevention), including Alzheimer's and multi-infarct dementia (LeBars et al. 1997). (See chapter 1.) It may work as well as prescription medications, such as Aricept (donepezil), which is commonly prescribed for Alzheimer's disease, although further studies are needed (Birks, Grimley, and Van Dongen 2002).

What is the recommended dose of ginkgo? The usual dose is 120 to 240 mg a day in two to three divided doses. The ultimate dose depends on the individual and how she responds to it.

What are the possible problems with taking ginkgo? In general, ginkgo is well tolerated. It may increase bleeding, especially when used with blood thinners. If you are on Coumadin (warfarin), talk to your doctor before you even *think* about taking ginkgo. Also, if you're planning to have surgery in the future, let your surgeon know you're taking it. Ginkgo may produce an additive effect to both MAO inhibitor drugs (a type of antidepressant) and SSRI antidepressants drugs such as Prozac (fluoxetine) and Paxil (paroxetine). Make sure your doctor knows you plan to take ginkgo before you start taking one of these medications.

Should you take Ginkgo? **Bottom line:** I don't typically recommend ginkgo biloba to my patients with claudication because conventional medications work better. However, it would be reasonable to try it for memory enhancement if you have the occasional "brain fade" (and who among us doesn't?). Of course, you have to remember to take it!

Turmeric

There has been increasing interest in turmeric for its medicinal properties. It is a plant in the ginger family that is widely used as food coloring, and as a principal ingredient of curry powder.

For which conditions has turmeric been used? It has been used for centuries in Ayurvedic and Chinese medicine as an anti-inflammatory, as well as to treat digestive problems. Recent studies have shown that people living in rural India, where turmeric is abundant in the diet, have a much lower incidence of Alzheimer's disease than other populations (Ringman, Frautschy, and Cole 2005). Animal studies have found that it has powerful anti-inflammatory properties that also may help in the treatment of various cancers, including those of the prostate, breast, skin, and colon (Aggarwal, Kumar, and Bharti 2003).

What is the recommended dose? Turmeric comes in the form of a supplement or can be used to flavor food. Studies have used from 750 mg to 1.5 grams of turmeric in three to four divided doses per day. In India, most people consume between 2.2 and 5 grams a day. This corresponds to 60 to 200 mg of curcumin (found in turmeric) per day. The curcumin in turmeric gives curry powder its yellow color.

What are the possible problems with taking turmeric? The possible adverse effect of turmeric is thought to occur only when used in the medicinal form; the concern is that theoretically it could increase the blood-thinning effect of Coumadin (warfarin) and aspirin. This is not an issue with curry powder since it is usually used in such small amounts. If you are on Coumadin and taking turmeric in the medicinal form, you will need to have your blood monitored closely. If you are on Coumadin and use a lot of turmeric or curry powder in your food, be sure to let your clinician know.

Should you take turmeric? Bottom line: Using turmeric or curry powder as a regular spice in your food may help to prevent dementia, and it will enhance the taste of your food. I think more will be heard about the benefits of turmeric in the coming years.

Coenzyme Q10 (CoQ10)

Coenzyme Q10 (CoQ10) is normally found in your body and is necessary for the functioning of your cells. CoQ10 levels decrease with age and are low in patients with chronic diseases such as heart disease, Parkinson's disease, cancer, diabetes, and HIV/AIDS.

For which conditions has CoQ10 been used? Recent studies have found that supplemental CoQ10 may cause small decreases in blood pressure (Hodgson et al. 2002), although the standard dose for this purpose has not been determined. If you are already on high blood pressure medicine, and wish to try CoQ10, you may be able to use less of your antihypertensive medication. It may help patients with angina by improving exercise tolerance. In one study, CoQ10 given to patients within three days of a heart attack reduced deaths, abnormal heart rhythms, and second heart attacks (Singh et al. 1998). We discuss the benefit of CoQ10 when it is taken with statin drugs in the section on reducing blood lipids in chapter 3. There has been some promising research on the use of CoQ10 in slowing the progression of dementia in Alzheimer's patients (Gutzmann and Hadler 1998), and it may also slow the progression of Parkinson's disease (Shults et al. 2002). And as mentioned in chapter 9, CoQ10, also known as idebenone, is effective in treating some of the signs of aging when contained in a skin cream.

What is the recommended dose? The recommended starting dose is 60 mg per day. Note that there is a particular form of CoQ10 that you should buy; the recommended form is the soft gel or emulsified form. These are better absorbed. You should take CoQ10 with a fat-containing meal or snack.

What are the possible problems with taking CoQ10? There are few side effects of CoQ10. Very rarely CoQ10 may cause nausea, heartburn, a rash, dizziness, or flu-like symptoms, all of which are mild and brief, and go away once the supplement is stopped.

Should you take CoQ10? Whether taking CoQ10 is of benefit remains controversial, and studies are ongoing. (Are you picking up a theme here?) **Bottom line:** I recommend CoQ10 to all of my patients who are taking statin drugs or red yeast rice to lower blood lipids. I also prescribe it for my patients with Alzheimer's disease, Parkinson's disease, and coronary artery disease (CAD) as a complement to their standard medication. There is great potential benefit with little risk.

Deglycyrrhizinated Licorice

Licorice is not just a candy made from the plant; it has medicinal uses as well.

For what conditions has licorice been used? Licorice root has been used for centuries to treat digestive disorders. It can also soothe chancre sores. However, at high doses it can be dangerous, as it causes high blood pressure, loss of potassium, and swelling, all due to a component in licorice called glycyrrhizic acid. When this component is removed, what remains is called deglycyrrhizinated licorice (DGL), which has no side effects.

What is the recommended dose? DGL is usually taken as a tablet or wafer. It is most effective if two tablets or wafers are chewed slowly before or between meals. It can also be found in a powder form that, when used as a paste, can soothe chancre sores.

What are the possible problems with DGL? As mentioned above, whole licorice root with glycyrrhizic acid can cause high blood pressure, alter hormone levels, cause fluid retention, and interfere with a variety of medications. It is very important to make sure that there is no glycyrrhizic acid in whatever preparation you use.

Dr. R's Story

My mother loves to eat licorice. One day many years ago, she found this gourmet black licorice that was so irresistible that she had to eat the whole bag. The next day, she looked like someone had pumped her up with a hose. She was terribly swollen. It was the glycyrrhizic acid in the licorice that got her. That was the last time she ate that much licorice in one sitting!

Should you take DGL? Bottom line: This may be a reasonable alternative for women who have heartburn and do not want to take conventional medications. I have had several patients for whom the proton pump inhibitor drugs (such as Nexium and Prevacid) and the H_2 blocker drugs (such as Zantac) did not help. DGL was a successful treatment for them. It is also a very good treatment for painful chancre sores.

S-Adenosylmethionine (SAMe)

SAMe is a synthetic form of a chemical that is found naturally in our body. It acts as an antioxidant and protects the body from environmental damage.

For what conditions has SAMe been used? We talked about the use of SAMe in the treatment of osteoarthritis and fibromyalgia in chapter 8. Additionally, in multiple studies it significantly improved depression. It has also been found to improve the itching of cholestasis, a condition in which bile cannot flow to the bowel from the liver; instead the bile remains in the liver. This occurs in some people who have liver disease, and can also occur during pregnancy (AHRQ 2002).

What is the recommended dose? The dose varies between 400 and 1,600 mg a day. SAMe is usually taken at a dose of 200 to 600 mg for osteoarthritis, and at doses from 400 to 1,600 mg for depression.

What are the possible problems with taking SAMe? Because SAMe increases serotonin levels, it should not be used with SSRI antidepressants and should not be used by people with bipolar disorder. Also, because it may decrease the effectiveness of medications used to treat Parkinson's disease, patients with this disorder should avoid it.

Should you take SAMe? Bottom line: If you have osteoarthritis or mild depression or cholestasis and you want to go the herbal route for treatment, this is a reasonable alternative, as long as your doctor monitors you.

Black Cohosh

We discussed black cohosh in chapter 10, and I will elaborate on it here.

For what conditions has black cohosh been used? Black cohosh is primarily used to help with symptoms of menopause, although its safety and effectiveness have been studied only for durations of up to six months. Most of the studies for this use are weak, and, in fact, no one is really sure how it works. Personally, it did work in getting rid of my hot flashes.

What is the recommended dose? The recommended dose to help alleviate menopausal symptoms is 20 to 40 mg twice a day. Start with the lower dose and try it for one to two weeks; if you don't notice a response, then increase to the higher dose.

What are the possible problems with taking it? Black cohosh contains a small amount of salicylic acid and should be used with caution by those allergic to aspirin. There probably is not enough of this chemical present in most products to raise concerns about bleeding. Black cohosh may lower blood pressure and should be used with caution in people on beta-blockers or calcium channel blockers (Blumenthal, Goldberg, and Brinkman 2000). One of the concerns about black cohosh has been that it may increase the chance of developing breast cancer. However, a study published in the *International Journal of Cancer* found that the use of black cohosh was associated with a 61 percent *reduction* of breast cancer risk (Rebbeck et al. 2007) in the group of over 2,000 women studied. More research needs to be done.

Should you take it? **Bottom line:** Black cohosh is a relatively safe product that is a reasonable alternative to hormones for symptoms of menopause. Again, it is very important to let your clinician know that you are on this supplement.

Echinacea

Did you know that echinacea is a member of the daisy family? So much for that famous line "Please don't eat the daisies."

For what conditions has echinacea been used? Historically, it has been used to treat colds, tonsillitis, wound infections, snakebites, and a wide variety of other conditions. Although older studies done in Germany suggest that it may decrease the duration and severity of colds, recent studies have not confirmed this—that is, until a very recent paper looked at the combined results from many studies and found that echinacea can shorten the duration of a cold by one and a quarter days and can reduce the chances of getting a cold by half (Shah 2007). One of the problems in studying echinacea is that there is such variability when it comes to the preparation. There are three different species used for medicinal purposes, and their preparation methods are extremely variable. More well-designed studies are needed.

What is the recommended dose? The dosage in capsules (containing powdered herb) for treatment of upper respiratory tract infections is 500 to 1,000 mg by mouth three times daily for five to seven days.

What are the possible problems with taking echinacea? There are usually few side effects from taking this herb. The main ones are nausea, diarrhea, constipation, and a skin rash when used topically. However, there have been reported episodes of anaphylaxis (a potentially fatal allergic reaction) and severe asthma with its use. People with a history of allergy to plants in the daisy family should not take it. Because it may affect the immune system, patients with HIV/AIDS and those with autoimmune disorders need to avoid echinacea.

Should you take it? **Bottom line:** As long as you don't have an allergy to plants in the daisy family or problems with your immune system, echinacea may be of benefit to you if you feel a cold coming on, or if you have been exposed to someone who has one. Be sure to let your primary care provider know you are taking it.

Astragalus

Astragalus is a traditional Chinese medicine, made from a plant native to the area, which has been used for thousands of years.

For what conditions has astragalus been used? It was originally used to promote endurance, lower blood pressure, and improve urinary function. More recently, it has been found to improve immunity in those with compromised immune systems due to chemotherapy for colorectal cancer (Taixiang, Munro, and Guanjian 2005). It also may help in the general strengthening of normal immune systems (Tan and Vanitha 2004). I take it instead of echinacea when I feel a cold starting, and suggest it to friends who travel a lot. One friend, who used to have colds and upper respiratory infections all winter, has not had even one cold since he's been taking astragalus.

What is the recommended dose? Various doses of astragalus have been used or studied, including 250 to 500 mg of extract taken four times daily; 1 to 30 grams of dried root taken daily (doses as high as 60 grams have been reported); or 500 to 1,000 mg of root capsules taken three times daily. Dosing with the tinctures or the fluid extracts depends on the preparation. The dosage recommendations should be on the bottles. For preventing colds, I usually recommend one to two of the 500 mg capsules a day. If you still get a cold, increase it to one to two capsules, three times a day.

What are the possible problems with taking astragalus? There are no known side effects. However, astragalus may increase the effect of certain antiviral medicines such as acyclovir (Zovirax) and interferon. If you are taking these medications, talk to your doctor before considering using astragalus. In addition, it may counteract the immune-suppressing effects of cyclosporine, which is used in organ transplant patients, and thus may increase the risk of organ rejection. For that reason, people who have had organ transplants should not take it. Finally, if you have an autoimmune disease such as lupus, Crohn's disease, or ulcerative colitis, you should not use astragalus, as it may cause a flare-up in the disease.

Should you take astragalus? Bottom line: Astragalus is relatively safe. If you do not have an autoimmune disease, are not on antiviral medication or interferon, and want to give it a try to prevent or treat a cold, it may help.

Korean Pine Nut Oil

Pinolenic acid is an extract made from pine nut oil. Either name may appear on product labels.

For what conditions has Korean pine nut oil been used? When a capsule of the extract is taken one hour before a meal, it stimulates hunger-suppressing hormones. In a study presented at the American Chemical Society national meeting in 2006, subjects had increased levels of these hormones for over four hours after taking 3 grams of Korean pine nut oil extract and eating a small breakfast of carbohydrates (Causey 2006).

What is the recommended dose? The recommended dose is 1,000 mg one hour before eating.

What are the possible problems? There are no reported side effects.

Should you take Korean pine nut oil? Bottom line: For weight loss, the key is to eat less and exercise more. Korean pine nut oil may help some people to eat less. Again, discuss taking it with your doctor before you try it.

Valerian Root

Hippocrates, the "father" of Western medicine, prescribed valerian root for his patients who couldn't sleep. He described the aroma as pleasant, and it was used in perfumes. Because most people today would not describe the odor as Hippocrates did, my guess is that our smell receptors have become more refined through the ages.

For what conditions has valerian root been used? Historically, this herb was used as a diuretic and as an aid to digestion; it is currently used for insomnia. Valerian was also used as an official remedy by the U.S. military for shell shock during World War I, and as a sedative from 1820 until 1936. Valerian root, in fact, acts as a mild and effective sedative and can be used both as an occasional sleep aid and for chronic sleep problems.

What is the recommended dose? The generally recommended dose is 600 mg of the standardized extract taken one to two hours before sleep, and used over a month. It takes a while (meaning days to weeks) for this to work, so don't expect it to help immediately. Finding a standard extract of Valerian is a *must*; all reputable manufacturers will indicate on the label that theirs contains a standardized form.

What are the possible problems with valerian? The side effects are mild and infrequent, and are described as continued mild sedation in the morning or a mild headache.

Should you take valerian? Bottom line: For insomnia, this is a safe, natural way to get to sleep.

Green Tea

You probably know that green or black tea is one of the most widely consumed beverages in the world. In addition to being used to make the drink, green tea is now sold as an extract.

What exactly is green tea? White, green, and black teas all come from the leaves of a plant known as *Camellia sinensis*. The difference in the three teas lies in the degree to which they are treated. Picking the leaves and air-drying them produce white tea. Picking the leaves and then heating and drying them produces green tea. Adding another step involving oxidation produces black tea. All of the teas contain antioxidants, but because of the various steps in processing, white tea probably contains the most, as it is the least processed. The reason that green tea is more popular than white tea is simply a matter of cost. White tea is expensive.

For what conditions has green tea been used? It is helpful in reducing inflammation in those with arthritis. It can cause improvement in asthma patients, but this may be due to the caffeine in the tea. Green tea is highly touted in cancer prevention; there are ongoing studies testing it for the prevention of a wide variety of cancers including those of the stomach, colon, pancreas, esophagus, prostate, cervix, and breast (Dufresne and Farnworth 2001). It may also be beneficial in the treatment of estrogen receptor positive breast cancer (see chapter 12.) Regular green tea drinkers may have a reduced risk of heart attacks. It may lower cholesterol, improve memory and mental alertness, and prevent dental cavities. When applied to the skin, it may help wrinkles (Dufresne and Farnworth 2001). Lately, it has been touted to aid in weight loss. That's a lot of work for one little drink to do. More studies are needed.

What is the recommended dose? How much is needed on a daily basis for cancer prevention? We really don't know. Preliminary data has found that drinking four cups a day of decaffeinated green tea may decrease the amount of damage to DNA in heavy smokers (Hakim et al. 2004). If you want to take it in the form of an extract at an equivalent dose, it would be 300 to 400 mg a day.

What are the possible problems with taking green tea? The only downside to drinking a lot of green tea is that you may be visiting the bathroom more often. And if you are sensitive to caffeine, you may have a problem with the caffeinated green tea. If that's the case, then get decaffeinated green tea. The potential benefits are great and the downside is minimal. Of course, you can use the extract if you want to avoid the bathroom problem.

Should you take green tea? Bottom line: *Drink up!* But watch the caffeine.

Dr. R's Personal Regimen of Supplements

Whew! That's it. I hope that I've given you an idea of what is out there in the world of supplements. (And I only covered a few!) Remember: You must always weigh the risks and the benefits of each. It is also important to be forthcoming with your medical provider regarding what you are taking. Make sure you tailor what you want to what you really need. Because these supplements can be expensive, get the majority of the nutrients you need from your diet and then supplement only what you can't get in foods or beverages.

Here's what I take on a regular basis: First, I am impressed with the studies on turmeric and green tea, so I take a combination pill called Protandim. This contains five herbs: turmeric, milk thistle, and ashwagandha, bacopa, and green tea extracts. I also take 1 gram of Eskimo 3 fish oil daily, as well as 1,200 mg of liquid calcium, 300 mg of magnesium, and 2,000 IU of vitamin D. The one thing that noticeably improved my energy and overall well-being was the vitamin D. I also take 100 mg of CoQ10. I used to take a multivitamin, but I eat a healthy diet, so I stopped taking it. Selenium, which is easy to get in a vitamin, is usually tough to get in the diet. However, I found that I can get enough by eating two to three Brazil nuts each day. I have taken black cohosh for menopausal symptoms; it got rid of my hot flashes, and then I went on hormones. When I start to feel sick with an upper respiratory infection, I take astragalus and it has averted many a cold. I personally like it better than echinacea. Finally, only recently I started taking Brain Fog Lifter, containing ginkgo biloba, acetyl-L-carnitine, ginseng, bilberry, and small amounts of other herbs. That memory I had prior to menopause is starting to come back. A big indicator of that is I am remembering to take the Brain Fog Lifter!

THE DOCS CHAT ABOUT SUPPLEMENTS

DR. J: And you thought I use a lot of skin care products—I don't even begin to take the supplements you do! Just vitamin D, folic acid, and loads of green tea for me. (Don't chide me about taking calcium; I get the recommended amount in my diet through lots of yogurt and cheese.) What are some of the common problems that you see in your practice with patients who take a lot of supplements?

DR. R: I've seen many patients who are paying a lot of money, and are actually taking the same herbs in different preparations. Moreover, they often take way too much of some supplements. One patient was feeling horrible; when we looked at everything she was taking, we found she'd been consuming over 5,000 mg of calcium a day. (Boy was she constipated!) That's why it's so important for patients to bring all the supplements they take with them on their medical visits to evaluate them with their clinician.

DR. J: What if a patient's clinician doesn't know a lot about supplements?

DR. R: The patient must let her clinician know that she is interested in taking supplements. If the clinician doesn't have time to learn about them, the patient can go to an integrative medicine practitioner or find a clinician who has knowledge in the field.

DR. J: What should people do about their supplements if they are going to have surgery?

DR. R: It is so important to let the surgeon and anesthesiologist know if you are on supplements. Many of them can increase bleeding—including fish oil, ginkgo biloba, and even garlic. Most surgeons will have you stop your supplements at least two to three weeks prior to surgery.

PEARLS OF WISDOM FOR SUPPLEMENTING WISELY

○ Natural is not necessarily safe.

○ Tell your primary care clinician and your surgeon about all the supplements you take, and the dosages.

○ Better yet, take your supplements with you to your next medical appointment.

○ Become an informed consumer; know the benefits and risks of your supplements.

○ Try to get most of your nutrients from whole foods.

CHAPTER 14

Complementary and Alternative Medical (CAM) Therapies: How to Complement Wisely

There was a time when the entire traditional medical establishment in America considered the field of complementary and alternative medicine (CAM) to be *way* out there. No more. Today, many prestigious medical institutions have realized the value of these therapies and are not only doing research in the field, but also incorporating the therapies into their programs. Harvard, Johns Hopkins, the University of Arizona, Scripps Medical Center, and Sloan-Kettering are just a few of the institutions integrating many of these modalities into their treatments. The National Institutes of Health has an entire division devoted to the study of CAM, known as the National Center for Complementary and Alternative Medicine. What caused those in the field of traditional medicine to change their minds? You did! The public is driving this change in attitude. It is estimated that as many as 62 percent of Americans are using CAM therapies and spending $47 billion a year (Eisenberg et al. 1998).

What exactly is CAM? It is a varied group of medical health care systems, practices, and products that are not considered part of the conventional medical system…yet. This chapter discusses the most commonly used CAM therapies, including acupuncture, aromatherapy, chiropractic, guided imagery, biofeedback, hypnosis, massage therapy, meditation, prayer, and yoga. There are so many more, it would take another book to describe them. Vitamins and herbal supplements are discussed in chapter 13.

Authors' note: Because Robin has studied CAM and uses many of these therapies in her practice and as part of her life, she has written this chapter.

WHAT DO YOU NEED TO KNOW ABOUT CAM IN GENERAL?

Many of the same principles apply when you are deciding to use CAM therapies as when you are considering the use of supplements.

Buyer Beware

Just as with supplements, research the specific CAM therapy and the practitioner of that therapy. Be aware of the following issues.

Is the CAM therapy beneficial and safe for use with your medical problem? Not all CAM therapies are good or safe for all medical problems; neither are all CAM therapies good for every person. Ask your primary clinician what she knows about this. Call the offices of a few CAM practitioners and ask if they commonly treat your medical problem with their particular therapy. Ask friends about their experiences. See the Resources section for books and websites on CAM.

Is the CAM practitioner qualified? Equally as important, find a practitioner who is qualified. Some of the CAM therapies have organizations that certify the practitioner as being competent and qualified. Also, in some of the CAM fields such as acupuncture, hypnosis, and chiropractic, state licensing is required. The best ways to find out if the practitioner you are considering is qualified include asking your primary clinician; calling the state health department for practitioners in fields that require licensing; or calling a university medical center near you and asking if there is a CAM department, and if not, who you can speak to about recommendations for CAM practitioners.

How do you pay for the CAM therapy? Find out if the CAM therapy you are considering is covered by your insurance for your particular medical problem. Some CAM therapies are covered by insurance; many others are not. Do not be surprised by having to pay at the time of your appointment; research this issue beforehand.

Who do you call if there is a problem after the treatment? Some CAM practitioners' are not available after office hours. Be sure to ask at the time of the appointment what you should do if there is a problem after the treatment has been completed. Always let your primary clinician know if you experience a problem after CAM therapy.

Be Sure Your Primary Care Clinician Knows About Your CAM Treatment

Just as with any supplements you may take, discuss your plans for CAM therapy with your clinician before you have it. Make sure she is comfortable with your having the treatment, especially in light of your medical history and current problems.

ACUPUNCTURE

Acupuncture is a health practice that began in China over 2,500 years ago.

What is it? *Acupuncture* is based on the idea that the body contains meridians or "lines" of energy known as qi (chi). When the energy is balanced, we are healthy. When there is imbalance, we become sick. Acupuncturists use fine needles (both sterile and disposable) that they place in specific points corresponding to different areas of the body. When stimulated, the needles help to move the qi, or energy, in those areas. For instance, if you have a headache, a needle may be placed in a specific spot on your hand because its placement there has been found to relieve headaches. For help in stopping smoking, a spot on your ear may be used for the same reason.

What is it used for? Acupuncture can help with a wide variety of conditions, including smoking cessation, recovery from various addictions, stroke rehabilitation, nausea after an operation or chemotherapy, fibromyalgia, menstrual cramps, irritable bowel, and headaches (NIH Consensus Panel 1997). There is even a relatively new subspecialty within the field called cosmetic acupuncture. This is done on the face; by improving overall health, it improves the appearance of the skin. It is not a face-lift, but it can firm skin tone, soften deep wrinkles, and erase fine lines. Acupuncture has been found to help urge incontinence as well (see chapter 7). A study of eighty-five women found that one treatment a week for four weeks decreased symptoms in nearly 60 percent of the women treated with acupuncture, as opposed to 40 percent treated with placebo. Urgency and urinary frequency were also reduced (Emmons and Otto 2005).

Is it safe? The Food and Drug Administration has approved disposable, sterile needles for acupuncture. Complications are very rare; infection at the site of the needle and punctured organs are possible but not likely, especially when a qualified, licensed acupuncturist does it. Be sure your acupuncturist is using only sterile, disposable needles.

My experience. I've had several acupuncture treatments. I was reluctant at first, because I hate needles! (I know, I'm a doctor and shouldn't have a problem, and I don't when it comes to sticking other people, but I hate having it done to me.) However, when acupuncture is done properly, the needles really don't hurt. For me, when the needle first went in, I felt a little crampy sensation at the puncture site, and then the feeling of a type of release in that part of the body being treated.

For instance, I have shoulder pain, and when the needle went in the acupuncture point, I felt the pain begin to go away. I had a treatment before my hysterectomy, and I felt very calm and relaxed the day of the surgery; I'm sure that the acupuncture had something to do with it. One wonderful side effect of acupuncture is that several days after a treatment I feel happier. I have been told that is due to the endorphin release that comes with the movement of qi.

Should you try it? Based on my experience with acupuncture, and that of my patients, as well as the research and the minimal associated risks, I can strongly recommend it for the following conditions: migraine headaches, hormone issues, nausea related to chemotherapy, fibromyalgia, smoking cessation, osteoarthritis of the knee, and back pain.

AROMATHERAPY

The use of aromatic oils has been around for thousands of years. However, the term "aromatherapy" has been used only since 1920, when a scientist working in a perfume factory in France accidentally set his arm on fire. Looking for the closest cool liquid to put his arm in, he found a vat of lavender oil. He noticed that he had very little pain and healed very quickly with minimal scarring. He devoted the rest of his career to studying the healing properties of essential oils.

What is it? *Aromatherapy* is the use of essential oils to treat various conditions. It is most often used along with massage. An essential oil is an oil containing the aroma of a plant. You might know them as oils of lavender, rose, sweet orange, sandalwood, bergamot, jasmine, and eucalyptus, to name a few. In France, this is a part of conventional medicine. Oils are regulated, and some even require a prescription. However, here in the U.S. aromatherapy has been looked upon with skepticism, and the quality of the oils is not regulated.

What is it used for? Although aromatherapy is mainstream medicine in France and Japan, it is rarely used medically in America. However, several studies have shown the value of its use. A study done at Sloan-Kettering in 1994 found that patients undergoing an MRI who were treated with a vanilla scent experienced two-thirds less anxiety than those who were given no scent (Redd and Manne 1995). A recent study done in Japan found that a thirty-minute aromatherapy massage with lavender, sandalwood, and sweet orange oils twice a week, for four weeks, reduced anxiety and boosted the immune systems of breast cancer patients as measured by an increase in natural killer cells, special white blood cells that the body makes to attack cancer cells (Imanishi et al. 2007). Past studies found that massage alone did not reduce anxiety, but that it did relieve anxiety when done in combination with aromatherapy (Wilkinson et al. 1999).

Essential oils in the U.S. have been used as insect repellents, such as citronella and bergamot. Eucalyptus oil is often added to steam treatments for colds. Lavender oil can soothe headaches and can be very calming. Tea tree oil is an antimicrobial agent that can treat small skin infections. These oils are considered to be excellent moisturizers for dry skin, which is an added benefit to using them.

Is it safe? Some of the essential oils are very potent. They can cause skin irritation and have more serious consequences if too much is absorbed, such as seizures and liver damage. Some of the citrus oils can cause a skin reaction with sun exposure in some individuals. One time, a friend of mine picked limes in the sun and got juice all over herself. The next day she had blisters on all the skin that had been exposed to sun and lime juice. It's important to let your doctor know if you are using aromatherapy.

My experience. I probably don't need to say much about this, because most of us have experienced how different smells make us feel. That said, I've used lavender oil for years to help with my sleep and my children's sleep. I used to place a small drop of oil on the underside of their pillows. It helped them to sleep, and then became a bedtime ritual. Of course, that stopped when they became teenagers, but it really was sweet! I've also used tea tree oil regularly for cuts that look as though they are getting infected. It works great for small nail infections as well; however, if you use it for this purpose and the infection doesn't clear up within a few days, or it gets worse, you need to be seen by a medical practitioner. Finally, jasmine and sandalwood are my favorite scents. I recently found out that they are supposed to act as aphrodisiacs. Now I know why I like them so much.

Should you try it? Yes, definitely! There is very little downside (unless you have extremely sensitive skin), and a lot of potential benefit. I would recommend that you start aromatherapy with lavender oil for relaxation.

CHIROPRACTIC

The word "chiropractic" comes from the Greek words *cheir* (hand) and *praxis* (action). Hippocrates in ancient Greece was the first to describe the practice of spinal manipulation. Daniel David Palmer, a healer from Iowa, started the modern practice of chiropractic. He believed that in order for the organs of the body to maintain normal function, they needed to receive normal nerve impulses. For this to happen, he thought that the spine needed to be aligned properly.

What is it? *Chiropractic* is an alternative medical system that uses spinal manipulation to improve body function. The philosophy behind chiropractic is that the body, when given the opportunity and proper alignment, is able to heal itself. Chiropractic must be practiced by a trained, licensed individual. Chiropractors go through a four-year training program after college and earn a Doctor of Chiropractic (DC) degree when they are done. Their focus is on the body structure and how it relates to health. They use adjustments or manipulations; they may also use heat, ultrasound, electrical stimulation, and diet therapy in their practice. However, they are not medical doctors. Neither are they doctors of osteopathy (DO), who are trained at osteopathic medical schools where the focus is on the importance of the musculoskeletal system in general health. Despite a focus similar to chiropractors, doctors of osteopathy are trained in the function of the entire body and can specialize, prescribe, and practice just as medical doctors do.

What is it used for? As discussed in chapter 8, Americans rack up millions of visits to the chiropractor each year. Most of these visits are for back and neck pain. Many people also go to chiropractors for sports injuries, headaches, and joint strains.

Is it safe? The treatments are relatively safe; however, there have been a few reported cases of stroke after neck manipulations (Jeret and Bluth 2002). Some traditional medical doctors worry about the possibility that the adjustments could cause fractures in patients with severe osteoporosis. That is why it is important that you first discuss the advisability of seeing a chiropractor with your regular clinician. If you get an okay, ask your primary care practitioner for recommendations for specific chiropractors whose abilities are known.

My experience. I've been to a chiropractor only a few times. I went for that shoulder and neck pain I mentioned. It really helped me. The chiropractor was very gentle, but his movements were very fast. After each adjustment, I burst out laughing hysterically. He told me that was not that unusual, but I bet they heard me in the next county! Oftentimes it will bring out a burst of emotion. Some people even cry. If I had neck or back pain that was due to strain, I would do it again. (I would also give the chiropractor earplugs next time!)

Should you try it? Yes, but discuss with your regular clinician the specific complaint for which you want to see a chiropractor, and make sure that there are no other health issues that might make the manipulation dangerous for you.

GUIDED IMAGERY, HYPNOSIS, AND BIOFEEDBACK

Although guided imagery, hypnosis, and biofeedback all use the many abilities of our minds, they are very different from each other in how they work and how they're used.

Guided imagery

This is a practice that guides your thoughts and imagination in a way that allows you to relax. When you focus on something specific and imagine and visualize it as though it were real, it can help your mind relax. This may be followed by the sensation that what you are visualizing actually *is* real. For instance, think about the tastiest chocolate you've ever eaten. See it with your mind's eye, notice its consistency, imagine how it smells, how it feels on your tongue, and how it tastes going down. I'll bet you start to salivate a little! A guided imagery specialist can take you to a relaxing place in your mind, including all the surrounding details. When this happens, your whole body relaxes and you can imagine yourself healed, relaxed, pain free, or however you need to feel. Many studies have shown that with cancer patients, guided imagery can help both the quality and length of life (Shrock, Palmer, and Taylor 1999). It can help lower blood pressure, reduce stress, and reduce the side effects of chemotherapy (Astin et al. 2003).

Hypnosis

We've all seen the TV shows where a hypnotist gets people to squawk like chickens. That's showbiz and really isn't hypnosis. When you are hypnotized, you are in a daydreamlike state in which you can hear everything going on around you. The hypnotist is actually speaking to your subconscious. You are relaxed enough that your mind is open to suggestion; however, it is important to know that, even under hypnosis, no one can be made to do anything she doesn't want to do. Hypnosis has been a help to many people for a variety of problems, including smoking cessation, addictions, chronic pain, stress, and anxiety. Hypnosis has an interesting history. It was first used formally by scientists in the late 1700s and was introduced by Dr. Franz Mesmer. He called what he did "mesmerism." He thought that the hypnotic state was something magical that flowed from the therapist. His theory went by the wayside and the term "hypnosis" took over. However, the term "to mesmerize" stuck.

Biofeedback

Biofeedback helps you to regulate your body's functions with the aid of monitoring devices. It has been approved by the National Institutes of Health for the treatment of chronic pain, tension headaches, and some forms of insomnia. With the help of a biofeedback specialist, you can alter the way you think, reduce your pulse rate and muscle tension, and change your body temperature. Biofeedback devices monitor these functions and let you know, through the use of sound or images, when you have achieved your target response. We discuss the use of biofeedback in the treatment of urinary incontinence in chapter 7.

Are these treatments safe? Guided imagery, hypnosis, and biofeedback are all relatively safe. However, once again it is important to go to a trained therapist. Many psychologists, therapists, and even some doctors are trained in these modalities. Check with your primary care clinician to find a qualified therapist.

My experience. I have experienced all of these treatments. I had a guided imagery session prior to my hysterectomy in which I envisioned myself on a beach, totally relaxed, healed, and pain free. I listened to the fifteen-minute tape that the therapist made for me every day for a week before the surgery. After the operation, I was pain free and healed very quickly. I was back to my regular three-mile exercise walk in two weeks. Was it the guided imagery that helped me? I really believe it did.

Hypnosis has also helped me to fall back asleep in the middle of the night. The hypnotherapist taught me to visualize myself going down ten steps to the beach. With each step I become more relaxed. Once on the beach, I feel the warm sand on my feet as I walk to a comfortable beach chair and listen to the waves. Since I ended my hypnotherapy sessions, when I wake up in the middle of the night I go through that script in my head and see myself going down the steps. It used to take me getting all the way to the beach before I fell asleep; now I take only one or two steps and I am back in dreamland.

I also used a computer biofeedback program to lower my pulse rate. In this program, I had to move a balloon on the computer screen by lowering my pulse. I watched the computer screen and had a little pulse monitor wrapped around my finger that was connected to the computer. It wasn't easy, but after several tries I got that puppy off the ground and sailing through the sky!

Should you try one, or all, of these? Yes, but the usual warnings apply: Discuss it with your clinician and make sure that you see a qualified, experienced practitioner.

MASSAGE

Although massage therapy is thousands of years old, it is as "hot" a treatment now as it's ever been. Just look at how many spas offer massages these days. Because massage therapy is so widespread, I will mention only a few things about it.

What is it? *Massage* is defined as the manipulation of soft tissue and muscles, and should be administered by a licensed or certified therapist. There are more than eighty different types of massage; some use light touch and others use very deep pressure.

What is it used for? It is used to relax the muscles and relieve stress, and as therapy for symptoms of certain diseases, like fibromyalgia, in which it can improve pain, stiffness, and sleep disturbances. It is also used with cancer patients because it can help with their nausea, anxiety, depression, and fatigue.

Is it safe? Massage is relatively safe, although there are certain conditions where it is not advised, including deep venous thrombosis (blood clot in the leg), a bleeding problem (and taking the blood thinner Coumadin, or warfarin), a fever, a recent fracture, or an open wound. If you have severe osteoporosis, you should let the massage therapist know. Also, if you have swelling in your legs, make sure your primary clinician okays your having a massage; sometimes leg swelling (especially if it's in only one leg and has occurred only recently) can be caused by a blood clot.

My experience. What can I say? Who doesn't love a massage?

Should you try it? Absolutely, and take a few friends.

MEDITATION

Meditation has been around for thousands of years. Some forms of meditation are part of certain religious practices. Other forms, such as mindfulness meditation, are oriented toward stress reduction and healing.

What is it? *Meditation* is a technique that helps to quiet the mind and results in a relaxation response. The meditator generally finds a quiet place and a comfortable position. She then may focus on a word or mantra (Transcendental Meditation) or her breath flowing in and out (mindfulness meditation). When doing this, she can allow her thoughts to flow by, as in a stream or on a highway high above her head. This allows the meditator to be in a state of what is called "relaxed alertness" or "awareness." By meditating daily for anywhere from fifteen minutes to an hour, certain physiologic changes in the body have been noted. I've mentioned just two types of meditation. There are many more techniques.

What is it used for? There have been quite a few studies of the physiologic effects of Transcendental Meditation and mindfulness meditation. One study of patients on blood pressure medication found that those who meditated daily using Transcendental Meditation were able to significantly lower their blood pressure and discontinue some of their blood pressure medicine more often than those who were given general relaxation tips (Parati and Steptoe 2004). A study of forty-eight workers at a biotech company found that those who meditated using mindfulness meditation, six days a week for four months, were able to boost their immune response to the flu vaccine. They also exhibited increased positive brain wave activity when compared to workers who didn't meditate (Davidson et al. 2003). Meditation has been used for stress reduction, anxiety and depression, chronic pain, cancer, HIV/AIDs, and sleep disorders (Bonadonna 2003).

Is it safe? Meditation is safe. The only harm there might be is if it was used instead of seeking medical attention for health problems.

My experience. I meditate twice daily using Transcendental Meditation. If for some reason I forget to do it, I can really tell. First of all, it helps me to relax. Since I've been meditating regularly, I am calmer overall. What used to get me really agitated doesn't get me that upset anymore. I feel healthier and more energetic. In addition, my blood pressure has gone down each year to the point that my doctor has to keep checking it because she doesn't believe how low it is.

Should you try it? Definitely, it is so good for your overall health and well-being! But don't use it for a medical problem first; see your clinician for medical advice.

PRAYER

A survey of more than 31,000 people conducted in 2004 by the National Center for Health Statistics in association with the National Center for Complementary and Alternative Medicine found that when it comes to prayer, almost half of those surveyed used prayer for health reasons (Barnes et al. 2004). Hospitals routinely employ professionally trained chaplains because of the widespread belief that attending to the spiritual needs of patients is an important part of overall health care.

What is it used for? Many consider prayer to be both comforting and healing. Recently, researchers have been interested in the health benefits of prayer—for the individual who is ill and prays for herself, and for the same ill individual when she is prayed for by others (called *intercessory* prayer). An early study found that those patients admitted to the coronary care unit over a ten-month period who were prayed for did better than patients who were not prayed for. In the prayed-for group, fewer patients required cardiopulmonary resuscitation; overall, these patients required fewer medications (Byrd 1988). Since then, some studies have confirmed the health benefits of intercessory prayer; others showed no benefit (Roberts, Ahmed, and Hall 2000). How about the effect of prayer on the individual? Prayer can help some people to find meaning, and improve the spiritual sense of well-being for those with a terminal disease (McClain, Rosenfeld, and Breitbart 2003). A study that followed 5,000 people over twenty-eight years found that women who attended religious services once a week or more had a 35 percent lower mortality rate than those women who did not attend regular religious services (Strawbridge et al. 1997). Clearly, for some people, faith and prayer are extremely important and provide comfort, a sense of well-being, and improvements in their health, and possibly the health of others through intercessory prayer.

Is it safe? Prayer is safe. The same caution applies to prayer as with any of the modalities we have discussed. It is a wonderful complement to medical treatment, but it shouldn't interfere with getting conventional medical care quickly if there is a problem to be addressed. Prayer can be used along with traditional medical therapies.

The actual experience. Prayer is something we each do in our own way. This is one type of therapy that needs no explanation about how it feels because it is so individual, and the odds are good that most of us have done it at some point in our lives.

YOGA

Yoga originated in India as a part of Hinduism.

What is it? *Yoga* is a group of spiritual and physical practices that allow the individual doing it to find peace and understanding. There are a variety of poses and breathing techniques that aid in furthering these goals, but the practice of yoga as part of Hinduism involves diet, meditation, and behaviors in addition to the poses and exercises. In the U.S., most people who practice yoga focus on the poses and breathing, which is called "hatha yoga." Although most of us think of yoga classes, in which the positions and techniques are taught, as complex and hard to do, there are classes available for varying levels of skill. For instance, some classes may focus mostly on the breathing. A good yoga instructor will be able to design a program that fits the individual's skill level, and should be able to work with any disability. Be sure that you take a class at the appropriate level of difficulty for your abilities. (And don't be embarrassed to change to an easier one if you need it.)

What is it used for? We talked about how yoga can help breast cancer patients in chapter 12. It can also help patients with heart disease. A recent study done at Yale University took patients with and without heart disease and gave them yoga and meditation instruction for one and a half hours, three times a week for six weeks. For all of those who participated in yoga there was a reduction in blood pressure, heart rate, and body mass index (BMI, referring to body weight). For those with coronary artery disease there was almost a 70 percent improvement in the ability of their blood vessels to open in order to provide more blood flow to the body (Sivasankaran, Pollard-Quintner, and Sachdeva 2006). When practiced regularly, it can decrease anxiety, help with relaxation, and provide a sense of well-being. It is also useful for improving strength, flexibility, and balance. (See chapter 11.)

Is it safe? For the most part, yoga is safe. However, since some of the poses are complicated, it is a type of practice that must be learned in stages, otherwise you can get injured. The key is to find a good teacher who can supervise your poses and ensure you are doing them correctly and not overdoing it.

The actual experience. Gynecologist and integrative medicine physician Joanne Perron, MD, describes what yoga has meant to her.

Should you try it? Yes, but with the usual cautions.

Breath and Breast, or How Yoga Guided My Breast Cancer Journey
By Joanne Perron, MD

The radiologist was performing an ultrasound of my breast and waiting for me to recognize what she already knew. I saw the distorted mass, cursed in my usual truck driver fashion, and held my breath. "Yep, you have breast cancer and you'll need to get a mastectomy." In that instant, I felt like I had been pushed out of a plane without my parachute. Where was my breath? I knew how to breathe. I was a certified yoga teacher and a physician trained in integrative medicine. My mind took control and the mental quagmire began. Sobbing, shallow breath, heart thumping, another shallow breath, "Yoga, where are you?" I thought, for only a brief instant. Then, as my mind raced down the labyrinth of possible scenarios and outcomes, I smashed into my mortality imagining my last breath.

After a few days of nonstop nail-biting and nights of sleeplessness, I realized that whatever life I had left living with cancer had to become more peaceful and present. I simply could not continue letting my mind imagine the drama of cancer. So starting in a child's pose I began to find and observe my breath again. My mantra was "inhale healing, exhale toxicity." Again and again I returned to this as I climbed each hill of multiple surgeries and rounds of chemotherapy.

Yoga is about taking nonreactivity and equanimity cultivated during asana (pose) practice off the mat and into everyday experience. While the asanas make my body feel alive, it is the knowledge that my life unfolds breath by breath that I treasure the most.

THE CAM WRAP-UP

Complementary therapies can be a wonderful adjunct to conventional medical care; however, it is important to go to a reputable and qualified practitioner who understands your medical history. It is also important to let your primary care clinician know about all the complementary therapies that you are doing. Please, please remember that these should *complement* your medical treatments. They are not meant to replace them.

THE DOCS CHAT ABOUT CAM

DR. J: You covered a lot of territory! Of all the CAM methods that you discuss, I've only had massage therapy (though I love that)! And I've always been impressed at the effects of different scents on my moods. But I'll now try more. And I'm so excited because the clinic where I work is adding a wellness center that will offer many of the CAM therapies to our patients. I know you practice integrative medicine. Could you explain what an integrative medicine physician is?

DR. R: An integrative medicine specialist is a clinician who treats the whole person (mind, body, and spirit) and forms a partnership with each patient. The treatments recommended are based on an individual's needs and beliefs and may involve traditional and complementary therapies.

DR. J: How do you decide which type of treatment, traditional or complementary, to recommend for a patient's symptoms or illness?

DR. R: I spend a fair amount of time obtaining a history from my patients, and after examining them and doing whatever diagnostic tests I think are important, I'll come up with a healing plan based on my evaluation. This may involve traditional medicine, complementary, or both. I use an evidence-based approach, meaning that I prescribe treatments that have a scientific foundation, be they traditional or complementary.

DR. J: What's an example of a condition when you might recommend CAM therapy first?

DR. R: Chronic pain. Some patients with chronic pain have tried everything, from pain medications to surgery to physical therapy, and weren't able to get rid of their pain completely. I might recommend acupuncture, hypnosis, guided imagery, or biofeedback, but I won't necessarily tell that patient to stop her medications if they may be bringing her some relief. The important thing here is that the CAM treatment actually *complements* the traditional therapy and doesn't replace it. It becomes integrated. Eventually, that patient may be able to stop her pain medications because of the relief the CAM treatment has given her, but initially I rarely advise that a patient stop her traditional medications.

PEARLS OF WISDOM FOR CAM THERAPIES

○ Complementary therapies can be very helpful when used in concert with conventional medical care.

○ Always tell your doctor when you are using complementary treatments.

○ Find licensed, experienced therapists.

○ For medical issues, seek out your traditional medical clinician first and complement later.

○ Most of all, enjoy!

CHAPTER 15

Putting It All Together:
How to Enjoy Being a
Twenty-first-Century Woman

Here we are at the end of our book, and there is so much more information we'd like to share with you! We said in the introduction that the hardest part of writing this book was having *too many* topics we wanted to discuss. In this chapter we'll summarize a few of those topics that we think are especially important, and then refer you to our Resources section for more information. In addition, we're going to show what your health maintenance schedule should look like so you'll have your own road map for taking care of yourself and feeling good.

SELF-MEDICATING WITH (OR OVERUSE OF) COMMON SUBSTANCES

When you saw the section head above, did you immediately think this will be about a dangerous habit that leads to addiction, and that this section doesn't apply to you? No one ever wants to believe that she might be doing anything to endanger her health. But think about it. Taking an Advil or aspirin for your tennis elbow or a Tylenol for a tension headache, putting Bacitracin ointment on your scraped arm, and even using Preparation H for those pesky hemorrhoids or the bags under your eyes (neat trick actually)—all these behaviors are considered self-medication. Now, we're not saying that any of these behaviors, especially if done only occasionally, is particularly dangerous. But these habits can eventually become a problem.

How Self-Medicating Gets Out of Control

To see how taking just a few meds now and then, and/or using alcohol or nicotine, can spiral out of control, open your medicine cabinet and count the number of nonprescription (also called over-the-counter, or OTC) medicines. Then, to that number of OTC drugs, add all the prescription meds that were given to you with instruction to take "only as needed," such as lorazepam (Ativan) or alprazolam (Xanax) for anxiety, propranolol (Inderal) for nervousness before a presentation, hydro-codone (Lortab) or Tylenol #3 (with codeine) for those headaches that plain Tylenol doesn't touch, and zolpidem (Ambien) or eszopiclone (Lunesta) for those nights you just cannot shut off your mind and sleep. Now, also add the ampicillin or ciprofloxacin (Cipro) left over from your recent urinary tract infection that you saved to have on hand for your next sore throat. Don't stop counting yet. Add to the above the one or two glasses of wine or beer, or Scotch and soda, that begin those business or social dinners; those three cigarettes smoked in rapid succession when your mother-in-law comes to visit; and the three double espressos needed to stay up all night while sitting with your mother in the ER as she has her chest pain evaluated.

Any and all of these activities are forms of self-medication. As with all else in life, if done in moderation, they won't be problematic. The difficulty arises when you take too many different pills and substances, even if each individual one is taken in small numbers; or when you take one or two of the pills or substances more often, or take too many of the pills or substances at one time. Eventually, these habits may lead to addiction, particularly if you have one of the risk factors, such as a hereditary tendency or the presence of depression.

Related Issues

There are several related issues to be aware of. The first is that some of the OTC meds have addictive drugs in them, although in small doses, such that if you take a lot of them, you will be getting an addictive amount of these ingredients. The second related issue is the fact that aging slows down our ability to metabolize medications, so that they stay in our body longer than they might have years ago. Because of this, you can see how too many substances put into the body can make us feel ill. In fact, when mature adults come into our offices with the complaint of "just not feeling well" or "overwhelming fatigue," one of the first things we do is to review in detail all of the drugs, substances, and especially supplements they're taking. Often, their symptoms are due to the conglomeration of ingredients; weeding out the less necessary substances resolves the symptoms.

The third issue concerns antibiotics. Can they be addictive? No, we mention them for a different reason. You've probably heard about the increasing problem known as antibiotic resistance. This occurs when we overuse a particular antibiotic. The bacteria that the antibiotic was used against can mutate successfully (thus their nickname "superbugs") so that the antibiotics no longer kill the bug(s) when used in the future (Bancroft 2007). Perhaps you've heard of the antibiotic-resistant bacteria known as MRSA (methicillin-resistant *Staphylococcus aureus*). It's a huge problem, both in hospitals and in the community (Klevens et al. 2007). When you save your antibiotics and pop them at a later date for the same or another illness without professional medical input, you too are contributing to the problem.

What's so terrible about infectious agents becoming resistant to some of the antibiotics? The concern is that one day we will run out of antibiotics that work against the organisms that cause certain illnesses; in other words we won't be able to treat an infection. Then, we'll be right back where we were before antibiotics were invented, and more people will die of previously common infections.

How to Deal with Self-Medication

We hope that our discussion of the issue of self-medication will make you think about it—before it becomes a major problem. So, count the OTC meds that you take and keep track of how many cups of caffeinated coffee or cigarettes you use each day. Especially keep track of how much alcohol you drink each day. Doing this will make it easier to discuss these issues accurately with your primary care clinician at your next office visit, and will also help you to think twice before popping that sleeping pill or antianxiety tablet. Please see chapter 14 on CAM (complementary and alternative medicine) for healthy alternatives to some of these substances. Four more general warnings about medications: Take them *exactly* as prescribed. Do not share your prescription medications with anyone else or vice versa. If you order your prescription drugs from another country, make sure your primary care clinician knows. And don't forget to regularly check the expiration dates on all your meds, whether prescription or OTC.

HOW TO STOP SMOKING CIGARETTES

Cigarette smoking is the leading cause of preventable illnesses and death in the U.S. (Okuyemi, Nollen, and Ahluwali 2006). We've deliberately chosen to give you more information on this particular substance because it is a major risk factor for so many of the debilitating diseases of aging, including heart disease, stroke, lung disease, several cancers, gum disease, and age-related macular degeneration of the eye. In various parts of the book, we've stated that stopping smoking can actually lower your risk for a specific disease—and for death from that disease. For instance, a patient who has had a heart attack and gives up smoking decreases the risk of further heart problems by 35 to 50 percent (Critchley and Capewell 2003). Also, when you stop smoking, you reduce the risks posed by secondhand smoke to those around you.

We know how difficult it is to stop smoking. Because there are many reasons that it is so difficult (possible addiction to the nicotine, genetics making you prone to addiction, psychological factors like anxiety or low self-esteem, to name but a few), we will discuss several different ways to stop smoking. You may find that combining these methods offers the best chance of success.

Lifestyle Changes

Before you think about how you're going to quit smoking, you must be ready to stop. If there's too much else going on in your life, then put smoking cessation off, but not for too long. The following suggestions are quite like those for losing weight.

Change your mind-set. Decide that you are going to stop smoking. Make a list of all the reasons you have to quit.

Talk to your primary clinician. Set up an appointment just to discuss this issue. If unable to arrange that within a reasonable time period, ask for a phone consultation.

Set a date. Going "cold turkey" doesn't work for too many people. It's best to set a date in the near future, perhaps two weeks or one month, to stop smoking. Prior to that date, get everything you'll need ready: get rid of your cigarettes and ashtrays, clean your clothes that smell of tobacco, get your medications if you plan to go that route, and so on.

Talk to everyone else in your household who smokes. Although it would obviously be best for other people in your house to also stop smoking, if that's not the case, others must find a private place to smoke—out of your sight—and must let you know where it is so that you can avoid it.

Tell a buddy. Make sure someone close to you knows that you are doing this, so that person can encourage you through the rough spots. The first two weeks after quitting are the most difficult because that's when nicotine withdrawal symptoms may occur. The first two weeks also predict whether you will succeed in the long term; therefore, that time period is very important. Also, the chances of stopping permanently are increased tenfold if you don't cheat on the first day (Okuyemi, Nollen, and Ahluwali 2006). Let your buddy know when that day will be.

Consider joining a support group. This can be done either online or in person. We know that this is the one of the tools that really works to stop drinking alcohol and for weight loss.

Find a substitute activity. Whether it is going for a walk or looking at your favorite website, have one or two activities ready to do instead of smoking, especially when you feel a craving.

Avoid your routines for smoking. If you're used to having a nice long drag with your coffee after dinner on the porch, don't go out to the porch after dinner. If you're used to smoking after sex, try chewing gum, nicotine or plain. (We're not sure how attractive that will be to a new partner, but it is better than smoking, and certainly better than the nicotine nasal spray.)

Reward yourself. Think of a few things you really want, and after the first week, get some for yourself! Do the same thing after the second week. Then make a schedule for rewarding yourself regularly in the long term. It's not a splurge. You are taking steps to save your own life; this is a big deal!

Exercise. Continue your exercise routine, or start it before you stop smoking. Not only will you feel better by doing this, but you also will avoid the five pounds or more of weight gain that some women get when they quit smoking.

Maintain a healthy diet. Nothing bolsters your energy and sense of well-being like eating nutritiously. And the better you feel, the more likely you are to stay with the plan.

Medications

There are currently seven medications approved by the FDA for smoking cessation, including five nicotine substitutes, one antidepressant that reduces the cravings for nicotine, and a new medication that combines these effects.

Nicotine replacements. These products provide low doses of nicotine that don't contain the other contaminants found in cigarette smoke. The biggest problem we've seen is with patients who use the nicotine replacement products and still continue to smoke. The five nicotine substitutes are nicotine gum, nicotine patch, nicotine lozenge, nicotine inhaler, and nicotine nasal spray.

Bupropion (Zyban, Wellbutrin). This is an antidepressant medication that also reduces nicotine cravings. Wellbutrin is the form of bupropion prescribed originally for depression; Zyban is the identical product with a different name, prescribed for smoking cessation. You can safely take either of these or their generic form. Because this is a prescription drug, talk to your primary clinician about the pros and cons of taking this in your particular case.

Varenicline tartrate (Chantix). This drug was approved by the FDA in May 2006. It acts at sites in the brain that nicotine affects, providing relief from withdrawal symptoms and blocking the effects of nicotine if you smoke while on the medication. Because of many reports of serious mood and behavior symptoms (including attempted and completed suicide) associated with taking it, the FDA issued a Public Health Advisory on February 1, 2008, to alert patients and caregivers to new safety warnings about this drug. Discuss with your clinician any present or past psychiatric history you have before you start Chantix.

Complementary and Alternative Therapies (CAM)

The two CAM therapies that have been shown to help with quitting smoking are hypnosis and acupuncture. These two also work well when used in combination with some of the other therapies. Speak to your primary clinician about what might work specifically for you.

DEPRESSION AND ANXIETY DISORDERS

In our lifetimes, we've witnessed dramatic changes in the attitudes toward, approach to, and treatment of what used to be called mental illnesses and, thankfully, are now known as mood disorders. We now know that these diseases are not caused by demonic possession or a weak character, but are biochemical disorders, just like diabetes. We've seen the change from institutionalizing patients and performing radical brain surgery on those with mood disorders (think *One Flew Over the Cuckoo's Nest*) to treating them with medications. We aren't talking about just "the blues" here, but rather clinical depression, which may also have physical symptoms, such as fatigue, difficulty sleeping, or a change in eating patterns.

One in ten adults experiences depression each year, women being affected twice as often as men; even worse, two thirds of these don't get the help they need. And even though more of us get depressed as we age, depression, like dementia, is not a normal or expected part of aging. Therefore, you need to know that the risk factors for becoming depressed are a complex mix. Some of these include family history (although not everyone with a family history of mood disorders gets depression, and people without such a family history do get depressed); dysfunction of certain brain biochemicals; and environmental stressors, such as a significant loss, a difficult relationship, a life pattern change (changing or losing your job, coming out for a gay person, or moving from a place you know well and have lived in for ages to one where you know no one).

Much the same can be said of anxiety disorders, though many of us think we know how to handle those symptoms—Ativan (lorazepam) and Valium (diazepam). But remember, these are substances that can become addictive and that can interact with the other medications and substances you consume. Therefore, it's much better to get to the root of the anxiety (maybe it isn't really anxiety at all, but depression showing up with occasional anxious symptoms) than to self-medicate. For both of these problems, have a conversation with your primary care clinician about what you think may be depression or anxiety, and don't be surprised if your physical symptoms are diagnosed as due to a mood disorder.

SLEEP

Do you remember how, in our younger days, many of us considered sleep a waste of time? We saw it as a bodily enforced period away from what was really important: taking your son to school, taking your mother to the doctor, having an early morning meeting with your boss, teaching a class, going to yoga class, arguing a case in court. Back then, all sleep did was interrupt our lives. (Though Dr. J admits that she always loved to sleep, especially to nap, she just never had time for it.)

Today, it's a different story for both the medical profession and for us maturing women. The biggest indication that it's now a hot health topic is the sheer number of advertisements on TV for sleep aids. Sleep is one of those topics that in just a few years has gone from being a nonsubject in medical texts and conversations about health (except by pediatricians reassuring new moms that eventually the baby would do it) to a multidisciplinary specialty complete with funded research, professional organizations, and texts solely devoted to it.

The National Sleep Foundation's "2003 Sleep in America" poll found that two-thirds of adults over the age of sixty-five had sleep complaints; of these only 13 percent had actually been formally diagnosed with a sleep problem (Foley et al. 2007). We also know that the number of people with insomnia increases with age, and that insomnia occurs more often in women, those with certain medical illnesses, and those with depression or an anxiety disorder—and that rest and sleep are essential for our health and well-being. (Your mother was right, yet again.)

Sleeping for a short duration has been found in recent years to be a risk factor for obesity, diabetes, and cardiovascular disease. A recent study in the U.K. with over 6,500 participants, 1,567 of whom were women, found that the women who slept less than five hours a night were twice as likely to suffer from high blood pressure as those whose slept more than that amount. This was not found in the men (Cappuccio 2007). This finding caused the lead investigator to recommend that women get at least five hours or more of sleep every night.

Moreover, instead of just two problems related to sleep (not getting enough and getting too much), we now know that there are several types of sleep disorders, each with different treatments. We know that persistent or recurring difficulties with either falling asleep or staying asleep may be an indication of an illness. So even if your primary clinician doesn't ask you about your sleep, bring it up and discuss any sleep issues you may have with her.

DOMESTIC VIOLENCE

Although 22 percent of women are, or will be, physically assaulted by a partner or a date in their lifetime, it is not a subject in the forefront of women's health issues. But it should be. According to a National Violence Against Women Survey reported by the American Psychiatric Association, it is estimated that there are more than 5 million women over eighteen who are assaulted by an intimate partner, resulting in at least 1,300 deaths and 2 million injuries each year in the U.S. alone (Tjaden and Thoennes 2000). Domestic violence crosses all boundaries of race, ethnicity, and socioeconomic levels. It is insidious and potentially deadly. Not only is it dangerous to the victim's health because of physical and emotional injuries, but it has been shown that victims of domestic violence are more prone to poor general health and disability than those not exposed, and this includes many serious diseases and risky behaviors (Black, Breiding, and NCIPC 2008).

The usual story starts with a man who appears to be charming and caring, who sometimes sweeps his partner off her feet. Then, little things start to happen. He doesn't want her going out with her friends or family. He becomes "protective," wants to know where she is at all times, and may not want her to work or to go out without him knowing where and with whom. Little by little, she loses her independence. He takes over her funds, her car keys, and her life. If she does something to displease him, he may verbally abuse her, and then, typically, the violence escalates into full-blown battering. She will make excuses to her friends and family for her bruises and he will apologize. Then he will do it again. And again. He will tell her that it is her fault that she causes him to become angry with her. Eventually, she will want to leave, but she can't because she has no control over her finances and no money, and there may be children involved. Domestic violence happens slowly and often catches the victim unaware until she finds herself trapped in a web dominated by her abuser. It is all about power and control. What can a woman do? There are many things, including the following:

- Know that you are not alone.

- Talk to a friend, family member, minister, counselor, your doctor, or even an ER doctor. Over the past few years, many hours of training have been devoted to helping doctors recognize domestic violence victims and teaching them how to help those victims.

- Come up with a plan. This may involve storing car keys, money, and important documents in a safe, easily accessible place if you are in immediate danger and need to run.

- Call the National Domestic Violence Hotline (1-800-799-SAFE). There are county and statewide agencies that can help as well. Even if you aren't ready to leave the situation, the hotline services can help you.

THE HEALTH MAINTENANCE SCHEDULE: YOUR ROAD MAP TO GOOD HEALTH

Because we've given you so much information about how to take care of yourself, we thought it would be a good idea for you to have an actual schedule of how often to have preventive and screening exams, immunizations, and your home health maintenance routine. We've divided them into three categories: screening checkups and tests you get at a medical office, recommended immunizations, and home screening and care. If you are unable to have all of the following recommended tests at once, then first do those tests that are relevant to your own medical history. For instance, if your mother had breast cancer, a big risk factor for you, make sure you get a baseline and yearly mammogram. But do try to eventually do all the screening tests on a regular basis.

Screening Checkups and Tests at the Medical Office

Dental care. See your dentist at least every six months or more often, as the dentist recommends, for checkups and professional cleaning.

Vision care. Have a full eye exam, including vision testing, dilated eye exam, and measurement of intraocular pressure for glaucoma, every one to two years, depending on your medical history and the advice of your eye doctor.

Hearing care. Have a baseline audiogram in your early fifties. You should repeat this if you notice diminished hearing.

Full physical exam. Get a regular physical exam every one to two years, based on your risk factors and current medical condition, including (but not limited to) blood pressure check, weight and height check, baseline memory testing, and a full exam of your organ systems.

Breast exams. Have at least one breast exam done by a professional each year. If you see a gynecologist for your pelvic exams rather than having your primary care clinician do a pelvic at the time of your full physical, then schedule your visit to your gynecologist four to six months apart from your full physical exam. Schedule your mammogram four months apart from the other two exams (six months apart if your primary care clinician does your pelvic exams). This will allow you to have your breasts professionally checked two or three times a year.

Pelvic exam and Pap smear. You need to have a pelvic exam by your primary clinician or gynecologist every year to look for cancers of the reproductive tract. You need to have a Pap smear to look for cervical cancer every one to three years based on her advice as well.

Tests for sexually transmitted infections. Discuss with your clinician your risk factors for, or concerns about, sexually transmitted infections. Consider having baseline testing during the pelvic exam, including the HPV test, and blood tests including those for HIV, hepatitis B and C, and syphilis. Also, consider having these done before beginning a new sexual relationship.

Blood and urine tests. Have your clinician order baseline blood tests including fasting lipid panel, fasting glucose, kidney and liver tests, blood count, vitamin D level, thyroid tests (especially TSH), and a urinalysis. Based on the results and the advice of your clinician, continue to have these as necessary, but at least every one to two years.

EKG. It is important to have a baseline EKG by age fifty at the latest, depending on your risk factors and medical condition, and regular ones thereafter.

Cardiac testing. If you have risk factors or symptoms suspicious for cardiac disease, you should have a baseline test assessing your heart's function during and after exercise, such as a thallium stress test.

Mammograms or breast MRI. Get a mammogram (or breast MRI if advised by your doctor) to screen for breast cancer every year. See "Breast exams" above for scheduling tips.

Colonoscopy. Get a baseline colonoscopy looking for colon cancers at age fifty, or earlier if you have positive risk factors. Then get one regularly thereafter, every ten years, or as often as your doctor recommends.

Bone density scan (DEXA). A baseline bone density scan at age fifty is recommended if you have positive risk factors for osteoporosis or have broken a bone. Otherwise, current recommendations are that you have the initial one between the ages of sixty and sixty-five. (We both had baseline bone density scans in our early fifties.)

Professional skin exam. Everyone should see a dermatologist for a baseline full skin exam at age fifty or earlier. The dermatologist will recommend how often you should get follow-up exams.

Test for TB exposure. Have a baseline test, then depending on your risk factors, another every one to two years.

Recommended Immunizations for Women over Fifty

Immunizations are especially important at our age because the functioning of the immune system declines as we grow older, making us less able to successfully fight off some infections (ACIP 2007). For that reason, it's better to prevent them altogether. Before receiving any of the following vaccinations, you should talk to your clinician about all of your current medications and medical conditions. Some immunizations may be dangerous for you if you have certain conditions.

Tetanus/diphtheria (Td) vaccines. If you don't recall when you had your last Td vaccine, have one dose as soon as possible, and then every ten years thereafter. If you do recall, then have the next one ten years after the most recent Td. *If you step on a nail or a piece of glass, or otherwise break the skin anywhere on your body, particularly if you do this with a dirty object, and you don't recall when your last tetanus shot was, or if it was longer than ten years ago, you need to get a tetanus shot immediately; go to the nearest ER.* (Note: Another form of this vaccine also includes protection against pertussis. This is fine to have here instead of the Td vaccine.)

Influenza vaccine. Get one dose every year.

Pneumococcal vaccine (for pneumococcal pneumonia). Have one to two doses (about five years apart) by the time you are fifty-five, and another single dose at age sixty-five.

Varicella vaccine (for chicken pox). If you don't recall ever having had chicken pox, if you've never had shingles, and if your blood tests show no immunity to this virus, you should get the two doses (the second to follow four to eight weeks after the first) in your fifties or sixties.

Hepatitis A vaccine and hepatitis B vaccine. Ask your clinician if you should have either or both of these vaccines based on your risk factors and current medical diseases.

Meningococcal vaccine (for meningococcal meningitis). If you've had surgery to remove your spleen, if your spleen isn't working due to a disease, or if you have a disorder of the specific part of the immune system known as the complement system, you will want to get this vaccine before age fifty-five. Discuss this with your clinician, as well as the need for revaccination.

Zoster vaccine (to prevent shingles). Whether you've had shingles or not, have a single dose of this vaccine at the age of sixty or older.

Health Maintenance at Home: Screening and Care

The following are our recommendations for you to do at home.

Breast self-exam. Do this monthly. Remember to check your nipples for changes and for fluid, and check under your arms for lumps.

Skin self-exam. Depending on your skin type and your dermatologist's advice, examine your skin every one to three months and more often if you have many skin lesions or freckles.

Dental. Practice oral hygiene, including brushing and flossing, twice daily.

Vision. Avoid prolonged exposure to bright sunlight. Wear the appropriate sunglasses any time you are outside. (See chapter 2.)

Hearing. Turn down that loud music and/or TV! Keep earplugs handy for the times when you can't control the volume, such as at loud concerts.

Skin. Wear sunblock anytime you are outside, and when sitting by a window inside. Make sure it's active against both UVA and UVB rays of sunlight. Moisturize dry skin frequently.

Physical activity. Do aerobic exercise at least thirty minutes daily, five days a week; do strength exercises two days a week; and balance and flexibility exercises one to two days a week.

Diet. Make it colorful and fresh (and we don't mean by eating jelly beans or M&Ms). Avoid simple carbs like cake, cookies, candy, ice cream, and white breads.

THE DOCS CHAT ABOUT PUTTING IT ALL TOGETHER

DR. J: What one thing that we haven't mentioned in the book thus far would you tell our readers is important to do?

DR. R: Learn CPR (cardiopulmonary resuscitation). It saves lives! And it is now easier to do since you no longer have to breathe into a victim's mouth to get a good result. That's why it is now called "hands only CPR." (See the website in the Resources section.) What about you?

DR. J: Get a pet. They are great for keeping you active and keeping your stress level down. Okay. It's time to put away all the serious stuff and chat about what we really think about growing older. Let's start with the funny side. What bothers you most about growing older?

DR. R: Cellulite! I hate cellulite and I can do nothing about the "cottage cheese" look of my thighs! I've never been able to figure out why dimples on a baby's thighs are so cute and why they are so ugly on mine. What about you?

DR. J: I hate that I can't wear those shoes with high wedges anymore (I loved being taller!) due to knee issues, balance issues, and looking-ridiculous-wearing-them issues. And what serious aspects of aging do you hate?

DR. R: I do not like that what used to pop into my head automatically (names, information, you name it) doesn't do that anymore. On the flip side, it's very liberating to be experienced and to feel that I've earned the right to say whatever I want to say! How about you?

DR. J: I can deal with most everything having to do with aging so far, except I hate being old enough that it's more commonplace for loved ones and friends to pass away (although I know one can be any age and have that happen). But life is good at this age, especially because we're in this fabulous group of women born in the twentieth century!

DRS. R AND J: We hope that by reading this book, you, our readers, will have learned how to better take care of yourselves so that you can live healthy long lives. We wish you our absolute best. And don't forget the four A's: awareness, alertness, action, and advocacy!

Resources

RECOMMENDED READING

American Medical Association. 2007. *American Medical Association Guide to Preventing and Treating Heart Disease: Essential Information You and Your Family Need to Know About Having a Healthy Heart.* New York: John Wiley and Sons.

Brizendine, L. 2006. *The Female Brain.* New York: Broadway Books.

Brown, B., with M. C. Katigbak-Sillick. 2007. *Bobbi Brown Living Beauty.* New York: Springboard Press.

Downie, J., and F. Cook-Bolden, with B. N. Taylor. 2004. *Beautiful Skin of Color: A Comprehensive Guide to Asian, Olive, and Dark Skin.* New York: HarperCollins.

Ephron, N. 2006. *I Feel Bad About My Neck: And Other Thoughts on Being a Woman.* New York: Knopf.

Foltz-Gray, D. 2006. *The Arthritis Foundation's Guide to Good Living with Osteoarthritis.* 2nd ed. Atlanta, Georgia: Arthritis Foundation.

Gershon, M. 1999. *The Second Brain: A Groundbreaking New Understanding of Nervous Disorders of the Stomach and Intestine.* New York: HarperCollins.

McKhann, G., and M. Albert. 2002. *Keep Your Brain Young: The Complete Guide to Physical and Emotional Health and Longevity.* Somerset, New Jersey: John Wiley and Sons.

Newman, D. K., and A. J. Wein. 2003. *Overcoming Overactive Bladder: Your Complete Self-Care Guide.* Oakland, California: New Harbinger Publications.

Northrup, C. 2006. *Women's Bodies, Women's Wisdom.* New York: Bantam Books.

Northrup, C. 2006. *The Wisdom of Menopause.* New York: Bantam Books.

Nuland, S. B. 2007. *The Art of Aging: A Doctor's Prescription for Well-Being.* New York: Random House.

Pettus, M. 2006. *It's All In Your Head: Change Your Mind—Change Your Health*. Herndon, Virginia: Capital Books, Inc.

Rossman, M. 2000. *Guided Imagery for Self-Healing*. Tiburon, California: H. J. Kramer.

Siegel, B. 1998. *Love, Medicine and Miracles*. New York: Harper & Row.

Silver, J. 2006. *After Cancer Treatment: Heal Faster, Better, Stronger*. Baltimore: Johns Hopkins Press.

Snowdon, D. 2002. *Aging with Grace: What the Nun Study Teaches Us About Leading Longer, Healthier, and More Meaningful Lives*. New York: Bantam Books.

Teitelbaum, J. 1996. *From Fatigued to Fantastic! A Manual for Moving Beyond Chronic Fatigue and Fibromyalgia*. New York: Avery Publishing Company.

Weil, A. 2007 *Healthy Aging: A Lifelong Guide to Your Physical and Spiritual Well-Being*. New York: Knopf.

WEBSITES AND PHONE NUMBERS

Women's Health Topics:
U.S. Department of Health and Human Services: www.4woman.gov
Phone: 1-888-994-9662
Centers for Disease Control and Prevention: www.cdc.gov/women/
(includes extensive information on sexually transmitted infections)

Diseases of Aging:
The National Institutes of Health: www.nihseniorhealth.gov

Cancer:
National Cancer Institute Cancer Information Service: www.cancer.gov
Phone: 1-800-4-CANCER

Domestic Violence:
U.S. Department of Agriculture, Safety, Health and Employee Welfare Division: www.usda.gov/da/shmd/aware.htm
The National Domestic Violence Hotline: 1-800-799-SAFE (7233); 1-800-787-3224 (TTY)

Smoking Cessation:
The American Lung Association, Freedom from Smoking: www.ffsonline.org
Phone: 1-800-LUNG-USA

CAM and Supplements:
The Center for Complementary and Alternative Medicine: http://nccam.nih.gov
Natural Standard: www.naturalstandard.com

Cardiopulmonary Resuscitation (CPR):
www.americanheartassociation.com/presenter.jhtml?identifier=3011764

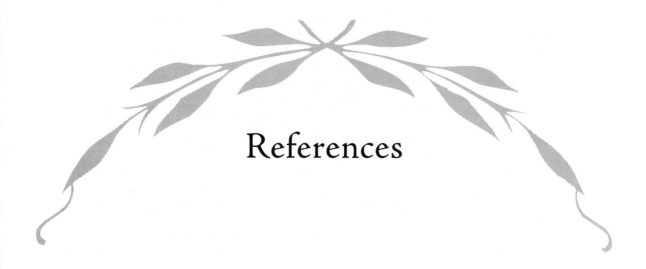

References

AADA/SID (American Academy of Dermatology Association and the Society for Investigative Dermatology). 2005. *The Burden of Skin Diseases.* Dayton, Ohio: The Lewin Group.

Abraham, A. G., N. A. Condon, and E. W. Gower. 2006. The new epidemiology of cataract. *Ophthalmology Clinics of North America* 19(4):415-425.

ACS (American Cancer Society). 2007a. Statistics 2000 through 2007. Available at www.cancer.org/docroot/ stt/stt_0.asp. Accessed February 14, 2008.

———. 2007b. What are the key statistics for breast cancer? www.cancer.org/docroot/cri/content/cri_2_4_1x_ what_are_the_key_statistics_for_breast_cancer_5.asp. Accessed April 24, 2008.

———. 2007c. What are the key statistics for colorectal cancer? www.cancer.org/docroot/cri/content/cri_2_4_1x_ what_are_the_key_statistics_for_colon_and_rectum_cancer.asp. Accessed March 27, 2008.

Adams, P. F., G. E. Hendershot, and M. A. Marano. 1999. Current estimates from the National Health Interview Survey, 1996. *Vital Health Statistics. Series 10, Data from the National Health Survey* 200:1-203.

ACIP (Advisory Committee on Immunization Practices). 2007. Recommended adult immunization schedule—United States, October 2007 to September 2008. *Morbidity and Mortality Weekly Report* 56:Q1-4.

Aggarwal, B. B., A. B. Kumar, and C. Bharti. 2003. Anticancer potential of curcumin: Preclinical and clinical studies. *Anticancer Research* 23:363-398.

AHA (American Heart Association). 2007. Heart Disease and Stroke Statistics. 2007 Update At-a-Glance. www.americanheart.org/presenter.jhtml?identifier=3000090. Accessed March 21, 2008.

AHRQ (Agency for Healthcare Research and Quality). 2002. S-Adenosyl-L-Methionine for treatment of depression, osteoarthritis, and liver disease: Summary. Evidence Report/Technology Assessment No. 64. www.ahrq.gov/clinic/epcsums/samesum.htm. Accessed March 21, 2008.

Amend, K., D. Hicks, and C. B. Ambrosone. 2006. Breast cancer in African-American women: Differences in tumor biology from European-American women. *Cancer Research* 66:8327-8330.

American College of Gastroenterology. 2006. Understanding some of the medications often prescribed for GERD and ulcers. www.acg.gi.org/patients/cgp/cgpvol1.asp#medication.www.acg.gi.org/patients/cgp/ cgpvol1.asp#medication. Accessed March 24, 2007.

American Lung Association. 2006. *Trends in Asthma Morbidity and Mortality.* www.lungusa.org/atf/cf/ {7A8D42C2-FCCA-4604-8ADE-7F5D5E762256}/ASTHMA06FINAL.PDF. Accessed March 23, 2008.

Andres, R. 1995. Body weight and age. In *Eating Disorders and Obesity: A Comprehensive Handbook*, edited by K. D. Brownell and C. G. Fairburn. New York: Guilford Press.

AREDS (Age-Related Eye Disease Study Research Group). 2001. A randomized, placebo-controlled clinical trial of high-dose supplementation with vitamins C and E, beta carotene, and zinc for age-related macular degeneration and vision loss. AREDS report no. 8. *Archives of Ophthalmology* 119:1417-1436.

Arias, E. 2006. United States life tables, 2003. *National Vital Statistics Reports* 54(14):1-40.

Astin, J. A., S. L. Shapiro, D. M. Eisenberg, and K. L. Forys. 2003. Mind-body medicine: State of the science, implications for practice. *Journal of the American Board of Family Practice* 16:131-147.

Autier, P., and S. Gandini. 2007. Vitamin D supplementation and total mortality. *Archives of Internal Medicine* 167:1730-1737.

Bach, P., J. Jett, U. Pastorino, M. S. Tockman, S. J. Swensen, and C. B. Begg. 2007. Computed tomography screening and lung cancer outcomes. *Journal of the American Medical Association* 297:953-961.

Bailey, J. V. 2004. Sexually transmitted infections in women who have sex with women. *Sexually Transmitted Infections* 80:244-246.

Bance, M. 2007. Hearing and aging. *Canadian Medical Association Journal* 176(7):925-927.

Bancroft, E. A. 2007. Antimicrobial resistance: It's not just for hospitals. *Journal of the American Medical Association* 298:1802-1804.

Barabasi, A.-L. 2007. Network medicine—from obesity to the "diseasome." *New England Journal of Medicine* 357:404-407.

Barnes, P. M., E. Powell-Griner, K. McFann, and R. L. Nahin. 2004. Complementary and alternative medicine use among adults: United States, 2002. *Advance Data* 343:1-19. Available at nccam.nih.gov/news/report.pdf. Accessed February 19, 2008.

Baron, J. A. 2005. Dietary fiber and colorectal cancer: An ongoing saga. *Journal of the American Medical Association* 294:2904-2906.

Barr, E. L. M., P. Z. Zimmet, T. A. Welborn, D. Jolley, D. J. Magliano, D. W. Dunstan, et al. 2007. Risk of cardiovascular and all-cause mortality in individuals with diabetes mellitus, impaired fasting glucose, and impaired glucose tolerance. The Australian Diabetes, Obesity, and Lifestyle Study. *Circulation* 116:151-157.

Barter, P., A. M. Gotto, D. Phil, J. Larosa, J. Maroni, M. Szarek, et al. 2007. HDL cholesterol, very low levels of LDL cholesterol, and cardiovascular events. *New England Journal of Medicine* 357:1301-1310.

Bell, D. B., and J. Nappi. 2000. Myocardial infarction in women: A critical appraisal of gender differences in outcomes. *Pharmacotherapy* 20:1034-1044.

Beresford, S. A. A., K. C. Johnson, C. Ritenbaugh, N. L. Lasser, L. G. Snetselaar, H. R. Black, et al. 2006. Low-fat dietary pattern and risk of colorectal cancer: The Women's Health Initiative randomized controlled dietary modification trial. *Journal of the American Medical Association* 295:643-654.

Berman, B. M., L. Lao, P. Langenberg, W. L. Lee, A. M. K. Gilpin, and M. C. Hochberg. 2004. Effectiveness of acupuncture as adjunctive therapy in osteoarthritis of the knee: A randomized, controlled trial. *Annals of Internal Medicine* 141:901-910.

Bialek, S. R., and N. A. Terrault. 2006. The changing epidemiology and natural history of hepatitis C virus infection. *Clinics in Liver Disease* 10(4):697-715.

Birks, J., E. V. Grimley, and M. Van Dongen. 2002. *Ginkgo biloba* for cognitive impairment and dementia. *Cochrane Database of Systematic Reviews* 4:CD003120.

Black, M. C., M. J. Breiding, and NCICP (National Center for Injury Prevention and Control). 2008. Adverse health conditions and health risk behaviors associated with intimate partner violence—United States, 2005. *Morbidity and Mortality Weekly Report* 57(5):113-117.

Blaser, M. 1990. *Helicobacter pylori* and the pathogenesis of gastroduodenal inflammation. *Journal of Infectious Diseases* 161:626-633.

Blumenthal, M., A. Goldberg, and J. Brinckman, eds. 2000. *Herbal Medicine: Expanded Commission E Monographs*. Newton, Massachusetts: Lippincott, Williams, and Wilkins.

Boiko, S. 2001. Aging and sun damage. In *Women's Dermatology: From Infancy to Maturity*, edited by L. C. Parish, S. Brenner, and M. Ramos-e-Silva. London and New York: Parthenon Publishing Group.

Bonadonna, R. 2003. Meditation's impact on chronic illness. *Holistic Nursing Practice* 17:309-319.

Bonow, R. O., and M. Gheorghiade. 2004. The diabetes epidemic: A national and global crisis. *American Journal of Medicine* 116(suppl 5A):2S-10S.

Bray, G. A. 2004. Medical consequences of obesity. *Journal of Clinical Endocrinology and Metabolism* 89(6):2583-2589.

———. 2007. The missing link—lose weight, live longer. *New England Journal of Medicine* 357:818-820.

Brenn, L. 2004. Joint Replacement: An Inside Look. *FDA Consumer* 38(2):12-19. Available at www.fda.gov/fdac/features/2004/204_joints.html. Accessed March 25, 2008.

Buccolo, L. S. 2005. Viral hepatitis. *Clinics in Family Practice* 7(1):105-125.

Bump, R. C., W. G. Hurt, J. A. Fantyl, and J. F. Wyman. 1991. Assessment of Kegel pelvic muscle exercise performance after brief verbal instruction. *American Journal of Obstetrics and Gynecology* 165:322-329.

Busch, A., C. L. Schachter, P. M. Peloso, and C. Bombardier. 2002. Exercise for treating fibromyalgia syndrome. *Cochrane Database of Systematic Reviews* 3:CD003786.

Byrd, R. C. 1988. Positive therapeutic effects of intercessory prayer in a coronary care unit population. *Southern Medical Journal* 81:826-829.

Calle, E. E., C. Rodriguez, K. Walker-Thurmond, and M. J. Thun. 2003. Overweight, obesity, and mortality from cancer in a prospectively studied cohort of U.S. adults. *New England Journal of Medicine* 348:1625-1638.

Cappuccio, F. P., S. Stranges, N. B. Kandala, M. A. Miller, F. M. Taggart, M. Kumari, et al. 2007. *Hypertension* 50:693-700.

Carmichael, M. 2007. Stronger, faster, smarter. *Newsweek*, March 26, 38-46.

Castelo-Branco, C., F. Figueras, M. J. Martinez de Osaba, and J. A. Vanrell. 1998. Facial wrinkling in postmenopausal women: Effects of smoking status and hormone replacement therapy. *Maturitas* 29:75-86.

Causey, J. L. 2006. Korean pine nut fatty acids (pinolenic acid) induce satiety-producing hormone release in overweight human volunteers. Paper presented at the American Chemical Society National Meeting and Exposition, March 26-30, 2006, Atlanta, Georgia.

CDC (Centers for Disease Control and Prevention). 2001. New asthma estimates: Tracking prevalence, health care and mortality. National Center for Health Statistics. www.cdc.gov/asthma/brfss/default.htm. Accessed March 29, 2008.

———. 2007a. Cervical cancer: Gynecologic cancer awareness. www.cdc.gov/cancer/cervical/gynecologic.htm. Accessed November 4, 2007.

———. 2007b. Prehospital and hospital delays after stroke onset—United States, 2005-2006. *Morbidity and Mortality Weekly Report* 56(19):474-478.

———. 2007c. STD Surveillance 2006. www.cdc.gov/STD/stats/toc2006.htm. Accessed April 24, 2008.

———. 2008a. HIV and AIDS in the United States. A Picture of today's epidemic. www.cdc.gov/hiv/topics/surveillance/unitedstates.htm. Accessed April 30, 2008.

———. 2008b. National STD Prevention Conference. www.cdc.gov/STDConference/2008/media/release-12march2008.htm. Accessed April 30, 2008.

CDC Divisions of HIV/AIDS Prevention. 2006. HIV/AIDS among women who have sex with women. www.cdc.gov/hiv/topics/women/resources/factsheets/wsw.htm. Accessed July 4, 2007.

Christakis, N. A., and J. H. Fowler. 2007. The spread of obesity in a large social network over 32 years. *New England Journal of Medicine* 357:370-379.

Clark, L. C., G. F. Combs, B. W. Turnbull, E. H. Slate, D. K. Chalker, J. Chow, et al. 1997. Effects of selenium supplementation for cancer prevention in patients with carcinoma of the skin. *Journal of the American Medical Association* 276:1957-1963.

Clegg, D., D. J. Reda, C. L. Harris, M. A. Klein, J. R. O'Dell, M. H. Hooper, et al. 2006. Glucosamine, chondroitin sulfate, and the two in combination for painful knee osteoarthritis. *New England Journal of Medicine* 54:795-808.

Clemons, T. E., R. C. Milton, R. Klein, J. M. Seddon, and F. L. Ferris III; Age-Related Eye Disease Study Research Group. 2005. Risk factors for the incidence of advanced age-related macular degeneration in the Age-Related Eye Disease Study. AREDS report no. 19. *Ophthalmology* 112:533-539.

Cohen, L., J. Gerner, and W. B. Baile. 2000. Complementary programs for patients with cancer: Implications for quality of life, treatment response, and survival. *Lancet Oncology* 1:55-56.

Collaborative Group on Epidemiological Studies of Ovarian Cancer. 2008. Ovarian cancer and oral contraceptives: Collaborative reanalysis of data from 45 epidemiological studies including 23,257 women with ovarian cancer and 87,303 controls. *Lancet* 371:303-314.

Conen, D., P. Ridker, J. Buring, and R. J. Glynn. 2007. Risk of cardiovascular events among women with high normal blood pressure or blood pressure progression: Prospective cohort study. *British Medical Journal* 335:432.

Critchley, J. A., and S. Capewell. 2003. Mortality risk reduction associated with smoking cessation in patients with coronary heart disease. *Journal of the American Medical Association* 290:86-97.

Crofford, L. J., M. C. Rowbotham, and P. J. Mease. 2005. Pregabalin for the treatment of fibromyalgia syndrome: Results of a randomized, double-blind, placebo-controlled trial. *Arthritis and Rheumatism* 52:1264-1273.

Danforth, K. N., S. S. Tworoger, J. L. Hecht, B. A. Rosner, G. A. Colditz, S. E. Hankinson, et al. 2007. Breast feeding and risk of ovarian cancer in two prospective cohorts. *Cancer Causes and Control* 18:517-523.

Davidson, R. J., J. Kabat-Zinn, J. Schumacher, M. Rosenkranz, D. Muller, S. F. Santorelli, et al. 2003. Alterations in brain and immune function produced by mindfulness meditation. *Psychosomatic Medicine* 65:564-570.

Dickman, R., E. Schiff, A. Holland, C. Wright, S. R. Sarella, B. Han, et al. 2007. Clinical trial: Acupuncture vs. doubling the proton pump inhibitor dose in refractory heartburn. *Alimentary Pharmacology and Therapeutics* 26:1333-1344.

Dormier, S., and C. Howham. 2007. The effect of dietary intake on hot flashes in menopausal women. *Journal of Obstetric, Gynecologic, and Neonatal Nursing* 36:255-262.

Drachman, D. A. 2005. Do we have brain to spare? *Neurology* 64:12.

———. 2006. Aging of the brain, entropy, and Alzheimer's disease. *Neurology* 67:1340-1352.

Dufresne, C. J., and E. R. Farnworth. 2001. A review of latest research findings on the health promotion properties of tea. *Journal of Nutritional Biochemistry* 12:404-421.

Dunne, E. F., E. R. Unger, M. Sternberg, G. McQuillan, D. C. Swan, S. S. Patel, et al. 2007. Prevalence of HPV infection among females in the United States. *Journal of the American Medical Association* 297:813-819.

Einstein, A. J., M. J. Henzlova, and S. Rajagopalan. 2007. Estimating risk of cancer associated with radiation exposure from 64-slice computed tomography coronary angiography. *Journal of the American Medical Association* 298:317-323.

Eisenberg, D. M., R. B. Davis, S. L. Ettner, S. Appel, S. Wilkey, M. Van Rompay, et al. 1998. Trends in alternative medicine use in the United States, 1990-1997: Results of a follow-up national survey. *Journal of the American Medical Association* 280:1569-1575.

Ellwein, L. B., and C. J. Urato. 2002. Use of eye care and associated charges among the Medicare population: 1991-1998. *Archives of Ophthalmology* 120:804-811.

Emmons, S., and L. Otto. 2005. Acupuncture for overactive bladder: A randomized controlled trial. *Obstetrics and Gynecology* 106:138-143.

Epel, E. S., B. McEwen, T. Seeman, K. Matthews, G. Castellazzo, K. D. Brownell, et al. 2000. Stress and body shape: Stress-induced cortisol secretion is consistently greater among women with central fat. *Psychosomatic Medicine* 62:623-632.

Ernster, V. L., D. Grady, R. Miike, D. Black, J. Selby, and K. Kerlikowske. 1995. Facial wrinkling in men and women, by smoking status. *American Journal of Public Health* 85:78-82.

Eskandari, F., P. E. Martinez, S. Torvik, T. M. Phillips, E. M. Sternberg, S. Mistry, et al. 2007. Low bone mass in premenopausal women with depression. *Archives of Internal Medicine* 167:2329-2336.

Espey, D. K., X.-C. Wu, J. Swan, C. Wiggins, M. A. Jim, E. Ward, et al. 2007. Annual report to the nation on the status of cancer, 1975-2004, featuring cancer in American Indians and Alaska natives. *Cancer* 110:2119-2152.

Esposito, K., M. Ciotola, F. Giugliano, B. Schisano, R. Autorino, S. Iuliano, et al. 2007. Mediterranean diet improves sexual function in women with the metabolic syndrome. *International Journal of Impotence Research* 19:486-491.

Evans, A. L., A. J. Scally, S. J. Wellard, and J. D. Wilson. 2007. Prevalence of bacterial vaginosis in lesbians and heterosexual women in a community setting. *Sexually Transmitted Infections* 83(6):470-475.

Evans, R. W. 2006. Headache. In *ACP Medicine*, edited by D. Dale and D. Federman. New York: WebMD.

Ezzo, J., A. Vickers, M. A. Richardson, C. Allen, S. L. Dibble, B. F. Issell, et al. 2005. Acupuncture-point stimulation for chemotherapy-induced nausea and vomiting. *Journal of Clinical Oncology* 23:7188-7198.

Farris, P. K. 2005. Topical vitamin C: A useful agent for treating photoaging and other dermatologic conditions. *Dermatologic Surgery* 31(7 pt 2):814-817.

FDA (Food and Drug Administration). 2007a. FDA news: FDA issues dietary supplements final rule. www.fda.gov/bbs/topics/NEWS/2007/NEW01657.html. Accessed February 22, 2008.

———. 2007b. FDA proposes new rule for sunscreen products. www.fda.gov/bbs/topics/NEWS/2007/NEW01687.html. Accessed September 19, 2007.

Felson, D. T., Y. Zhang, J. M. Anthony, A. Naimark, and J. J. Anderson. 1992. Weight loss reduces the risk for symptomatic knee osteoarthritis in women. *Annals of Internal Medicine* 116:535-539.

Feskanich, D., W. C. Willett, M. J. Stampfer, and G. A. Colditz. 1997. Milk, dietary calcium, and bone fractures in women: A 12-year prospective study. *American Journal of Public Health* 87:992-997.

Fine, S. L. 2005. Age-related macular degeneration 1969-2004: A 35-year personal perspective. *American Journal of Ophthalmology* 139:405-420.

Fischer, A., F. Sananbenesi, X. Wang, and M. Dobbin. 2007. Recovery of learning and memory is associated with chromatin remodeling. *Nature* 447:178-182.

Fito, M., M. Guxens, D. Corella, G. Saez, R. Estruch, R. de la Torre, et al. 2007. Effect of a traditional Mediterranean diet on lipoprotein oxidation: A randomized controlled trial. *Archives of Internal Medicine* 167:1195-1203.

Flegal, K. M., B. I. Graubard, D. F. Williamson, and M. H. Gail. 2007. Cause-specific excess deaths associated with underweight, overweight, and obesity. *Journal of the American Medical Association* 298:2028-2032.

Foley, D. J., M. V. Vitiello, B. L. Bliwise, S. Anconi-Israel, A. A. Monjan, and J. K. Walsh. 2007. Frequent napping is associated with excessive daytime sleepiness, depression, pain, and nocturia in older adults: Findings from the National Sleep Foundation "2003 Sleep in America" poll. *American Journal of Geriatric Psychiatry* 15:344-350.

Ford, E. S., U. A. Ajani, J. B. Croft, J. A. Critchley, D. R. Labarthe, T. E. Kottke, et al. 2007. Explaining the decrease in U.S. deaths from coronary disease. *New England Journal of Medicine* 356:2388-2398.

Ford, E. S., W. H. Giles, and W. H. Dietz. 2002. Prevalence of the metabolic syndrome among U.S. adults: Findings from the third National Health and Nutrition Examination Survey. *Journal of the American Medical Association* 287:356-359.

Franco, O. H. 2007. Associations of diabetes mellitus with total life expectancy with and without cardiovascular disease. *Archives of Internal Medicine* 167:145-151.

Freedman, R. R., and S. Woodward. 1992. Behavioral treatment of menopausal hot flashes: Evaluation by ambulatory monitoring. *American Journal of Obstetrics and Gynecology* 167:436-439.

Freeman, E. W., M. D. Sammel, H. Lin, C. R. Gracia, G. W. Pien, D. B. Nelson, et al. 2007. Symptoms associated with menopausal transition and reproductive hormones in midlife women. *Obstetrics and Gynecology* 110:230-240.

Fu, J. B., T. Y. Kau, R. K. Severson, and G. P. Kalmekerian. 2005. Lung cancer in women: Analysis of the national surveillance, epidemiology, and end results database. *Chest* 127:768-777.

Gershon, M. 1999. *The Second Brain: A Groundbreaking New Understanding of Nervous Disorders of the Stomach and Intestine.* NewYork: Harper and Row.

Ghersetich, I., C. Comacchi, B. Bianchi, and T. M. Lotti. 2001. Structure and function of the skin. In *Women's Dermatology: From Infancy to Maturity,* edited by L. C. Parish, S. Brenner, and M. Ramos-e-Silva. London and New York: Parthenon Publishing Group.

Girardi, M., and H. R. Konrad. 2005. Imbalance and falls in the elderly. In *Otolaryngology: Head and Neck Surgery,* 4th ed., edited by C. Cummings, P. W. Flint, B. H. Haughey, K. T. Robbins, J. R. Thomas, L. A. Harker, et al. Philadelphia: Mosby.

Gold, E. B., J. Bromberger, S. Crawford, S. Samuels, G. A. Greendale, S. D. Harlow, et al. 2001. Factors associated with age at natural menopause in a multiethnic sample of midlife women. *American Journal of Epidemiology* 153:865-874.

Gold, E. B., B. Sternfeld, J. L. Kelsey, C. Brown, C. Mouton, N. Reame, et al. 2000. Relation of demographic and lifestyle factors to symptoms in a multi-racial/ethnic population of women 40-55 years of age. *American Journal of Epidemiology* 152:463-473.

Goldenberg, D. L., K. H. Kaplan, and M. G. Nadeau. 1994. A controlled study of a stress-reduction, cognitive-behavioral treatment program in fibromyalgia. *Journal of Musculoskeletal Pain* 2:53-66.

Goodman, G. E., M. D. Thornquist, J. Balmes, M. C. Cullen, F. L. Meyskens, G. S. Omenn, et al. 2004. The beta-carotene and retinol efficacy trial: Incidence of lung cancer and cardiovascular disease mortality during 6-year follow-up after stopping beta-carotene and retinol supplements. *Journal of the National Cancer Institute* 96:1729-1731.

Gordon, M. 2005. A conservative approach to the nonsurgical rejuvenation of the face. *Dermatology Clinics* 23:365-371.

Grbic, J. T., R. L. Landesberg, S-Q. Lin, P. Mesenbrink, I. R. Reid, P.-C. Leung, et al. 2008. Incidence of osteonecrosis of the jaw in women with postmenopausal osteoporosis in the health outcomes and reduced incidence with zoledronic acid once yearly pivotal fracture trial. *Journal of the American Dental Association* 139(1):32-40.

Greendale, G. A., B. A. Reboussin, A. Sie, H. R. Singh, L. K. Olson, O. Gatewood, et al. 1999. Effects of estrogen and estrogen-progestin on mammographic parenchymal density: Postmenopausal Estrogen/Progestin Interventions (PEPI) investigators. *Annals of Internal Medicine* 130:262-269.

Gregg, E. W. 2007. Mortality trends in men and women with diabetes, 1971-2000. *Annals of Internal Medicine* 147:1-8.

Griffiths, C. E. 1998. Assessment of topical retinoids for the treatment of Far-East Asian skin. *Journal of the American Academy of Dermatology* 39(2 pt 3):S104-S107.

Gupta, M. A., and B. A. Gilchrest. 2005. Psychosocial aspects of aging skin. *Dermatology Clinics* 23:643-648.

Gutzmann, H., and D. Hadler. 1998. Sustained efficacy and safety of idebenone in the treatment of Alzheimer's disease: Update on a 2-year double-blind multicentre study. *Journal of Neural Transmission. Supplementum* 54:301-310.

Gynecologic Cancer Foundation. 2007. Ovarian cancer symptoms consensus statement. www.wcn.org/ov_cancer_cons.html. Accessed February 2, 2008.

Hakim, I. A., R. B. Harris, H. H. Chow, M. Dean, S. Brown, L. U. Ali, et al. 2004. Effect of a 4-month tea intervention on oxidative DNA damage among heavy smokers: Role of glutathione S-transferase genotypes. *Cancer Epidemiology, Biomarkers and Prevention* 13:242-249.

Halder, R. M., and C. J. Ara. 2003. Skin cancer and photoaging in ethnic skin. *Dermatology Clinics* 21:725-732.

Hann, H.-W. L., R. S. Hann, and W. C. Maddrey. 2007. Hepatitis B virus infection in 6,130 unvaccinated Korean-Americans surveyed between 1988 and 1990. *American Journal of Gastroenterology* 102(4):767-772.

Hanna, F., A. J. Teichtahl, R. Bell, S. R. Davis, A. E. Wluka, R. O'Sullivan, et al. 2007. The cross-sectional relationship between fortnightly exercise and knee cartilage properties in healthy adult women in midlife. *Menopause* 14:830.

Henderson, V. W., J. R. Guthrie, E. C. Dudley, H. G. Burger, and L. Dennerstein. 2003. Estrogen exposures and memory at midlife: A population-based study of women. *Neurology* 60:1369-1371.

Hodgson, J. M., G. F. Watts, D. A. Playford, V. Burke, and K. D. Croft. 2002. Coenzyme Q10 improves blood pressure and glycaemic control: A controlled trial in subjects with type 2 diabetes. *European Journal of Clinical Nutrition* 56:1137-1142.

Holloway, V. L. 2003. Ethnic cosmetic products. *Dermatology Clinics* 21:743-749.

Holmes, D. M., A. R. Stone, and P. R. Barry. 1983. Bladder training 3 years on. *British Journal of Urology* 55:660-664.

Holschneider, C. H., and J. S. Berek. 2000. Ovarian cancer: Epidemiology, biology, and prognostic factors. *Seminars in Surgical Oncology* 19:3-10.

Howe, H. L., X. Wu, L. A. Ries, V. Cokkinides, F. Ahmed, A. Jemal, et al. 2006. Annual report to the nation on the status of cancer, 1975-2003, featuring cancer among U.S. Hispanic/Latino populations. *Cancer* 107:1711-1742.

Hsia, J., K. L. Margolis, C. B. Eaton, N. K. Wenger, M. Allison, L. Wu, et al. 2007. Prehypertension and cardiovascular disease risk in the Women's Health Initiative. *Circulation* 115:855-860.

Hu, F. B. 2007. Diet and cardiovascular disease prevention: The need for a paradigm shift. *Journal of the American College of Cardiology* 50:22-24.

Hu, S., R. M. Soza-Vento, D. F. Parker, and R. S. Kirsner. 2006. Comparison of stage at diagnosis of melanoma among Hispanic, black, and white patients in Miami-Dade County, Florida. *Archives of Dermatology* 142:704-708.

Hunsberger, J. G., S. S. Newton, A. H. Bennett, C. H. Duman, D. S. Russell, S. R. Salton, et al. 2007. Antidepressant actions of the exercise-regulated gene VGF. *Nature Medicine* 13:1476-1482.

Hye, A., S. Lynham, M. Thambisetti, M. Causevic, J. Campbell, H. L. Byers, et al. 2006. Proteome-based plasma biomarkers for Alzheimer's disease. *Brain* 129:3042-3050.

IELCAPI (International Early Lung Cancer Action Program Investigators). 2006. Women's susceptibility to tobacco carcinogens and survival after diagnosis of lung cancer. *Journal of the American Medical Association* 296:180-184.

Imanishi, J., H. Kuriyama, I. Shigemori, S. Wantanabe, Y. Aihara, M. Kita, et al. 2007. Anxiolytic effect of aromatherapy massage in patients with breast cancer. *Evidence Based Complementary and Alternative Medicine* 4:1-6.

Ito, T. Y., M. L. Polan, B. Whipple, and A. S. Trant. 2006. The enhancement of female sexual function with ArginMax, a nutritional supplement, among women differing in menopausal status. *Journal of Sex and Marital Therapy* 32:369-378.

Jackson, B. A. 2003. Cosmetic considerations and nonlaser cosmetic procedures in ethnic skin. *Dermatologic Clinics* 21:703-712.

Jensen, M. D. 2008. Obesity. In *Cecil Textbook of Medicine*, 23rd ed., edited by L. Goldman and D. Ausiello. Philadelphia: Saunders Elsevier.

Jeret, J. S., and M. Bluth, M. 2002. Stroke following chiropractic manipulation: Report of 3 cases and review of the literature. *Cerebrovascular Diseases* 13:210-213.

Jones, R., R. Latinovic, J. Charlton, and M. C. Gulliford. 2007. Alarm symptoms in early diagnosis of cancer in primary care: Cohort study using General Practice Research Database. *British Medical Journal* 334:1040-1050.

Kaelin, C. M. 2004. Paget's Disease. In *Diseases of the Breast*, 3rd ed., edited by J. R. Harris, M. E. Lippman, M. Morrow, and C. K. Osborne. Philadelphia: Lippincott, Williams, and Wilkins.

Kaidbey, K. H., P. P. Agin, R. M. Sayre, and A. M. Kligman. 1979. Photoprotection by melanin: A comparison of black and Caucasian skin. *Journal of the American Academy of Dermatology* 1:249-260.

Kashima, M. L., W. J. Goodwin, T. Balkany, and R. R. Casiano. 2005. Special considerations in managing geriatric patients. In *Otolaryngology: Head and Neck Surgery*, 4th ed., edited by C. Cummings, P. W. Flint, B. H. Haughey, K. T. Robbins, J. R. Thomas, L. A. Harker, et al. Philadelphia: Mosby.

Kasner, S. E., and L. B. Morganstern. 2006. Cerebrovascular disorders. In *ACP Medicine*, edited by D. Dale and D. Federman. New York: WebMD.

Keshavarz, H., S. D. Hillis, B. A. Kieke, and P. A. Marchbanks. 2002. Hysterectomy surveillance—United States, 1994-1999. *Morbidity and Mortality Weekly Report* 51(SS05):1-8.

Kikuchi, K., H. Kobayashi, T. Hirao, A. Ito, H. Takahashi, H. Tagami, et al. 2003. Improvement of mild inflammatory changes of the facial skin induced by winter environment with daily applications of a moisturizing cream. *Dermatology* 207:269-275.

King, D. E. 2007. Turning back the clock: Adopting a healthy lifestyle in middle age. *American Journal of Medicine* 120:598-603.

Klein, R., M. D. Knudtson, K. J. Cruikshanks, and B. E. K. Klein. 2008. Further observations on the association between smoking and the long-term incidence and progression of age-related macular degeneration. *Archives of Ophthalmology* 126:115-121.

Klevens, R. M., M. A. Morrison, J. Nadle, S. Petit, K. Gershman, S. Ray, et al. 2007. Invasive methicillin-resistant *Staphylococcus aureus* infections in the U.S. *Journal of the American Medical Association* 298:1763-1771.

Kligman, A. M., G. L. Grove, R. Hirose, and J. J. Leyden. 1986. Topical tretinoin for photoaged skin. *Journal of the American Academy of Dermatology* 15(4 pt 2):836-859.

Knopman, D. S. 2006. Alzheimer's disease and other major dementing illnesses. In *ACP Medicine*, edited by D. Dale and D. Federman. New York: WebMD.

———. 2008. Alzheimer's disease and other dementias. In *Cecil Textbook of Medicine*, 23rd ed., edited by L. Goldman and D. Ausiello. Philadelphia: W. B. Saunders.

Kochanek, K. D., S. L. Murphy, R. N. Anderson, and C. Scott. 2004. Deaths: Final data for 2002. *National Vital Statistics Reports* 53(5):1-115.

Kojic, A. M., and S. Cu-Uvin. 2007. Special care issues of women living with HIV-AIDS. *Infectious Disease Clinics of North America* 21(1):133-148.

Kolata, G. 2007. Lifesaving opportunities missed, before and after stroke. *New York Times*, May 28, A1.

Kris-Etherton, P., R. H. Eckel, B. V. Howard, S. St. Jeor, and T. L. Bazzarre. 2001. AHA Science Advisory: Lyon Diet Heart Study. Benefits of a Mediterranean-style, National Cholesterol Education Program/American Heart Association Step I dietary pattern on cardiovascular disease. *Circulation* 103:1823-1825.

Krishnan, S., L. Rosenberg, M. Singer, F. B. Hu, L. Djousse, L. A. Cupples, et al. 2007. Glycemic index, glycemic load, and cereal fiber intake and risk of type 2 diabetes in U.S. black women. *Archives of Internal Medicine* 167:2304-2309.

Kritz-Silverstein, D., E. Barrett-Connor, and D. L. Wingard. 1997. Hysterectomy, oophorectomy, and heart disease risk in older women. *American Journal of Public Health* 87:676-680.

Landefeld, C. S., B. J. Bowers, A. D. Feld, K. E. Hartmann, E. Hoffman, M. J. Ingbar, et al. 2008. National Institutes of Health state-of-the-science statement: Prevention of fecal and urinary incontinence in adults. *Annals of Internal Medicine* 148:449-458.

Lang, T., A. LeBlanc, H. Evans, Y. Lu, H. Genant, and A. Yu. 2004. Cortical and trabecular bone mineral loss from the spine and hip in long-duration spaceflight. *Mineral Research* 19:1006-1012.

Lappe, J. M., D. Travers-Gustafson, K. M. Davies, R. R. Recker, and R. P. Heaney. 2007. Vitamin D and calcium supplementation reduces cancer risk: Results of a randomized trial. *American Journal of Clinical Nutrition* 85:1586-1591.

Lautenschlager, S., H. Wulf, and M. Pittelkow. 2007. Photoprotection: A review. *Lancet* 370:528-537.

Lawrence, R. C., C. G. Helmick, F. C. Arnett, R. A. Deyo, D. T. Felson, E. H. Giannini, et al. 1998. Estimates of the prevalence of arthritis and selected musculoskeletal disorders in the United States. *Arthritis and Rheumatism* 41:778-799.

LeBars, P. L., M. M. Katz, T. M. Berman, A. M. Freedman, and A. F. Schatzberg. 1997. A placebo-controlled, double-blind, randomized trial of an extract of *Ginkgo biloba* for dementia. *Journal of the American Medical Association* 278:1327-1332.

Lesser, R. G., D. A. Darnley-Fisch, T. H. Kupin, and R. M. Schiffman. 2001. Glaucoma. In *Textbook of Primary Care Medicine*, edited by J. Noble. Philadelphia: Mosby.

Li, Y., D. Baer, G. D. Friedman, N. Vdaltsova, and A. L. Klatsky. 2007. Wine, liquor, beer and risk of breast cancer. *European Journal of Cancer Supplements* 5:161.

Lindau, S. T., L. P. Schumm, E. O. Laumann, W. Levinson, C. A. O'Muircheartaigh, and L. J. Waite. 2007. A study of sexuality and health among older adults in the United States. *New England Journal of Medicine* 357:762-774.

Livingston, E. H. 2005. Complications of bariatric surgery. *Surgical Clinics of North America* 85(4):853-868.

MacClellan, L. R., W. Giles, J. Cole, M. Wozniak, B. Stern, B. D. Mitchell, et al. 2007. Probable migraine with visual aura and risk of ischemic stroke: The stroke prevention in young women study. *Stroke* 38: 2438-2445.

Manson, J. E., M. A. Allison, and J. E. Rossouw. 2007. Estrogen therapy and coronary-artery calcification. *New England Journal of Medicine* 356:2591-2602.

Marchetti, G. F., and S. L. Whitney. 2005. Older adults and balance dysfunction. *Neurology Clinics* 23(3):785-805.

Marini, H., L. Minutoli, F. Polito, A. Bitto, D. Altavilla, M. Atteritano, et al. 2007. Metabolism in osteopenic postmenopausal women. *Annals of Internal Medicine* 146:839-847.

Martidis, A., and M. T. S. Tenant. 2004. Age-related macular degeneration. In *Ophthalmology*, 2nd ed., edited by M. Yanoff, J. S. Duker, J. J. Augsburger, D. T. Azar, G. R. Diamond, and J. J. Dutton. St. Louis: Mosby.

Martin, D. 2006. Improvement in fibromyalgia symptoms with acupuncture: Results of a randomized controlled trial. *Mayo Clinic Proceedings* 81:749-757.

Mayo Clinic Staff. 2006. Rosacea. www.mayoclinic.com/health/rosacea/DS00308/SECTION=1. Accessed September 17, 2007.

McClain, C. S., B. Rosenfeld, and W. Breitbart. 2003. Effect of spiritual well-being on end-of-life despair in terminally-ill cancer patients. *Lancet* 361:1603-1607.

McDaniel, D. H., B. A. Neudecker, J. C. DiNardo, J. A. Lewis II, and H. I. Maibach. 2005. Idebenone: A new antioxidant—part I. A relative assessment of oxidative stress protection capacity compared to commonly known antioxidants. *Journal of Cosmetic Dermatology* 4:10-17.

McSweeney, J. C., M. Cody, P. O'Sullivan, K. Elberson, D. Moser, and B. Garvin. 2003. Women's early warning symptoms of acute myocardial infarction. *Circulation* 108:1673-1675.

McTiernan, A., C. Kooperberg, E. White, S. Wilcox, R. Coates, L. L. Adams-Campbell, et al. 2003. Recreational physical activity and the risk of breast cancer in postmenopausal women: The Women's Health Initiative Cohort Study. *Journal of the American Medical Association* 290:1331-1336.

Menaker, J., D. M. Stein, and T. M. Scalea. 2007. Incidence of early pulmonary embolism after injury. *Journal of Trauma* 63:620-624.

Mensah, G. A., A. H. Mokdad, E. Ford, K. M. Narayan, W. H. Giles, F. Vinicor, et al. 2004. Obesity, metabolic syndrome, and type 2 diabetes: Emerging epidemics and their cardiovascular implications. *Cardiology Clinics* 22(4):485-504.

Messier, S. P., D. J. Gutekunst, C. Davis, and P. Devita. 2005. Weight loss reduces knee-joint loads in over-weight and obese older adults with knee osteoarthritis. *Arthritis and Rheumatism* 52:2026-2032.

Messina, M., and S. Barnes. 1991. The role of soy products in reducing risk of cancer. *Journal of the National Cancer Institute* 83:541-546.

Meyerhardt, J. A., D. Niedzwiecki, D. Hollis, L. B. Saltz, F. B. Hu, R. J. Mayer, et al. 2007. Association of dietary patterns with cancer recurrence and survival in patients with stage III colon cancer. *Journal of the American Cancer Society* 298:754-764.

Mitrou, P. N., V. Kipnis, A. C. M. Thiebaut, J. Reedy, A. F. Subar, E. Wirfalt, et al. 2007. Mediterranean dietary pattern and prediction of all-cause mortality in a U.S. population: Results from the NIH-AARP diet and health study. *Archives of Internal Medicine* 167:2461-2468.

Morita, Y., I. Iwamoto, N. Mizuma, T. Kuwahata, T. Matsuo, and M. Yoshinaga. 2006. Precedence of the shift of body-fat distribution over the change in body composition after menopause. *Journal of Obstetrics and Gynaecology Research* 32:513-516.

Mutrie, N., A. M. Campbell, F. Whyte, A. McConnachie, C. Emslie, L. Lee, et al. 2007. Benefits of supervised group exercise programme for women being treated for early stage breast cancer: Pragmatic randomized controlled trial. *British Medical Journal* 334:517-520.

Napoli, N., J. Thompson, R. Civitelli, and R. C. Armamento-Villareal. 2007. Effects of dietary calcium compared with calcium supplements on estrogen metabolism and bone mineral density. *American Journal of Clinical Nutrition* 85:1428-1433.

Narod, S. 2007. Ovarian cancer and HRT in the MillionWomen Study. *Lancet* 369:1667-1668.

NCEP (National Cholesterol Education Program) Expert Panel. 2002. Third Report of the National Cholesterol Education Program (NCEP) Expert Panel on Detection, Evaluation, and Treatment of High Blood Cholesterol in Adults (Adult Treatment Panel III) final report. *Circulation* 106:3189.

NHLBI (National Heart, Lung, and Blood Institute). 1998. Clinical Guidelines on the Identification, Evaluation, and Treatment of Overweight and Obesity in Adults: The Evidence Report. www.nhlbi.nih.gov/guidelines/obesity/ob_gdlns.htm. Accessed February 14, 2008.

———. 2004. Third Report of the Expert Panel on Detection, Evaluation, and Treatment of High Blood Cholesterol in Adults (Adult Treatment Panel III). www.nhlbi.nih.gov/guidelines/cholesterol/index.htm. Accessed March 21, 2008.

———. 2006. Better detection of pulmonary embolism. www.nih.gov/news/research_matters/june2006/06022006embolism.htm. Accessed March 22, 2008.

National Institute of Arthritis and Musculoskeletal and Skin Diseases. 2004. Fibromyalgia. www.niams.nig.gov/Health_Info/Fibromyalgia/default.asp#fib_b. Accessed April 23, 2008.

———. 2007. Osteoporosis overview. www.niams.nih.gov/Health_Info/Bone/Osteoporosis/default.asp.

National Institute on Aging. 2005. AgePage: Sexuality in later life. www.niapublications.org/agepages/sexuality.asp. Accessed July 1, 2007.

———. 2008. AgePage: HIV, AIDS, and Older People. www.nia.nih.gov/HealthInformation/Publications/hiv-aids.htm Accessed April 24, 2008.

NIH (National Institutes of Health) Consensus Panel. 1997. *Acupuncture: National Institutes of Health Consensus Development Conference Statement, November 3-5, 1997.* Accessed at http://consensus.nih.gov/1997/1997acupuncture107html.htm. Accessed February 18, 2008.

NLM (National Library of Medicine). 2008. Lumps in the breasts.www.nlm.nih.gov/medlineplus/ency/article/001502.htm. Accessed March 29, 2008.

National Osteoporosis Foundation. 2007. Fast facts. www.nof.org/osteoporosis/diseasefacts.htm. Accessed March 26, 2008.

Nelson, H. D., K. K. Vesco, E. Haney, R. Fu, A. Nedrow, J. Miller, et al. 2006. Nonhormonal therapies for menopausal hot flashes: Systematic review and meta-analysis. *Journal of the American Medical Association* 295:2057-2071.

Nelson, M. E., J. Rejeski, S. N. Blair, P. W. Duncan, J. O. Judge, A. C. King, et al. 2007. Physical activity and public health in older adults: Recommendation from the American College of Sports Medicine and the American Heart Association. *Circulation* 116:1094-1105.

News Staff. 2006. Breakthroughs of the year: The runners-up. *Science* 314:1850-1855.

Nir, Y., M. I. Huang, R. Schnyer, B. Chen, and R. Manber. 2007. Acupuncture for postmenopausal hot flashes. *Maturitas* 56:383-395.

Njolstad, I., E. Ameson, and P. G. Lund-Larsen. 1996. Smoking, serum lipids, blood pressure, and sex differences in myocardial infarction. *Circulation* 93:450-456.

Noel, M., and M. Reddy. 2005. Nutrition and aging. *Primary Care: Clinics in Office Practice* 32(2):659-669.

Nygaard, I. E., D. H. Thom, and E. A. Calho. 2004. Urinary incontinence in women. In *Urologic Diseases in America*, edited by M. S. Litwin and C. S. Saigal. U.S. Department of Health and Human Services. Public Health Service. National Institutes of Diabetes and Digestive and Kidney Diseases. Washington, D.C.: U.S. Government Publishing Office.

Okie, S. 2007. New York to trans fats: You're out! *New England Journal of Medicine* 356:2017-2021.

Okuyemi, K. S., N. L. Nollen, and J. S. Ahluwali. 2006. Interventions to facilitate smoking cessation. *American Family Physician* 74:262-271.

Palmer, J. R. 2006. Prenatal diethylstilbestrol exposure and risk of breast cancer. *Cancer Epidemiology, Biomarkers and Prevention* 15:1509-1514.

Parati, G., and A. Steptoe. 2004. Stress reduction and blood pressure control in hypertension: A role for Transcendental Meditation? *Journal of Hypertension* 22:2057-2060.

Parham, G. P., and M. L. Hicks. 2005. Racial disparities affecting the reproductive health of African-American women. *Medical Clinics of North America* 89:935-943.

Patel, J., P. Bach, and M. Kris. 2004. Lung cancer in US women a contemporary epidemic. *Journal of the American Medical Association* 291:1763-1768.

Patel, R., and A. Rompalo. 2005. Managing patients with genital herpes and their sexual partners. *Infectious Disease Clinics of North America* 19(2):427-438.

Payne, C. K. 2007. Conservative management of urinary incontinence: Behavioral and pelvic floor therapy, urethral and pelvic devices. In *Campbell-Walsh Urology*, 9th ed., edited by A. J. Wein, L. R. Kavoussi, A. C. Novick, A. W. Partin, and C. A. Peters. Philadelphia: Saunders Elsevier.

Pierce, J. P., M. L. Stefanick, S. W. Flatt, L. Natarajan, B. Sternfeld, L. Madlensky, et al. 2007. Greater survival after breast cancer in physically active women with high vegetable-fruit intake regardless of obesity. *Journal of Clinical Oncology* 25:2345-2351.

Pittler, M. H., and E. Ernst. 2000. *Ginkgo biloba* extract for the treatment of intermittent claudication: A meta-analysis of randomized trials. *American Journal of Medicine* 108:276-281.

Qureshi, A. A., F. Laden, G. A. Colditz, and D. J. Hunter. 2008. Geographic variation and risk of skin cancer in US women. Differences between melanoma, squamous cell carcinoma and basal cell carcinoma. *Archives of Internal Medicine* 168(5):501-507.

Ravdin, P. M., K. A. Cronin, N. Howlader, C. D. Berg, R. T. Chlebowski, E. J. Feuer, et al. 2007. The decrease in breast-cancer incidence in 2003 in the United States. *New England Journal of Medicine* 356:1670-1674.

Reardon, J. Z. 2007. Environmental tobacco smoke: Respiratory and other health effects. *Clinics in Chest Medicine* 28:559-573.

Rebbeck, T. R., A. B. Troxel, S. Norman, G. R. Bunin, A. DeMichele, M. Baumgarten, et al. 2007. A retrospective case-control study of the use of hormone-related supplements and association with breast cancer. *International Journal of Cancer* 120:1523-1528.

Redd, W., and S. Manne. 1995. Using aroma to reduce distress during magnetic resonance imaging. In *Compendium of Olfactory Research 1982-1994*, edited by A. Gilbert. Dubuque, Iowa: Kendall/Hunt Publishing, 47-52.

Reeves, G. K., K. Pirie, V. Beral, J. Green, E. Spencer, and D. Bull. 2007. Cancer incidence and mortality in relation to body mass index in the Million Women Study: Cohort study. *British Journal of Medicine* 335(7630):1134.

Resnick, N. M., and S. V. Yalla. 2007. Geriatric incontinence and voiding dysfunction. In *Campbell-Walsh Urology*, 9th ed., edited by A. J. Wein, L. R. Kavoussi, A. C. Novick, A. W. Partin, and C. A. Peters. Philadelphia: Saunders Elsevier.

Reynolds, G. 2007. For athletes, an invisible traffic hazard. *New York Times*, July 12. www.nytimes.com/2007/07/12/fashion/12Fitness.html. Accessed March 30, 2008.

Richman, A., and J. P. Witkowski. 2001. 7th Annual herb sales survey. *Whole Foods Magazine* 2001:23-30.

Ringman, J. M., S. A. Frautschy, and G. M. Cole. 2005. A potential role of the curry spice curcumin in Alzheimer's disease. *Current Alzheimer Research* 2:131-136.

Roberts, L., I. Ahmed, and S. Hall. 2000. Intercessory prayer for the alleviation of ill health. *Cochrane Database of Systematic Reviews* 2:CD000368.

Roberts, W. E. 2006. Dermatologic problems of older women. *Dermatology Clinics* 24:271-280.

Rocca, W. A., J. H. Bower, D. M. Maraganore, J. E. Ahlskog, B. R. Grossardt, M. de Andrade, et al. 2008. Increased risk of Parkinsonism in women who underwent oophorectomy before menopause. *Neurology* 70:200-209.

Rocca, W. A., J. H. Bower, D. M. Maraganore, J. E. Ahlskog, B. R. Grossardt, M. de Andrade, et al. 2007. Increased risk of cognitive impairment or dementia in women who underwent oophorectomy before menopause. *Neurology* 69:1074-1083.

Rosenberg, L., D. Boggs, L. L. Adams-Campbell, and J. R. Palmer. 2007. Relaxers not associated with breast cancer risk: Evidence from the Black Women's Health Study. *Cancer Epidemiology Biomarkers and Prevention* 16:1035-1037.

Rossouw, J. E., R. L. Prentice, J. E. Manson, L. Wu, D. Barad, V. Barnabei, et al. 2007. Postmenopausal hormone therapy and risk of cardiovascular disease by age and years since menopause. *Journal of the American Medical Association* 297:1465-1477.

Salm, M., D. Belsky, and F. A. Sloan. 2006. Trends in cost of major eye diseases to Medicare, 1991-2000. *American Journal of Ophthalmology* 142:976-982.

Scarabin, P. Y., E. Oger, and G. Plu-Bureau. 2003. Differential association of oral and transdermal oestrogen-replacement therapy with venous thromboembolism risk. *Lancet* 362:428-432.

Scarmeas, N., J. A. Luchsinger, R. Mayeux, and Y. Stern. 2007. Mediterranean diet and Alzheimer disease mortality. *Neurology* 60:1084-1093.

Schneider, E., M. K. Glynn, T. Kajese, and M. T. McKenna. 2006. Epidemiology of HIV/AIDS—United States, 1981-2005. *Morbidity and Mortality Weekly Report* 55(21):589-592.

Schneider, R. H., F. Staggers, C. N. Alexander, W. Sheppard, M. Rainforth, K. Kondwani, et al. 1995. A randomized controlled trial of stress reduction for hypertension in older African-Americans. *Hypertension* 26:820-827.

Schumacher, H. C., B. T. Bateman, B. Boden-Albala, M. F. Berman, J. P. Mohr, R. L. Schumacher, et al. 2007. Use of thrombolysis in acute ischemic stroke: Analysis of the nationwide inpatient sample 1999 to 2004. *Annals of Emergency Medicine* 50:99-107.

Shah, S. A. 2007. Evaluation of echinacea for the prevention and treatment of the common cold: A meta-analysis. *Lancet* 7:473-480.

Shamliyan, T. A., R. L. Kane, J. Wyman, and T. J. Wilt. 2008. Systematic review: Randomized, controlled trials of nonsurgical treatments for urinary incontinence in women. *Annals of Internal Medicine* 148:459-473.

Shantakurar, S., M. Terry, S. Teitelbaum, S. Britton, J. R. Milliken, P. Moorman, et al. 2007. Reproductive factors and breast cancer among older women. *Breast Cancer Research and Treatment* 102:365-374.

Shrock, D., R. F. Palmer, and B. Taylor. 1999. Effects of psychosocial intervention on survival among patients with stage I breast and prostate cancer: A matched case-control study. *Alternative Therapies in Health and Medicine* 5:49-55.

Shults, C. W., D. Oakes, K. Kieburtz, M. F. Beal, R. Haas, S. Plumb, et al. 2002. Effects of coenzyme Q10 in early Parkinson disease: Evidence of slowing of the functional decline. *Archives of Neurology* 59:1541-1550.

Shwayder, J. M. 2000. Pathophysiology of abnormal uterine bleeding. *Obstetrics and Gynecology Clinics of North America* 27(2):219-234.

Singh, M. A. F. 2004. Exercise and aging. *Clinics in Geriatric Medicine* 20(2):201-221.

Singh, R. B., G. S. Wander, A. Rastogi, P. K. Shukla, A. Mittal, J. P. Sharma, et al. 1998. Randomized, double-blind placebo-controlled trial of coenzyme Q10 in patients with acute myocardial infarction. *Cardiovascular Drugs and Therapy* 12:347-353.

Sivasankaran, S., S. Pollard-Quintner, and R. Sachdeva. 2006. The effect of a six-week program of yoga and meditation on brachial artery reactivity: Do psychosocial interventions affect vascular tone? *Clinical Cardiology* 29:393-398.

Sjostrom, L., K. Narbro, C. D. Sjostrom, K. Karason, B. Larsson, H. Wedel, et al. 2007. Effects of bariatric surgery on mortality in Swedish obese subjects. *New England Journal of Medicine* 357:741-752.

Sloane, P. D., R. Coeytaux, and R. S. Beck. 2001. Dizziness: State of the science. *Annals of Internal Medicine* 134:823-832.

Smith, D. K., L. A. Grohskopf, R. J. Black, J. D. Auerbach, F. Veronese, K. A. Struble, et al. 2005. Antiretroviral postexposure prophylaxis after sexual, injection-drug use, or other non-occupational exposure to HIV in the United States: Recommendations from the U.S. Department of Health and Human Services. *Morbidity and Mortality Weekly Report. Recommendations and Reports* 54(RR-2):1-20.

Smith-Warner, S. A., D. Spiegelman, S.-S. Yaun, P. A. Van den Brandt, A. R. Folsom, R. A. Goldbohm, et al. 1998. Alcohol and breast cancer in women: A pooled analysis of cohort studies. *Journal of the American Medical Association* 279:535-540.

Snowdon, D. 2003. Healthy aging and dementia: Findings from the Nun Study. *Annals of Internal Medicine* 139:450-454.

Sommer, A., J. M. Tielsch, J. Katz, H. A. Quigley, J. D. Gottsch, J. C. Javitt, et al. 1991. Racial differences in the cause-specific prevalence of blindness in East Baltimore. *New England Journal of Medicine* 325:1412-1417.

Spencer, F., D. Lessard, C. Emery, G. Reed, and R. Goldberg. 2007. Venous thromboembolism in the outpatient setting. *Archives of Internal Medicine* 167:1471-1475.

Spiegel, D., J. R. Bloom, H. C. Kraemer, and E. Gottheil. 1989. Effect of psychosocial treatment on survival of patients with metastatic breast cancer. *Lancet* 2:888-891.

Stearns, V., L. Ullmer, J. F. Lopez, Y. Smith, C. Isaacs, and D. Hayes. 2002. Hot flushes. *Lancet* 360:1851-1861.

Steinmetz, K. A. and J. D. Potter. 1991. Vegetables, fruit and cancer. I. Epidemiology. *Cancer Causes and Control* 2:325-357.

Stevens, J. A., K. A. Mack, L. J. Paulozzi, and M. F. Ballesteros. 2008. Self-reported falls and fall-related injuries among persons aged ≥65 years—United States, 2006. *Morbidity and Mortality Weekly Review* 57(09):225-229.

Stone, E. M. 2006. A very effective treatment for macular degeneration. *New England Journal of Medicine* 355:1493-1495.

Strander, B., A. Andersson-Ellstrom, I. Milsom, and P. Sparen. 2007. Long-term risk of invasive cancer after treatment for cervical intraepithelial neoplasia grade 3: Population based cohort study. *British Medical Journal* 335:1077-1080.

Strawbridge, W. J., R. D. Cohen, S. J. Sherma, and G. A. Kaplan. 1997. Frequent attendance at religious services and mortality over 28 years. *American Journal of Public Health* 87:957-961.

Subramanian, J., and R. Govindan. 2007. Lung cancer in never smokers: A review. *Journal of Clinical Oncology* 25:561-570.

Sui, X., M. J. LaMonte, J. N. Laditka, J. W. Hardin, N. Chase, S. P. Hooker, et al. 2007. Cardiorespiratory fitness and adiposity as mortality predictors in older adults. *Journal of the American Medical Association* 298:2507-2516.

Surtees, P. G., N. W. J. Wainwright, R. N. Luben, N. J. Wareham, S. A. Bingham, and K-T Khaw. 2008. Psychological distress, major depressive disorder, and risk of stroke. *Neurology* 70:788-794.

Taixiang, W., A. J. Munro, and L. Guanjian. 2005. Chinese medical herbs for chemotherapy side effects in colorectal cancer patients. *Cochrane Database of Systematic Reviews* 1:CD004540.

Takkouche, B., M. Etminan, and A. Montes-Martinez. 2005. Personal use of hair dyes and risk of cancer: A meta-analysis. *Journal of the American Medical Association* 293:2516-2525.

Tan, B. K., and J. Vanitha. 2004. Immunomodulatory and antimicrobial effects of some traditional Chinese medicinal herbs: A review. *Current Medicinal Chemistry* 11:1423-1430.

Theis, K., C. Helmick, and J. Hootman. 2007. Arthritis burden and impact are greater among U.S. women than men: Intervention opportunities. *Journal of Women's Health* 16:441-453.

Thompson, L. U., J. M. Chen, T. Li, K. Strasser-Weippl, and P. E. Goss. 2005. Cancer therapy: Clinical dietary flaxseed alters tumor biological markers in postmenopausal breast cancer. *Clinical Cancer Research* 11:3828-3835.

Thompson, R. L. 2003. Menopause and brain function. *Neurology* 61:9-10.

Thurman, D. J., J. A. Stevens, and J. K. Rao. 2008. Practice parameter: Assessing patients in neurology practice for risk of falls (an evidence-based review). *Neurology* 70:473-479.

Tinetti, M. E., D. I. Baker, G. McAvay, E. B. Claus, P. Garrett, M. Gottschalk, et al. 1994. A multifactorial intervention to reduce the risk of falling among elderly people living in the community. *New England Journal of Medicine* 331:821-827.

Tjaden, P., and N. Thoennes. 2000. Extent, nature, and consequences of intimate partner violence: Findings from the National Violence Against Women Survey. National Institute of Justice and the Centers for Disease Control and Prevention. www.ncjrs.gov/pdffiles1/nij/181867.pdf. Accessed March 31, 2008.

Touillaud, M. S., A. C. M. Thiebaut, A. Fournier, M. Niravong, M. C. Boutron-Ruault, and F. Clavel-Chapelton. 2007. Dietary lignan intake and postmenopausal breast cancer risk by estrogen and progesterone receptor status. *Journal of the National Cancer Institute* 99:475-486.

Towfighi, A., J. L. Saver, R. Engelhardt, and B. Ovbiagele. 2007. A midlife stroke surge among women in the United States. *Neurology* 69:1894-1895.

Trock, B. J., L. Hilakivi-Clarke, and S. Clarke. 2006. Meta-analysis of soy intake and breast cancer risk. *Journal of the Naional Cancer Insitute* 98:459-471.

Uemura, N., S. Okamoto, S. Yamamoto, N. Matsumura, S. Yamaguchi, M. Yamakido, et al. 2001. *Helicobacter pylori* infection and the development of gastric cancer. *New England Journal of Medicine* 345:784-789.

U.S. Consumer Product Safety Commission. 2000. Baby boomer sports injuries. www.cpsc.gov/LIBRARY/boomer.pdf. Accessed March 28, 2008.

USDHHS (U.S. Department of Health and Human Services). 2004. *The Health Consequences of Smoking: A Report of the Surgeon General*. Atlanta, Georgia: U.S. Department of Health and Human Services, Centers for Disease Control and Prevention, National Center for Chronic Disease Prevention and Health Promotion, Office on Smoking and Health. Available at www.cdc.gov/tobacco/data_statistics/sgr/sgr_2004/index.htm. Accessed March 24, 2008.

———. 2005. *Dietary Guidelines for Americans*, 6th ed. 2005. Washington DC: U.S. Government Printing Office.

Van der Worp, H. B., and J. van Gijn. 2007. Acute ischemic stroke. *New England Journal of Medicine* 357:572-579.

Villegas, R., S. Liu, Y. T. Gao, G. Yang, H. Li, W. Zheng, et al. 2007. Prospective study of dietary carbohydrates, glycemic index, glycemic load, and incidence of type 2 diabetes mellitus in middle-aged Chinese women. *Archives of Internal Medicine* 167:2310-2316.

Vitello, P. 2006. A ringtone meant to fall on deaf ears. *New York Times*, June 12. www.nytimes.com/2006/06/12/technology/12ring.html. Accessed March 22, 2008.

Vogel, V. G., J. P. Costantino, D. L. Wickerham, W. M. Cronin, R. S. Cecchini, J. N. Atkins, et al. 2006. Effects of tamoxifen vs. raloxifene on the risk of developing invasive breast cancer and other disease outcomes: The NSABP Study of Tamoxifen and Raloxifene (STAR) P-2 trial. *Journal of the American Medical Association* 295:2727-2741.

Vonk, J. M., H. Jongepier, C. I. M. Panhuysen, J. P. Schouten, E. R. Bleecker, and D. S. Postma. 2003. Risk factors associated with the presence of irreversible airflow limitation and reduced transfer coefficient in patients with asthma after 26 years of follow-up. *Thorax* 58:322-327.

Walker, L. G., M. B. Walker, K. Ogston, S. D. Heys, A. K. Ah-See, I. D. Miller, et al. 1999. Psychological, clinical and pathological effects of relaxation training and guided imagery during primary chemotherapy. *British Journal of Cancer* 80:262-268.

Wang, X., X. Qin, H. Demirtas, J. Li, G. Mao, Y. Huo, et al. 2007. Efficacy of folic acid supplementation in stroke prevention: A meta-analysis. *Lancet* 369:1876-1882.

Weber, P. 2001. Vitamin K and bone health. *Nutrition* 17:880-887.

Weinreb, R. N. 2006. Glaucoma. In *Conn's Current Therapy*, edited by R. E. Rakel and E. T. Bope. Philadelphia: W. B. Saunders (Elsevier).

Weinstock, H., S. Berman, and W. Cates Jr. 2004. Sexually transmitted diseases among American youth: Incidence and prevalence estimates, 2000. *Perspectives on Sexual and Reproductive Health* 36(1):6-10.

Welty, F. K., K. S. Lee, N. S. Lew, and J.-R. Zhou. 2007a. The association between soy nut consumption and decreased menopausal symptoms. *Journal of Womens Health* 16:361-369.

Welty, F. K., K. S. Lee, N. S. Lew, and J-R, Zhou. 2007b. Effect of soy nuts on blood pressure and lipid levels in hypertensive, prehypertensive, and normotensive postmenopausal women. *Archives of Internal Medicine* 167:1060-1067.

Whiteman, M. K., C. A. Staropoli, P. W. Langenberg, R. J. McCarter, K. H. Kjerulff, and J. A. Flaws. 2003. Smoking, body mass, and hot flashes in midlife women. *Obstetrics and Gynecology* 101:264-272.

Wilkinson, S., J. Aldridge, I. Salmon, E. Cain, and B. Wilson. 1999. An evaluation of aromatherapy massage in palliative care. *Palliative Medicine* 13:409-417.

Wittstein, I., D. R. Thiemann, J. Lima, K. L. Baughman, S. P. Schulman, and G. Gerstenblith. 2005. Neurohumoral features of myocardial stunning due to sudden emotional stress. *New England Journal of Medicine* 352:539-548.

Wolfe, F., K. Ross, J. Anderson, I. J. Russell, and L. Herbert. 2005. The prevalence and characteristics of fibromyalgia in the general population. *Arthritis and Rheumatism* 38:19-28.

WCRF/AICR (World Cancer Research Fund/American Institute for Cancer Research). 2007. Food, nutrition, physical activity, and the prevention of cancer: A global perspective. www.dietandcancer report.org/downloads/Second_Expert_Report.pdf. Accessed November 4, 2007.

Wood, C. E., T. C. Register, C. J. Lees, H. Chen, S. Kimrey, and C. J. Mark. 2007. Effects of estradiol with micronized progesterone or medroxyprogesterone acetate on risk markers for breast cancer in postmenopausal monkeys. *Breast Cancer Research and Treatment* 101:125-134.

Writing Group for the PEPI Trial. 1995. Effects of estrogen or estrogen/progestin regimens on heart disease risk factors in postmenopausal women. The Postmenopausal Estrogen/Progestin Interventions (PEPI) trial. *Journal of the American Medical Association* 273:199-208.

Writing Group for the Women's Health Initiative Investigators (WHI). 2002. Risks and benefits of estrogen plus progestin in healthy postmenopausal women: Principal results from the Women's Health Initiative randomized controlled trial. *Journal of the American Medical Association* 288:321-333.

Wu, A. H., M. C. Yu, C. C. Tseng, and M. C. Pike. 2003. Green tea and risk of breast cancer in Asian Americans. *International Journal of Cancer* 106:574-579.

Wu, C. M., K. McLaughlin, D. L. Lorenzetti, M. D. Hill, B. J. Manns, and W. A. Ghali. 2007. Early risk of stroke after transient ischemic attack: A systematic review and meta-analysis. *Archives of Internal Medicine* 167:2417-2422.

Yang, Y. X., J. D. Lewis, S. Epstein, and D. Metz. 2006. Long-term proton pump inhibitor therapy and risk of hip fracture. *Journal of the American Medical Association* 296:2947-2953.

Zellweger, M. J., R. H. Osterwalder, W. Langewitz, and M. E. Pfisterer. 2003. Coronary artery disease and depression. *European Heart Journal* 25:3-9.

Janet Horn, MD, is board-certified in internal medicine and infectious diseases, with training in obstetrics and gynecology. Much of her career was spent in solo private medical practice. For many years, she was a full-time faculty member at the Johns Hopkins University School of Medicine. Dr. Horn has authored many medical journal articles and several medical textbook chapters. Currently, she divides her time between medical writing and practicing medicine at the Shepherd's Clinic, which serves the uninsured.

Dr. Horn has been recognized by Baltimore Magazine and The Consumer's Guide to Top Doctors as one of the top doctors in Baltimore and in the United States. The Maryland Daily Record named her one of the top 100 women in Maryland in 1999.

Robin H. Miller, MD, is a board-certified internist and integrative medicine specialist who trained with Dr. Andrew Weil at the University of Arizona. She is founder and medical director of Triune Integrative Medicine, an innovative medical clinic in Medford, OR. Dr. Miller is also clinical assistant professor of medical informatics at the Oregon Health and Science University in Portland, OR. She is author of Kids Ask the Doctor.

Dr. Miller is an award-winning medical correspondent for KOBI, the NBC affiliate in southern Oregon and northern California, and can be seen on the Patient Channel on MSNBC.com. She writes a medical column for the Daily Courier in Grants Pass, OR, and a quarterly column for Ashland Magazine.

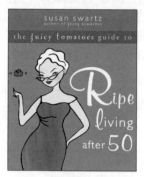
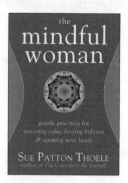
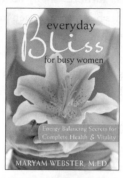
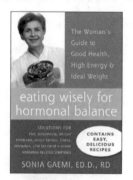
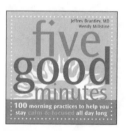
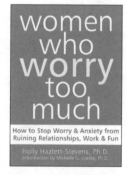